National Safety Council®

First Aid

Fourth Edition

Alton Thygerson, Ed.D.
Consultant/Medical Writer
National Safety Council

JONES AND BARTLETT PUBLISHERS
Sudbury, Massachusetts
BOSTON TORONTO LONDON SINGAPORE

JONES AND BARTLETT PUBLISHERS
40 Tall Pine Drive, Sudbury, MA 01776
978-443-5000
nsc@jbpub.com
http://nsc.jbpub.com

Jones and Bartlett Publishers Canada
2406 Nikanna Road
Mississauga, ON L5C 2W6
CANADA

Jones and Bartlett Publishers International
Barb House, Barb Mews
London W6 7PA
UK

National Safety Council®
First Aid Institute
1121 Spring Lake Drive
Itasca, IL 60143-3201
(630) 285-1121
(800) 621-7619
www.nsc.org

General Manager of Public Safety Group: Donna Siegfried

Production Credits
Chief Executive Officer: Clayton E. Jones
Chief Operating Officer: Donald W. Jones, Jr.
Executive V.P. and Publisher: Tom Manning
V.P. and Managing Editor: Judith H. Hauck
V.P., Sales and Marketing: Paul Shepardson
V.P., Production and Design: Anne Spencer
V.P., Manufacturing and Inventory Control: Therese Bräuer
Publisher, EMS & Aquatics: Lawrence D. Newell
Emergency Care Senior Acquisitions Editor: Tracy Foss
Director of Marketing, EMS and Health Sciences: Kimberly Brophy
Emergency Care Associate Editor: Jennifer Reed
Production Editor: Linda S. DeBruyn
Interactive Technology Director: W. Scott Smith
Text Design: Studio Montage
Typesetting and Editorial: Nesbitt Graphics
Illustrations: Rolin Graphics
Interior Photos: Richard Nye
Cover Design: Studio Montage
Cover Photographs (clockwise from top left):
© Brian Pieters, Masterfile;
© Wedgworth, Custom Medical Stock Photo;
Steve Ferry, P&F Communications;
Steve Ferry, P&F Communications
Printing and Binding: Courier Company

The first aid and CPR procedures in this book are based on the most current recommendations of responsible medical sources. The National Safety Council and the publisher, however, make no guarantee as to, and assume no responsibility for, the correctness, sufficiency or completeness of such information or recommendations. Other or additional safety measures may be required under particular circumstances.

Library of Congress Cataloging-in-Publication Data

First Aid/National Safety Council.—4th ed.
p. cm.
Includes index.
ISBN 0-7637-1321-X (alk. paper)
1. First aid in illness and injury—Popular works. I. National Safety Council. II. Title.
RC87.F475 2000
616.02'52–dc21 00-065547

Additional illustrations and photo credits appear on page 128, which constitutes a continuation of the copyright page.

Printed in the United States of America
05 04 03 02 01 10 9 8 7 6 5 4 3 2 1

About the National Safety Council Program

Congratulations on selecting the National Safety Council's First Aid and CPR program! You join good company, as the National Safety Council has successfully trained over 6 million people worldwide in first aid and cardiopulmonary resuscitation (CPR). The National Safety Council's training network of nearly 10,000 instructors at over 4,000 sites worldwide has established the National Safety Council programs as the standard by which all others are judged.

In setting the standards, the National Safety Council has worked in close cooperation with hundreds of national and international organizations, thousands of corporations, thousands of leading educators, dozens of leading medical organizations, and hundreds of state and local governmental agencies. Their collective input has helped create programs that stand alone in quality. Consider just a few of the National Safety Council's current collaborations:

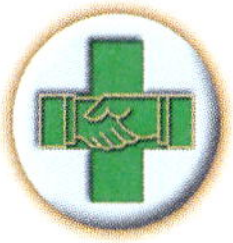

World's Leading Medical Organizations

The National Safety Council is currently working with both the American Academy of Orthopedic Surgeons (AAOS), Wilderness Medical Society (WMS), and the American Heart Association to help bring innovative, new training programs to the marketplace. The National Safety Council and the AAOS are developing a new First Responder program and the National Safety Council and the WMS are developing the first-of-its-kind wilderness first aid program.

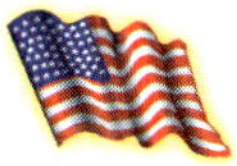

Spanning the Globe

Across the globe, from Boston to Bangkok, from Miami to Milan, from Seattle to Stockholm, people are trained with National Safety Council programs. National Safety Council first aid and CPR programs are already used in your area.

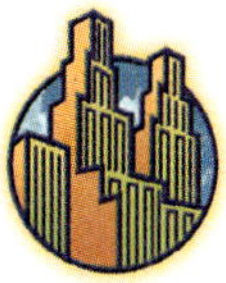

World's Leading Corporations

Thousands of corporations including Westinghouse, Exxon, General Motors, Ameritech, and U.S. West have selected many of the National Safety Council emergency care programs to train employees.

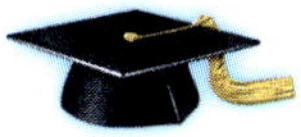

World's Leading Colleges and Universities

Hundreds of leading colleges and universities are working closely with the National Safety Council to fully develop and implement the Internet Initiative that will establish the National Safety Council as the leading online provider of emergency care programs.

Most importantly, in selecting the National Safety Council programs, you can feel confident that the programs are of the highest quality. You can rely on the National Safety Council. Founded in 1913, the National Safety Council is dedicated to protecting life, promoting health, and reducing accidental death. For nearly 90 years, the National Safety Council has been the world's leading authority on safety/injury education.

GREEN CROSS FOR SAFETY ®

National Safety Council ®

Table of Contents

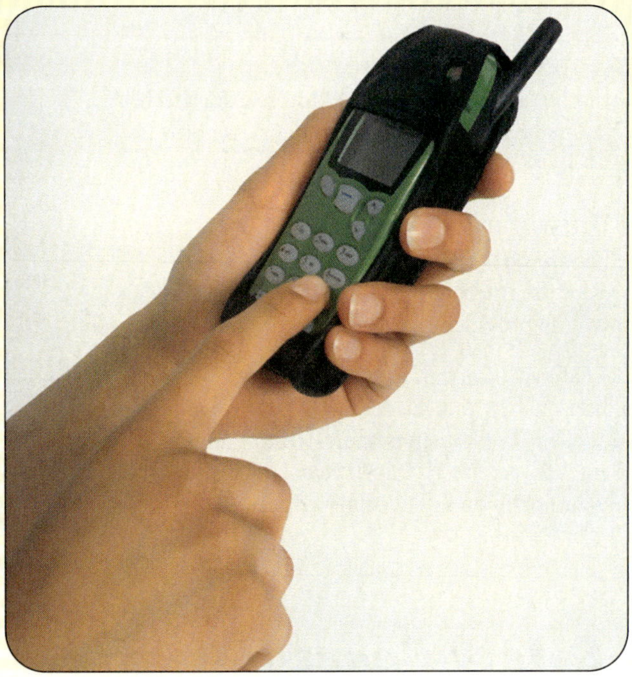

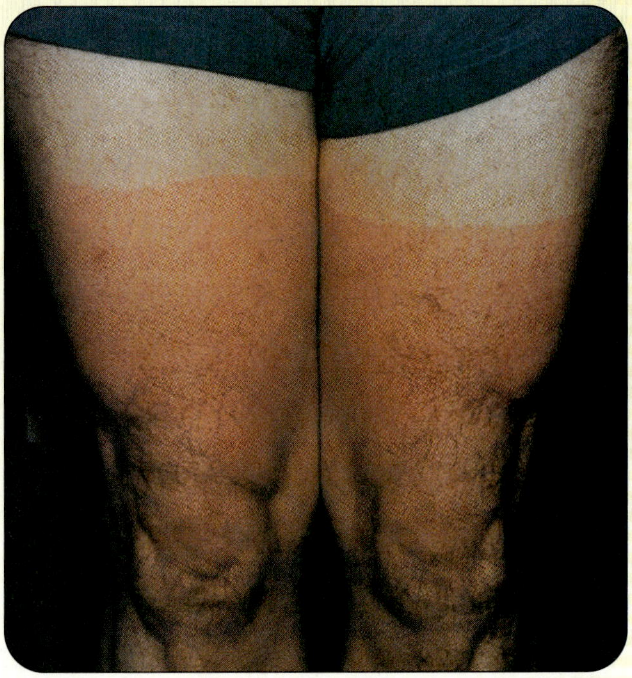

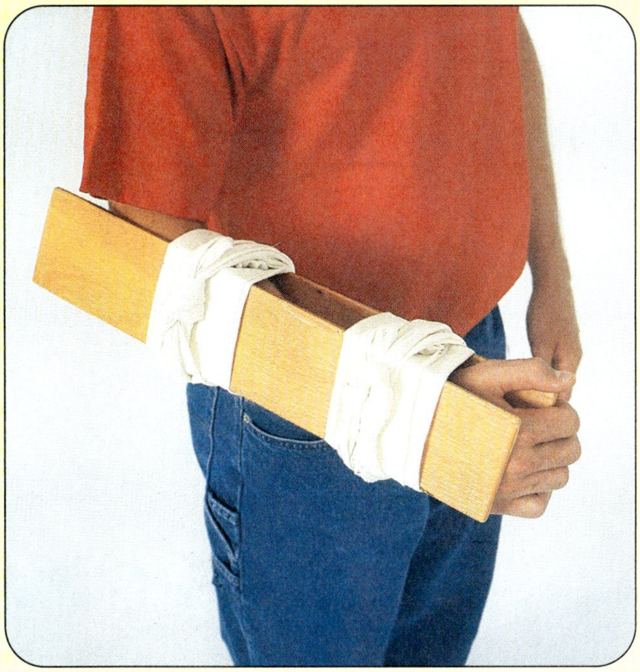

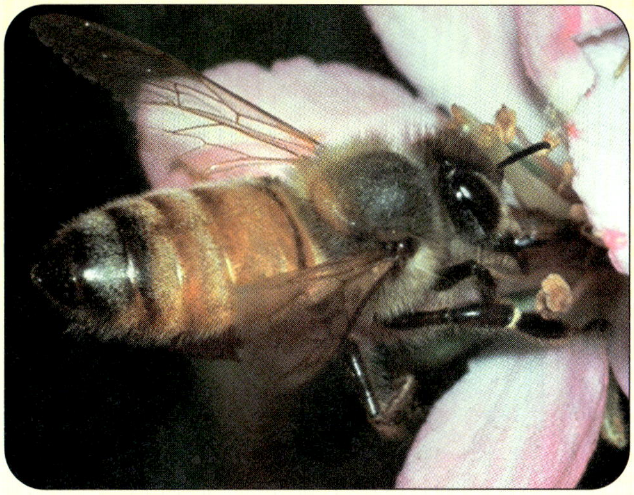

Your First Aid IQ

Test your current knowledge. Read each question and place your answer in the "Pre-check" column. After reading this manual and completing your course, read the questions again and place your answers in the "Post-check" column. Compare your answers and see what you have learned.

Question	Pre-check			Post-check		
1. Most communities use 9-1-1 as their emergency telephone number.	T	F	Uncertain	T	F	Uncertain
2. Most injured victims require a complete physical exam.	T	F	Uncertain	T	F	Uncertain
3. Direct pressure and elevation can control most injuries involving bleeding.	T	F	Uncertain	T	F	Uncertain
4. Heat should be applied quickly to any muscle, bone or joint injuries to reduce swelling.	T	F	Uncertain	T	F	Uncertain
5. Applying butter is an effective treatment for first degree burns.	T	F	Uncertain	T	F	Uncertain
6. An object impaled (stuck) in the body should removed so that bleeding can be controlled.	T	F	Uncertain	T	F	Uncertain
7. A splint is something used to stabilize (reduce movement) a broken bone.	T	F	Uncertain	T	F	Uncertain
8. Chest pain is one of the most frequent signals of a heart attack.	T	F	Uncertain	T	F	Uncertain
9. Sugar should be given to a responsive victim suspected of suffering a diabetic emergency.	T	F	Uncertain	T	F	Uncertain
10. Syrup of ipecac should be given to a person who has ingested a corrosive poisonous substance.	T	F	Uncertain	T	F	Uncertain
11. Ice should be applied to a snakebite wound.	T	F	Uncertain	T	F	Uncertain
12. Rub or massage a frostbitten part to quickly rewarm it.	T	F	Uncertain	T	F	Uncertain
13. Salt tablets should be given to victims of heat emergencies.	T	F	Uncertain	T	F	Uncertain
14. Hypothermia occurs only in subfreezing temperatures.	T	F	Uncertain	T	F	Uncertain
15. Extremely hot skin indicates heat exhaustion.	T	F	Uncertain	T	F	Uncertain

Chapter 1

Background Information

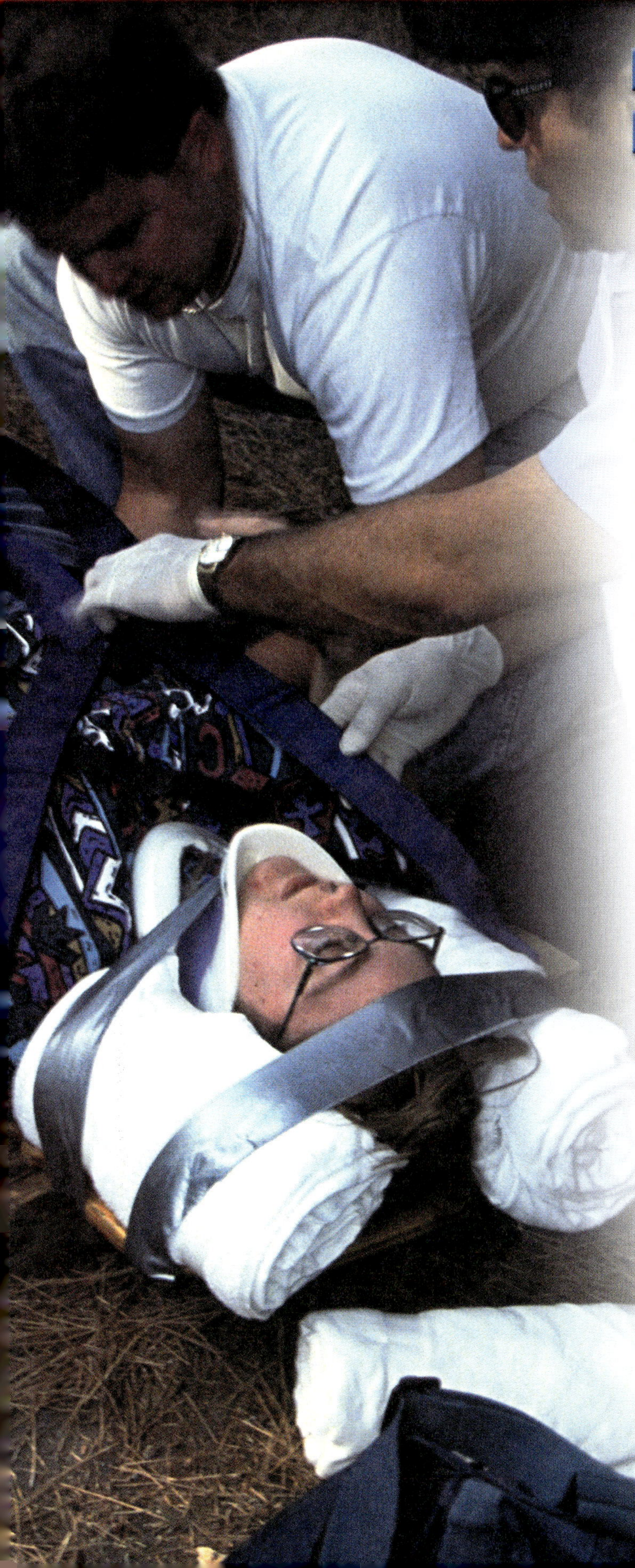

Need for First Aid Training

It's better to know first aid and not need it than to need it and not know it. Everyone should be able to perform first aid because most people will eventually find themselves in a situation requiring it, either for another person or for themselves.

A delay of as little as a few minutes when a person's heart stops can mean the difference between life and death. However, most injuries do not require life-saving efforts. During their entire lifetime, most people will see only one or two situations involving life-threatening conditions. While saving lives is important, knowing what to do for less severe injuries demands greater attention and more first aid training.

What Is First Aid?

First aid is one of those things you need to know—but never want to use. *First aid* is the immediate care given to an injured or suddenly ill person ▶Table 1. First aid does *not* take the place of proper medical treatment. Rather, it furnishes temporary assistance until the victim receives competent medical care, if needed, or until the chance for recovery without medical care is assured. Most injuries and illnesses do not require medical care.

Properly applied, first aid may mean the difference between life and death, between a rapid recovery and long hospitalization, or between temporary disability and permanent injury. First aid involves more than doing things for others; it also includes the things that people can do for themselves.

Recognizing a serious medical emergency and knowing how to get help may mean the difference between life and death. Recognition can be delayed because neither the victim nor bystanders know basic symptoms (eg, a heart attack victim may wait hours after the onset of symptoms before seeking help). Moreover, most people do not know first aid; even if they do, they may panic in an emergency.

Table 1: Leading Causes of Death

1. Heart Disease	> 700,000
2. Cancer	> 500,000
3. Stroke	> 150,000
4. Chronic Lung Disease	> 100,000
5. Unintentional Injury	> 90,000

Legal Considerations

Fear of lawsuits has made some people reluctant about getting involved at emergency scenes. First aiders, however, are rarely sued; those who are usually receive a favorable ruling from courts.

Consent

Before giving first aid, a first aider must have the victim's consent (permission). Touching another person without his or her permission or consent is unlawful (known as battery) and could be grounds for a lawsuit. Likewise, giving first aid without the victim's consent is unlawful.

Expressed Consent

Consent must be obtained from every conscious, mentally competent (able to make a rational decision) person of legal age. Tell the victim your name and that you have first aid training, and explain what you will be doing. Permission from the victim may be expressed either with words or with a nod of the head.

Implied Consent

Implied consent involves an unresponsive victim in a life-threatening condition. It is assumed or "implied" that an unresponsive victim would consent to lifesaving help. When a child is in a life-threatening situation, and the parent or legal guardian is not available for consent, first aid should be given based on implied consent. Do not withhold first aid from a minor just to obtain parental or guardian permission.

Abandonment

Abandonment means leaving a victim after starting to give help without ensuring someone else will continue the care at the same level or higher. Once you have started providing care, you must not leave a victim who still needs first aid until another competent and trained person takes responsibility for the victim.

Negligence

Negligence means not following accepted standards of care and causing injury to the victim. Negligence involves:

1. Having a duty to act
2. Breaching that duty (by giving substandard care)
3. Causing injury and damages

Duty to Act

No one is required to render first aid when no legal duty exists. Duty to act may occur in the following situations:

- *When your employment requires it.* If your employer designates you as responsible for rendering first aid to meet OSHA (Occupational Safety and Health Administration) requirements and you are called to an injury scene, you have a duty to act. Examples of occupations with job descriptions that include a duty to act include law enforcement officers, park rangers, athletic trainers, lifeguards, and teachers. ▼Figure 1

Figure 1

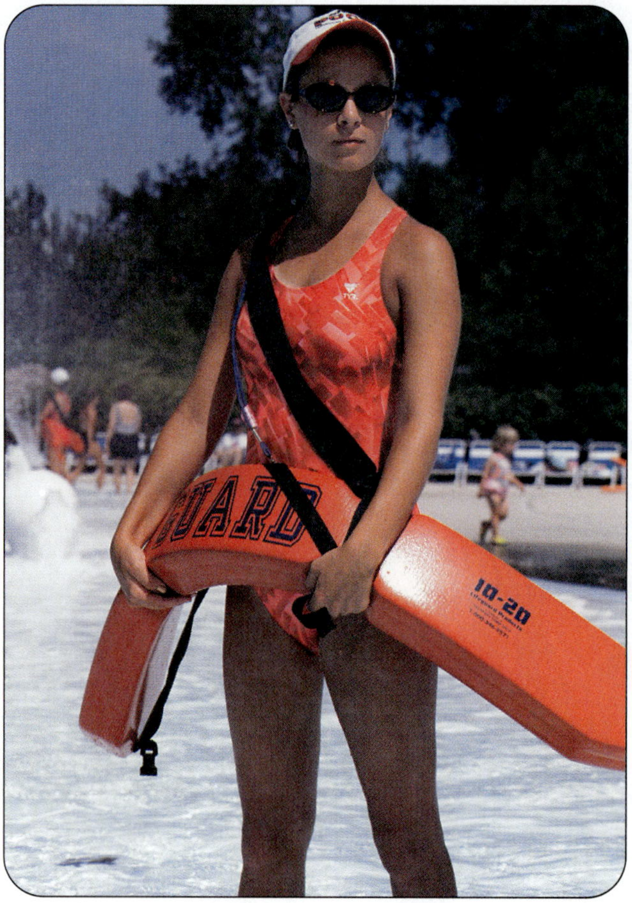

- *When a pre-existing responsibility exists.* You may have a pre-existing relationship with other persons that demands you be responsible for them, which means you must give first aid if they need it. Examples include a parent for a child, or a driver for a passenger.

Duty to act means following guidelines for standards of care. Standards of care ensure quality care and protection for injured or suddenly ill victims.

Breach of Duty

Generally, a first aider breaches (breaks) his or her duty to a victim by failing to provide the type of care that would be provided by a person having the same or similar training. One's duty can be breached by acts of omission or acts of commission. An *act of omission* is the failure to do what a reasonably prudent person with the same or similar training would do in the same or similar circumstances. An *act of commission* is doing something that a reasonably prudent person would *not* do under the same or similar circumstances. Forgetting to put on a dressing is an act of omission; cutting a snakebite site is an act of commission.

Injury and Damages Inflicted

Injury or damages must have resulted from a breach of duty. In addition to physical damage, injury and damage can include physical pain and suffering, mental anguish, medical expenses, and sometimes loss of earnings and earning capacity.

Good Samaritan Laws

In most emergencies, you are not legally required to give first aid. To encourage people to assist others needing help, Good Samaritan laws grant immunity against lawsuits. Although laws vary from state to state, Good Samaritan immunity generally applies only when the rescuer is (1) acting during an emergency, (2) acting in good faith, which means he or she has good intentions, (3) acting without compensation, and (4) not guilty of any malicious misconduct or gross negligence toward the victim (deviating from all rational first aid guidelines).

Good Samaritan laws are not a substitute for competent first aid or for keeping within the scope of your training.

To find out about your state's Good Samaritan laws, ask for information at your local library or an attorney.

Learning Activities

What Is First Aid?

Directions: Circle Yes if you agree with the statement, and circle No if you disagree.

Yes No **1.** In most locations, an ambulance can arrive within minutes. This quick response means that most people do not need to learn first aid.

Yes No **2.** Correct first aid can mean the difference between life and death.

Yes No **3.** Most injuries do not require life-saving first aid efforts.

Yes No **4.** You need to call for an ambulance and/or seek advanced medical care for all injured victims.

Yes No **5.** In most situations, before giving first aid, you must get consent (permission) from the victim.

Yes No **6.** If you ask a victim if you can help, and she says "No," you can ignore her and proceed to give first aid whether she likes it or not.

Yes No **7.** Employers can designate people as first aiders. This means that they must give first aid to injured employees while on the job.

Yes No **8.** First aiders who help injured victims are often sued.

Yes No **9.** Good Samaritan laws provide a degree of protection for first aiders who act in a rational manner during an emergency, in good faith, and without compensation.

Scenario: You are driving slowly looking for a house number in an unfamiliar residential area. You are attempting to deliver an important package to a customer. You see an elderly woman lying at the bottom of porch stairs outside of a house. You see no one else in the neighborhood, and you are alone. You quickly, but safely, stop your vehicle in front of the victim's house. As you approach the victim, you notice that her skin appears bluish, and she is motionless.

Yes No **10.** Do you have to stop to help her?

_______ **11.** If you stop and help, which type of consent would apply in this case?
A. expressed **B.** implied

Yes No **12.** If she does not respond to your tapping on her shoulders and shouting "Are you O.K.?" you can leave her and assume that someone else who is more competent or is a family member will arrive shortly to help her.

Yes No **13.** You decide to help. You straighten one of her legs, which causes a bone to protrude through the skin. Would this increase the likelihood of being sued?

Yes No **14.** For the situation in number 13, the Good Samaritan law protects you from being sued.

Yes No **15.** If the woman were your mother under your custodial care, you must give first aid to her.

Chapter 2

Action at an Emergency

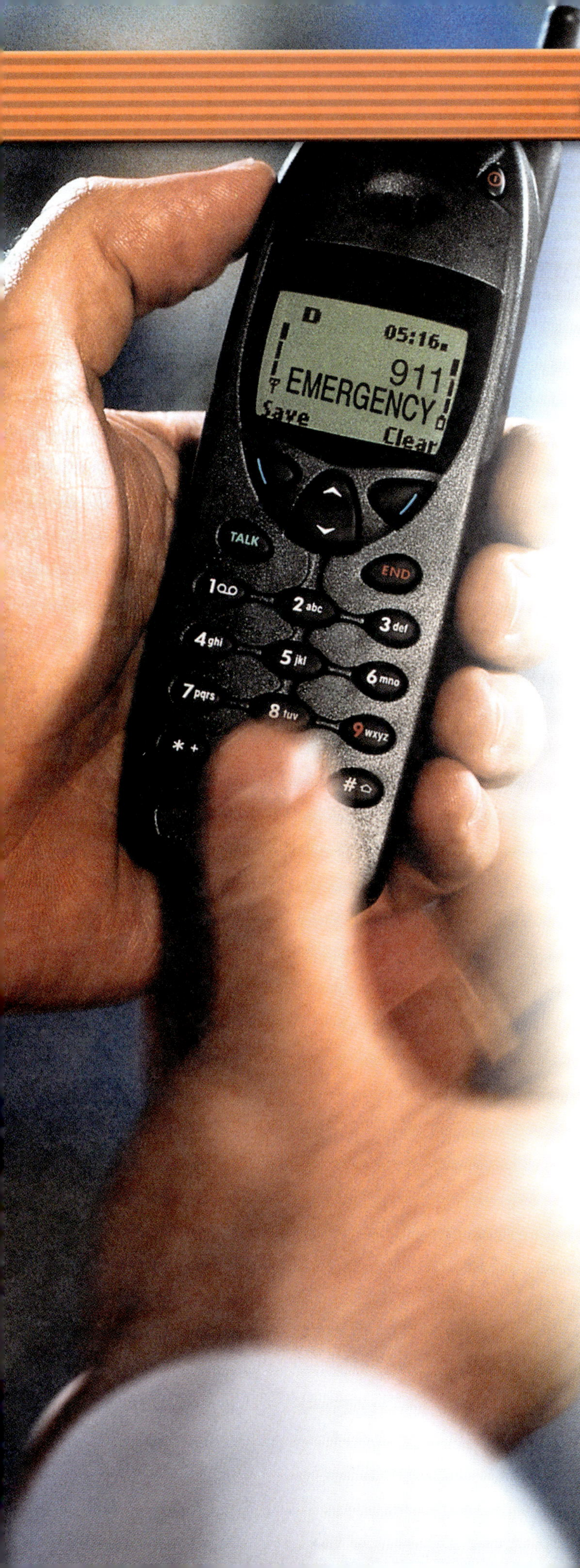

Bystander Intervention

The bystander is a vital link between the emergency medical service (EMS) and the victim. Typically it is a bystander who first recognizes a situation as an emergency and acts to help the victim. A bystander must perform the following actions quickly and reliably.

Recognize the Emergency

To help in an emergency, the bystander has to notice that something is wrong—usually a person's appearance or behavior or the surroundings suggesting something unusual has happened.

Decide to Help

At some time, everyone will have to decide whether to help another person. Making a quick decision to get involved at the time of an emergency is unlikely to occur unless the bystander has previously considered, the possibility of helping. Thus, **the most important time to make the decision to help is *before* you ever encounter an emergency.**

Deciding to help is an attitude about people, about emergencies, and about one's ability to deal with emergencies. It is an attitude that takes time to develop and is affected by a number of factors.

Call EMS, If Needed

People often make inappropriate decisions regarding calling EMS personnel. They delay calling for an ambulance until they are absolutely sure that an emergency exists, or they elect to bypass EMS personnel and transport the victim to medical care in a private vehicle. Such actions can present significant dangers to victims. Fortunately , most injuries and sudden illnesses that you will render care for will not require the need for advanced medical care—only first aid.

Assess the Victim

The bystander must decide if life-threatening conditions exist and what kind of help a victim needs immediately.

Provide Care

Often the most critical life-support measures are effective only if started immediately by the nearest available person. That person usually will be a layperson—a bystander.

Post-Care Reactions

After giving care for serious conditions, rescuers can feel an emotional "letdown," which is frequently overlooked. Discussing your feelings, fears, and reactions following the event can help prevent later emotional problems. You can talk to a trusted friend, a mental health professional, or a member of the clergy. Bringing out your feelings quickly helps to relieve personal anxieties and stress.

Scene Survey

If you are at the scene of an emergency situation, do a quick survey of the scene that includes looking for three things: (1) hazards that could be dangerous to you, the victim(s), or bystanders; (2) the cause (mechanism) of the injury or illness; and (3) the number of victims. This survey should only take a few seconds.

First, as you approach an emergency scene, scan the area for immediate dangers to yourself or to the victim. You cannot help another if you also become a victim. Always ask yourself: Is the scene safe to enter? (For details about specific hazards at an emergency scene, refer to Chapter 18.)

The second thing to do is to try to determine the cause of any injury or illness. Be sure to tell EMS personnel about your findings, so that they can fully recognize the extent of the problem.

Finally, determine how many people are involved. There may be more than one victim, so look around and ask about others involved.

Seek Medical Attention

Knowing when to call for an ambulance is important. To know when to call, you must be able to tell the difference between a minor injury or illness and a life-threatening one. For example, upper abdominal pain can be as minor as indigestion or as severe as a heart attack needing prompt medical care. Wheezing may be related to a person's asthma, for which the person can use his or her prescribed inhaler for quick relief, or it can be as serious as a severe allergic reaction from a bee sting.

Not every cut needs stitches, nor does every burn require medical attention. It is, however, always best to err on the side of caution.

According to the American College of Emergency Physicians (ACEP), if the answer to any of the following questions is yes, or if you are unsure, call 9-1-1 or your local emergency number (if other than 9-1-1) for help.

- Is the victim's condition life-threatening?
- Could the condition get worse and become life-threatening on the way to the hospital?
- Does the victim need the skills or equipment of emergency medical technicians or paramedics?
- Would distance or traffic conditions cause a delay in getting to the hospital?

ACEP also recommends that the following conditions are warning signs that require immediate transport to the hospital emergency department, either in an ambulance or car:

- fainting
- chest or abdominal pain or pressure
- sudden dizziness, weakness, or change in vision
- difficulty breathing, shortness of breath
- severe or persistent vomiting
- sudden, severe pain anywhere in the body
- suicidal or homicidal feelings
- bleeding that does not stop after 10 to 15 minutes of pressure
- a gaping wound with edges that do not come together
- problems with movement or sensation following an injury
- cuts on the hand or face
- puncture wounds
- the possibility that foreign bodies such as glass or metal may have entered a wound
- most animal bites and all human bites
- hallucinations and clouding of thoughts
- a stiff neck in association with a fever or a headache

- a bulging or abnormally depressed fontanel (soft spot) in infants
- stupor or dazed behavior accompanying a high fever that is not alleviated by acetaminophen or aspirin
- unequal pupil size, loss of consciousness, blindness, staggering, or repeated vomiting after a head injury
- spinal injuries
- severe burns
- poisoning
- drug overdose

When a serious situation occurs, call EMS (9-1-1 in most communities) *first*. Do *not* call your doctor, the hospital, a friend, relatives, or neighbors for help before you call EMS. Calling anyone else first only wastes time.

If the situation is not an emergency, call your doctor. However, if you are in *any* doubt as to whether the situation is an emergency, call EMS.

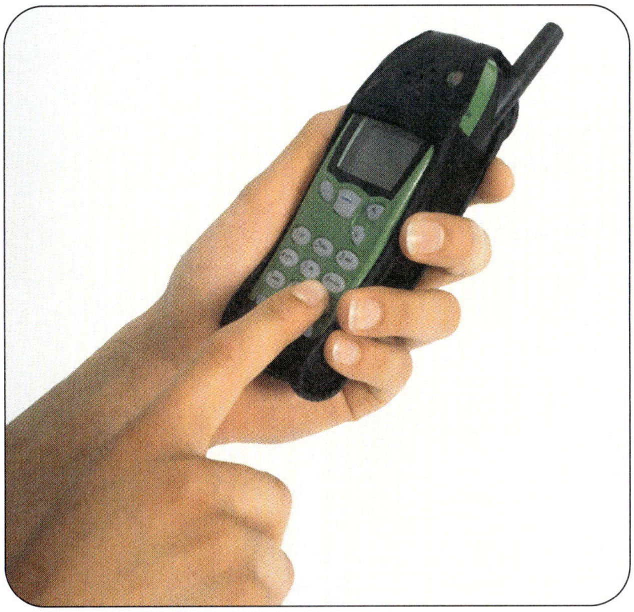

Figure 1 For help, phone 9-1-1 or the local emergency number.

How to Call EMS

To receive emergency assistance of every kind in most communities, you simply phone 9-1-1 **►Figure 1**. Check to see if this is true in your community. Emergency telephone numbers usually are listed on the inside front cover of telephone directories. Keep these numbers near or on every telephone. Call "0" (the operator) if you do not know the emergency number.

When you call EMS, the dispatcher will often ask for the following information. Speak slowly and clearly when you provide this information.

1. Your name and the phone number you are calling from. This prevents false calls and allows a dispatch center to call back if disconnected or for additional information if needed.
2. The victim's location. Give the address, names of intersecting roads, and other landmarks, if possible. Also, tell the specific location of the victim (eg, "in the basement").
3. What happened. State the nature of the emergency (eg, "My husband fell off a ladder and is not moving.").
4. Number of persons needing help and any special conditions.
5. Victim's condition (eg, "My husband's head is bleeding.") and any first aid you have provided (such as pressing on the site of the bleeding).

Do *not* hang up the phone unless the dispatcher instructs you to do so. Enhanced 9-1-1 systems can track a call, but some communities lack this technology or are still using a seven-digit emergency number. Since cell phones can not be tracked through enhanced 9-1-1, it is important that the number be provided to the dispatcher and that all information is conveyed. Also, the EMS dispatcher may tell you how best to care for the victim. If you send someone else to call, have the person report back to you so you can be sure the call was made.

Disease Precautions

First aiders must understand the risk of infectious diseases, which can range from mild to life threatening. The risk of getting a disease from a victim is very low. First aiders should know how to protect themselves against diseases carried by the blood and air. Precautionary measures help protect against infection from viruses and bacteria.

Bloodborne Disease

Some diseases are caused by microorganisms that are "borne" (carried) in a person's bloodstream. Contact with blood infected with such microorganisms may cause infection. Of the many bloodborne pathogens, three pose significant health threats to first aiders: hepatitis B virus (HBV), hepatitis C virus (HCV), and human immunodeficiency virus (HIV).

Hepatitis B

Hepatitis is a viral infection of the liver. Types A, B, and C are seen most often. Each is caused by a different virus.

A vaccine for hepatitis B is available and recommended for all infants and for adults who may have contact with carriers of the disease or with blood. Medical and laboratory workers, police, intravenous drug users, people with multiple sexual partners, and those living with someone who has a life-long infection are at high risk of hepatitis B (and hepatitis C as well). Vaccination is the best defense against HBV. There is no chance of developing hepatitis B from the vaccine. Federal laws require employers to offer a series of three vaccine injections free to all employees who may be at risk of exposure.

Without vaccination shots, exposure to hepatitis B may produce symptoms within two weeks to six months after the exposure. People with hepatitis B infection may be symptom free, but that does *not* mean they are not contagious. These people may infect others who are exposed to their blood. Symptoms of hepatitis B resemble those of the flu and include fatigue, nausea, loss of appetite, stomach pain, and perhaps a yellowing of the skin.

Hepatitis B starts as an inflammation of the liver and usually lasts one to two months. In a few people, the infection is very serious, and in some, mild infection continues for life. The virus may stay in the liver and can lead to severe damage (cirrhosis) and liver cancer. Medical treatment that begins immediately after exposure may prevent the infection from developing.

Hepatitis C

Hepatitis C is caused by a different virus from HBV, but both diseases have a great deal in common. Like hepatitis B, hepatitis C affects the liver and can lead to long-term liver disease and liver cancer. Hepatitis C varies in severity and there may not be any symptoms at the time of infection. Currently, there is no vaccine or effective treatment for hepatitis C.

HIV

A person infected with HIV can infect others, and HIV-infected persons almost always develop acquired immunodeficiency syndrome (AIDS), which interferes with the body's ability to fight off other diseases. No vaccine is available to prevent HIV infection, which eventually proves fatal. The best defense against AIDS is to avoid becoming infected.

Protection

In most cases, you can control the risk of exposure to bloodborne pathogens by wearing the proper Personal Protective Equipment (PPE) and by following some simple procedures.

Personal Protective Equipment (PPE)

Personal protective equipment (PPE) prevents an organism from entering the body. The most common type of protection is when a rescuer uses medical exam gloves. The Food and Drug Administration (FDA), the Centers for Disease Control and Prevention (CDC), and the Occupational Safety and Health Administration (OSHA) have stated that vinyl and latex medical exam gloves are equally protective. Some rescuers are allergic to latex, but can wear vinyl or Nitrile gloves. All first aid kits should have several pairs of medical exam gloves ▼Figure 2.

Protective eyewear and a standard surgical mask may be necessary at some emergencies; first aiders ordinarily will not have or need such equipment.

Mouth-to-barrier devices are recommended for rescue breathing and cardiopulmonary resuscitation (CPR). There are no documented cases of disease transmission to a rescuer as a result of performing unprotected CPR on an infected victim. Nevertheless, a mouth-to-barrier device should be used whenever possible ►Figure 3.

Universal Precautions and Body Substance Isolation Techniques

Individuals infected with HBV or HIV may not show symptoms and may not even know they are infectious. For that reason, all human blood and body fluids should be considered infectious, and precautions should be

Figure 2 Whenever possible, use gloves as a barrier.

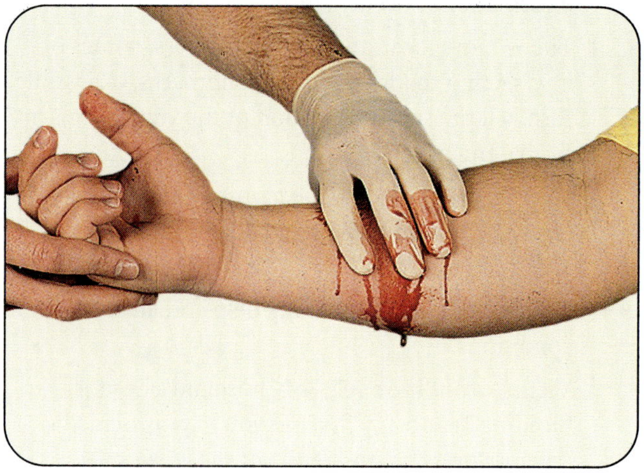

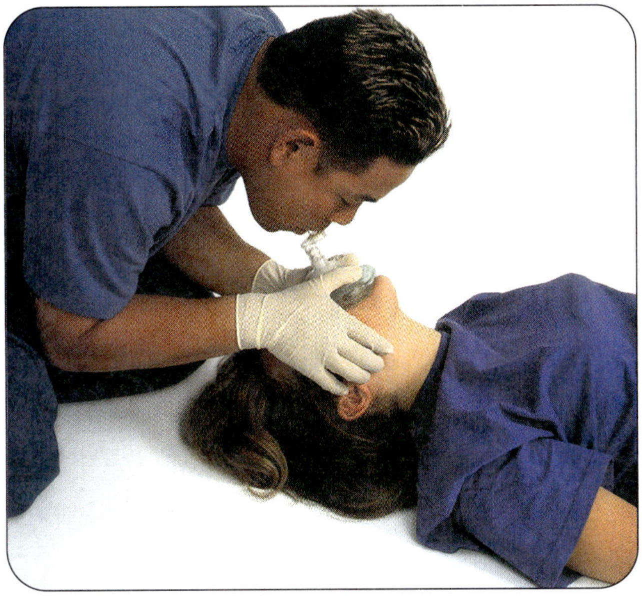

Figure 3 Pocket face mask, one-way valve

taken to avoid contact. The *body substance isolation* (BSI) technique assumes that *any* body fluid is a possible risk. EMS personnel routinely follow BSI procedures, even if blood or body fluids are not visible.

OSHA requires any company with employees who are expected to give first aid in an emergency to follow *universal precautions,* which assume that *all* blood and *certain* body fluids pose a risk for transmission of HBV and HIV. OSHA defines an employee who assists another with a nosebleed or a cut as a "Good Samaritan." Such acts, however, are not considered occupational exposure unless the employee who provided the assistance is a member of a first aid team or is designated or expected to render first aid as part of his or her job. In essence, OSHA's requirement excludes unassigned employees who perform unanticipated first aid.

Whenever there is a chance that you could be exposed to bloodborne pathogens, your employer must provide appropriate PPE, which might include eye protection, medical exam gloves, gowns, and masks. The PPE must be accessible, and your employer must provide training to help you choose the right PPE for your work.

While EMS personnel follow BSI procedures and OSHA requires designated worksite first aiders to follow universal precautions, what should a typical first aider do? It makes sense for first aiders to follow BSI procedures and assume that *all* blood and body fluids are infectious and follow appropriate protective measures.

Coping with Emergencies

When an injury occurs, first aiders can protect themselves and others against bloodborne pathogens by following these steps:

1. Wear appropriate PPE, such as gloves.
2. If you have been trained in the correct procedures, use absorbent barriers to soak up blood or other infectious materials.
3. Clean the spill area with an appropriate disinfecting solution, such as diluted bleach.
4. Discard contaminated materials in an appropriate waste disposal container.

If you have been exposed to blood or body fluids:

1. Use soap and water to wash the parts of your body that have been contaminated.
2. Report the incident to your supervisor, if the exposure happens while at work. Otherwise, contact your personal physician. Early action can prevent the development of hepatitis B and enable affected workers to track potential HIV infection.

The best protection against bloodborne disease is to use the safeguards described here. By following these guidelines, first aiders can decrease their chances of contracting bloodborne illnesses.

Airborne Disease

Infective organisms such as bacteria or viruses that are introduced into the air by coughing or sneezing are said to be "airborne." Droplets of mucus that carry those bacteria or viruses can then be inhaled by other individuals. The rate of tuberculosis (TB) has increased recently and is receiving much attention. TB, caused by bacteria, sometimes settles in the lungs and can be fatal. In most cases, a first aider will not know that a victim has TB. Assume that any person with a cough, especially one who is in a nursing home or a shelter, may have TB. Other symptoms include fatigue, weight loss, chest pain, and coughing up blood. If a surgical mask is available, wear it or wrap a handkerchief over your nose and mouth.

Learning Activities

Action at an Emergency

Directions: Circle Yes if you agree with the statement, and circle No if you disagree.

Yes No **1.** A scene survey should be done before giving first aid to an injured victim.

Yes No **2.** For a severely injured victim, call the victim's doctor before calling for an ambulance.

Yes No **3.** Most communities use the 9-1-1 telephone number for emergencies.

Yes No **4.** First aiders should assume that blood and all body fluids are infectious.

Yes No **5.** If you are exposed to blood while on the job, report it to your supervisor, and if off the job, your personal physician.

Yes No **6.** First aid kits should contain medical exam gloves.

Scenario: You are rushing parts to one of your largest customer's broken machines. Because "time is money," the customer is losing a lot for each hour its machine is down. It's beginning to rain. Suddenly, you see a motorcyclist skid off the highway, and end up in a ditch. You have a cellular telephone in your car.

7. Name the 5 actions that a bystander can take at an emergency.

a. ______________________ **d.** ______________________

b. ______________________ **e.** ______________________

c. ______________________

8. A scene survey consists of looking for what three things?

a. ______________________

b. ______________________

c. ______________________

9. When talking with an EMS dispatcher, what 5 items should you be prepared to provide?

a. ______________________ **d.** ______________________

b. ______________________ **e.** ______________________

c. ______________________

10. How would you protect yourself against bloodborne pathogens?

a. ______________________

b. ______________________

c. ______________________

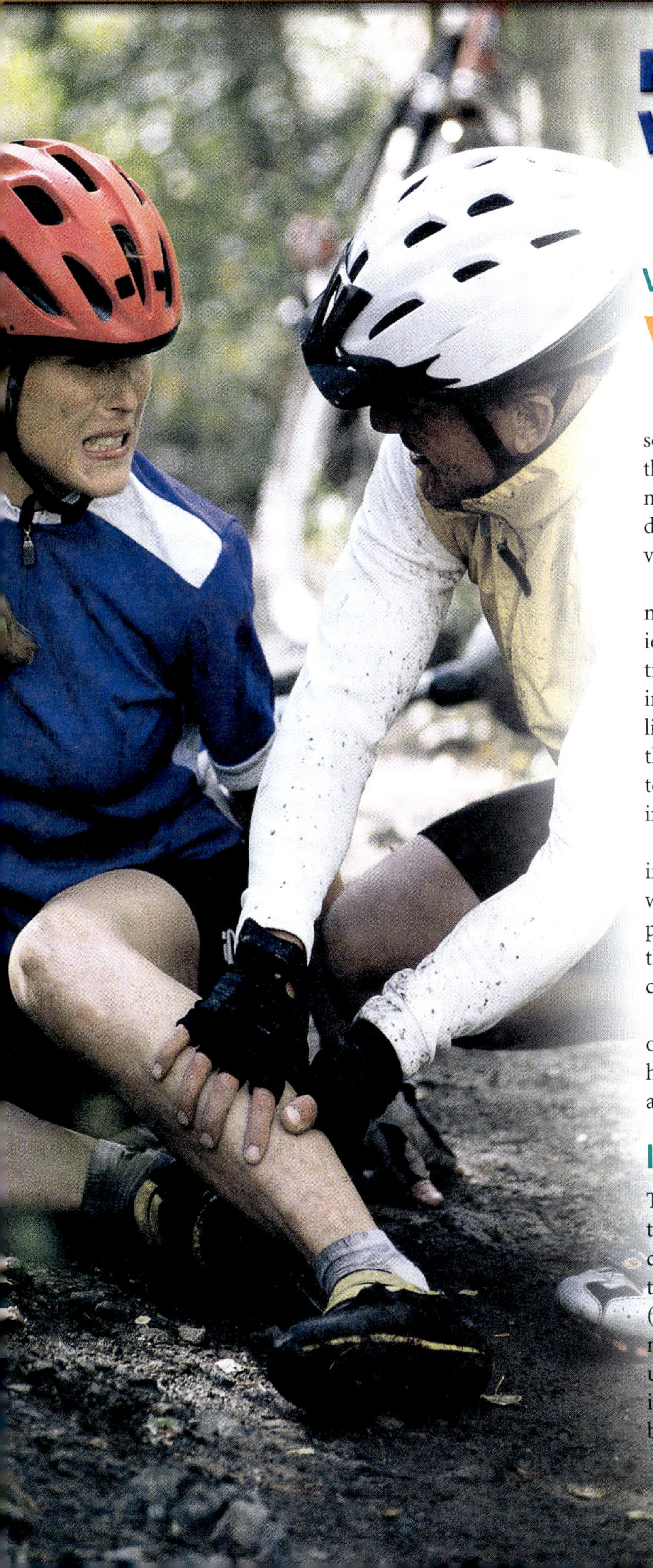

Chapter 3

Finding Out What's Wrong

Victim Assessment

Victim assessment is an important first aid skill. It requires an understanding of each assessment step as well as decision-making skills.

Every time you encounter a victim, first check out the scene. The scene survey determines the safety of the scene, the victim's cause of injury or nature of illness, and the number of victims. Without a scene survey, a potentially dangerous situation could result in further injury to the victim or to you and others.

The scene survey is followed by the initial victim assessment. During the initial victim assessment, the first aider identifies and corrects immediate life-threatening conditions involving problems with the victim's airway, breathing, and circulation (the ABCs). Victims with immediate life-threatening conditions can die within minutes unless their problems are quickly recognized and corrected. Determining the type of injury or illness is also part of the initial assessment.

A physical examination and medical history follow the initial assessment. These steps can reveal information that will help identify the injury or illness, its severity, and appropriate first aid. Detailed information is gained about the victim's injury (eg, painful ankle, bleeding nose) or chief complaint (eg, chest pain, itchy skin).

If two or more people are injured, attend to the quiet one first. A quiet victim might not be breathing or have a heartbeat. A victim who is talking, crying, or otherwise alert is obviously breathing.

Initial Assessment

The goal of the initial assessment is to determine whether there are life-threatening problems that require quick care ►Skill Scan. This assessment involves evaluating the victim's airway (A), breathing (B), and circulation (C). The following step-by-step initial assessment should not be changed. It takes less than a minute to complete, unless first aid is required at any point. By the end of the initial assessement, the victim's problem will most likely be identified as being an injury or an illness.

Skill Scan Initial Assessment

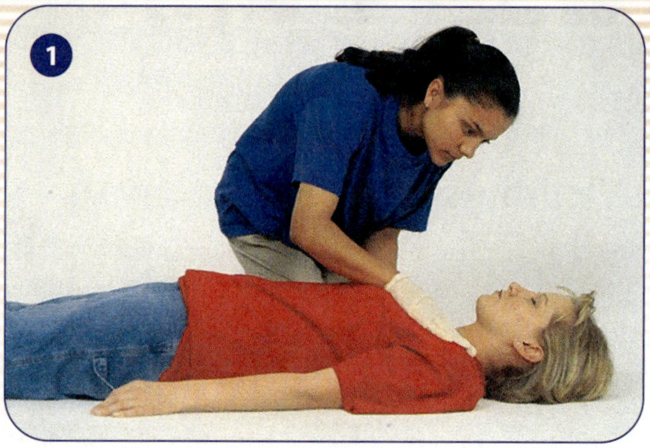

1. Responsive? Tap and shout.

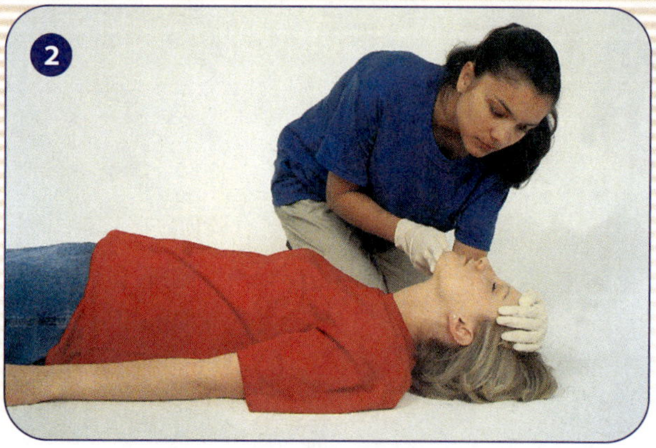

2. A = Airway open? Head-tilt/chin-lift.

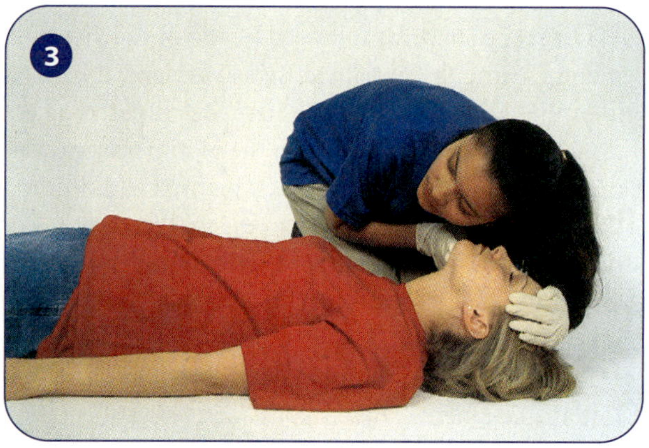

3. B = Breathing? Look, listen, and feel.

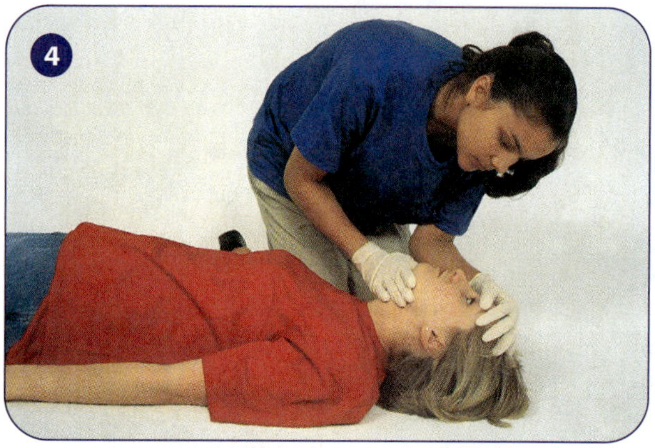

4. C = Circulation? Check for signs of circulation.

Check for responsiveness by speaking to the victim. If the person can talk, breathing and heartbeat are present. Check for orientation by asking their name, if they know where they are, and what happened. If the victim does not respond, tap his or her shoulder and ask, "Are you okay?" If there is no response, consider the victim as being unresponsive.

Immediate Threats to Life

A: Airway

The airway must be open for breathing. If the victim is speaking or crying, the airway is open. If a responsive victim cannot talk, cry, or cough forcefully, the airway is probably obstructed and must be checked and cleared. In this case, abdominal thrusts (Heimlich maneuver) can be given to clear an obstructed airway in a responsive adult victim.

In an unresponsive victim lying face up, the most common airway obstruction is the tongue. Snoring is evidence of this. If there is no suspected spinal injury, use the head tilt–chin lift method to open the airway.

Once the victim's airway is clear of obstruction, the initial assessment can continue.

B: Breathing

A breathing rate between 12 and 20 times per minute is normal for adults. Victims who are having difficulty moving air and who are breathing less than eight times per minute or more than 24 times per minute need care. Note any breathing difficulties or unusual breathing sounds such as wheezing, crowing, gurgling, or snoring. This step primarily focuses upon whether or not the victim is breathing and obvious breathing difficulties rather than the breathing rate.

Check for breathing in an unresponsive victim after opening the airway. Watch for the victim's chest to rise and fall as you place your ear next to the victim's mouth. "Look, listen, and feel" for about 10 seconds to check for breathing. If the victim is not breathing, keep the airway open and breathe two slow breaths into the victim. Whenever possible, use a mouth-to-barrier device (mask or face shield).

C: Circulation

After checking and correcting any airway and breathing problems, check the victim's circulation. This can be done by checking the signs of circulation—breathing, coughing, movement, noting the skin color and temperature, and searching for severe bleeding.

Signs of Circulation. The signs of normal circulation include breathing, coughing, movement, normal skin condition, and pulse.

Severe Bleeding Check for severe bleeding by looking over the victim's entire body for blood (blood-soaked clothing or blood pooling on the floor or the ground). Controlling bleeding requires the application of direct pressure or a pressure bandage. Avoid contact with the victim's blood, if possible, by using medical exam gloves or extra layers of dressings or cloth. Control any bleeding with pressure as described in Chapter 4.

Skin Condition A quick check of the victim's skin can also provide information about circulatory status. Check skin temperature, color, and condition (eg, moist, dry). Skin color, especially in light-skinned people, reflects the circulation under the skin as well as oxygen status. In darkly pigmented people, changes might not be readily apparent but can be assessed by the appearance of the nail beds, the inside of the mouth, and the inner eyelids. When the skin's blood vessels constrict or the pulse slows, the skin becomes cool and pale or cyanotic (blue-gray color). When the skin's blood vessels dilate or blood flow increases, the skin becomes warm.

You can get a rough idea of temperature by putting the back of your hand or wrist on the victim's forehead. If the victim has a fever, you should be able to feel it. Abnormal skin temperature will feel hot, cool, cold, or clammy (cool and moist).

If you suspect a spinal injury, do not move the victim. See Chapter 8 for the best way to immobilize a suspected spinal injury.

Physical Exam and SAMPLE History

The initial assessment is followed by a physical examination and the **SAMPLE** history. During this time you will note the victim's signs and symptoms:

- *Signs* = victim's conditions you can see, feel, hear or smell
- *Symptoms* = things the victim feels and is able to describe; known as the "chief complaint"

Physical Examination Check the victim's head, neck, chest, abdomen, pelvis, and extremities ▶Skill Scan. To help you evaluate these areas, look and feel for the following signs of injury: deformities, open injuries, tenderness, and swelling. The mnemonic **D-O-T-S** is helpful in remembering the signs of injury.

Skill Scan Physical Exam: Injury

Briefly Look and Feel for D-O-T-S Throughout the Body

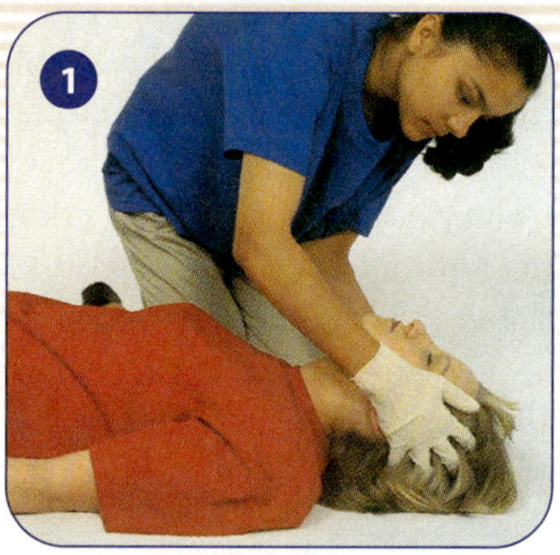

1. Head: Check the skull and scalp. Look and feel for D-O-T-S. Check for clear fluid in ears (cerebrospinal fluid).

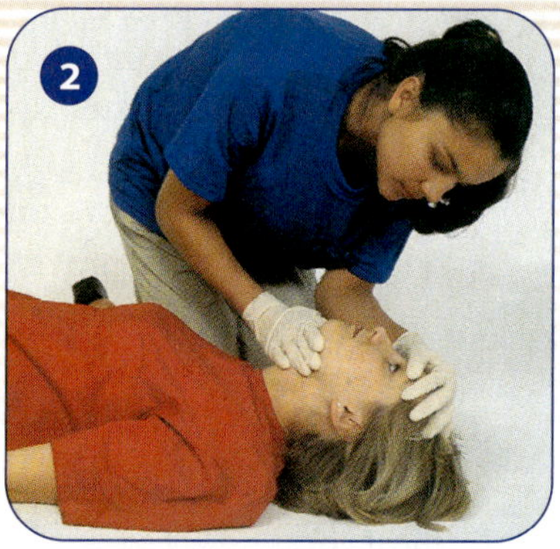

2. Eyes: Gently open both eyes and compare the pupils—they should be the same size. Check to see if they react to light.

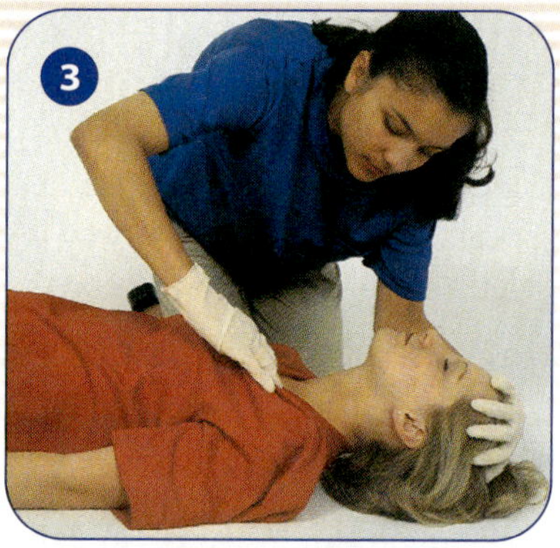

3. Neck: Look and gently feel for D-O-T-S. Check for a medical-alert necklace.

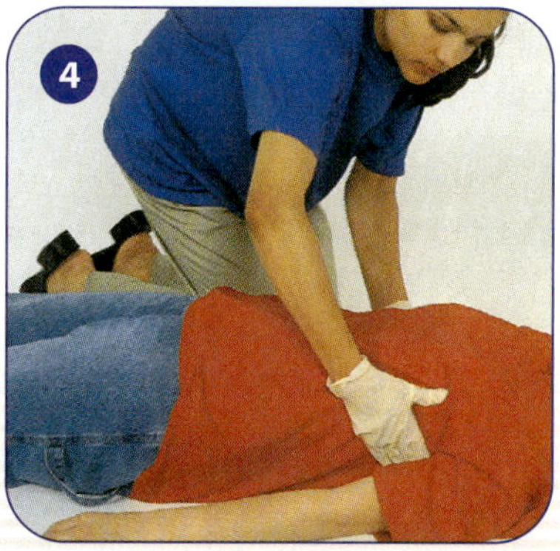

4. Chest: Check for D-O-T-S. Gently squeeze the chest for rib pain.

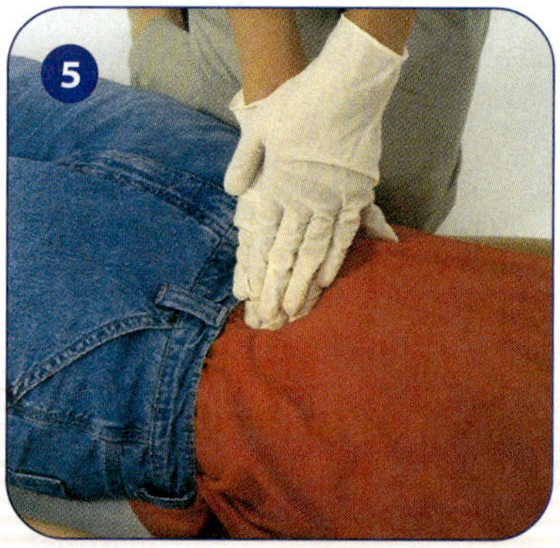

5. Abdomen: Check for D-O-T-S. Gently press the four abdominal quadrants.

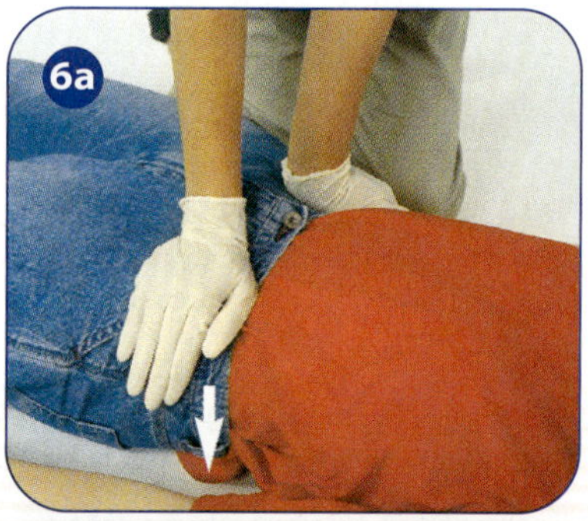

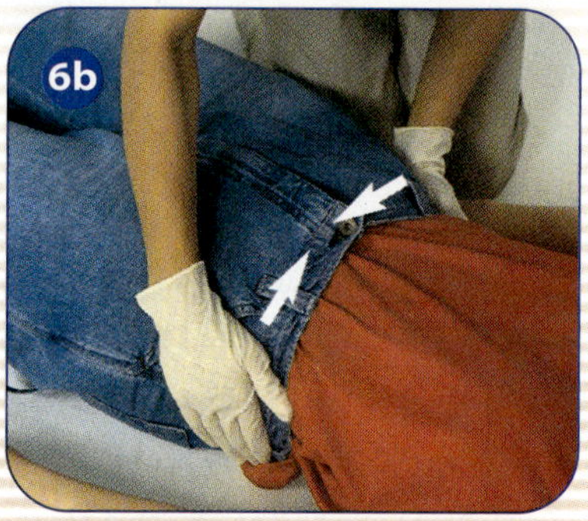

6. Pelvis: Check for D-O-T-S:
- **a.** Gently press downward on the tops of the hips for pain.
- **b.** Gently press towards each other for pain.

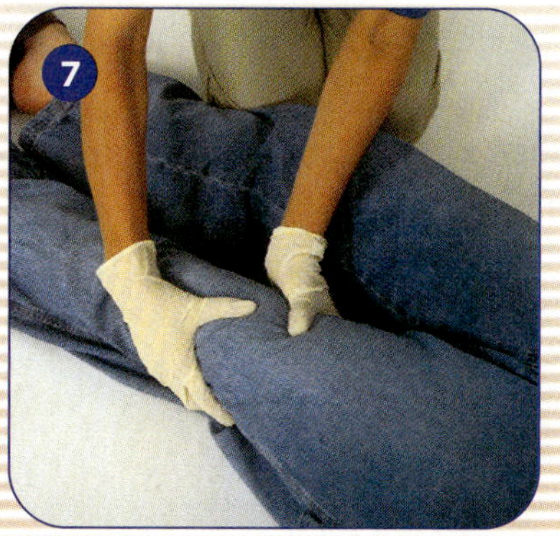

7. Extremities: Check the full length of both arms and legs for D-O-T-S. Check for CSM—circulation (pulse), sensation, movement.

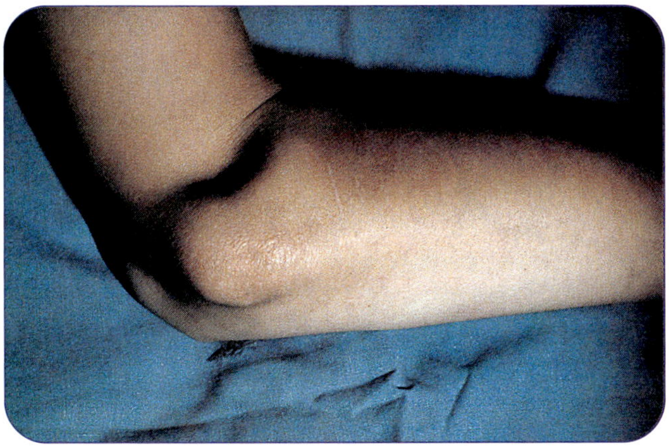

Figure 1 D = Deformity

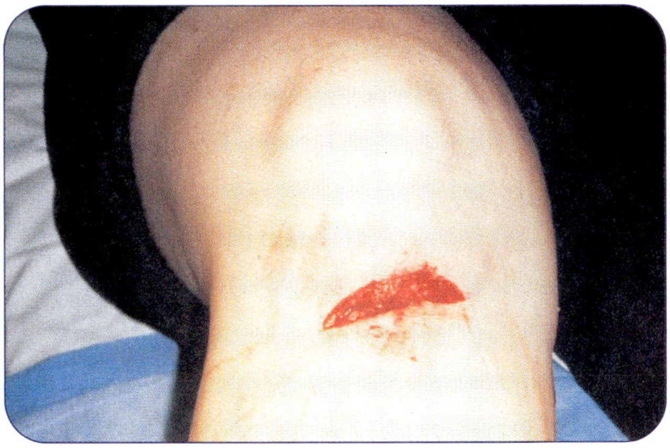

Figure 2 O = Open wounds

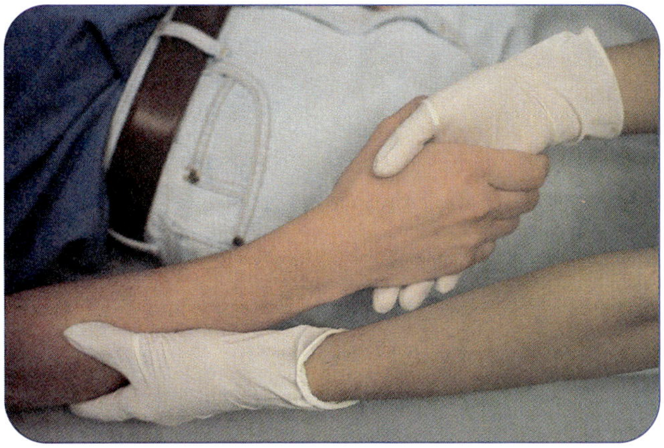

Figure 3 T = Tenderness

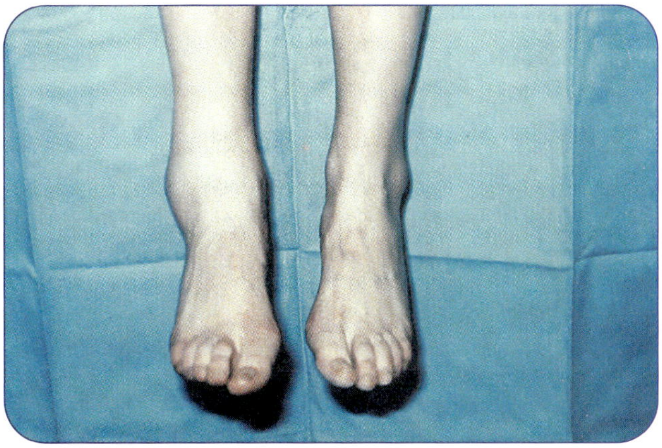

Figure 4 S = Swelling

Deformities occur when bones are broken, causing an abnormal shape.

Open wounds break the skin.

Tenderness is sensitivity to touch.

Swelling is the body's response to injury that makes the area look larger than usual

Here are some things you should look and feel for during the physical exam:

Head Have someone stabilize the victim's head and neck to keep it from moving. Look and feel for D-O-T-S over the entire head. Look for leakage of blood or fluid (cerebrospinal fluid) from the nose or ears.

Eyes Check the pupils of the eyes for equality and reactivity to light. Pupils should be of equal size when the brain is not injured. To check for reactivity to light, use a flashlight or cover and then uncover the victim's eyes with your hand. Pupils normally quickly constrict in response to light.

Neck Look and feel for D-O-T-S.

Chest Look and feel the entire chest for D-O-T-S. Squeeze or compress the sides together for rib pain.

Abdomen Look and feel for D-O-T-S. Gently press all four abdominal quadrants for rigidity and tenderness, using the pads of your fingers. If the victim complains of pain in a particular area, ask the victim to point to it; press that area last.

Pelvis Look and feel for D-O-T-S. Gently squeeze the hips inward together and gently press the hips downward.

Extremities Look and feel the entire length and girth of each extremity (arms and legs) for D-O-T-S. Check the **C**irculation, **S**ensation, and **M**ovement (use the mnemonic **CSM** as a way of remembering) of each extremity. Check for circulation in the arms by feeling for the radial pulse on the victim's thumb side of the wrist and check the circulation of the legs by feeling for the posterior tibial pulse between the inside of the ankle bone and the Achilles tendon. In a responsive victim, check for sensation by asking the victim whether he or she can feel you pinching his or her fingers and toes. To check for movement, ask the victim to wiggle his or her fingers and toes, to squeeze your hand with his or her hands, and to push his or her feet against your hand. Compare the responses of one extremity against the responses of the other for any differences. Lack of sensation or movement can indicate an injured extremity or spinal injury.

If you suspect a spinal injury, do not move the victim's head or neck. Stabilize the victim against any movement, and be sure to tell him or her not to move.

SAMPLE History The information in a **SAMPLE** history can affect the first aid you give. It is called a SAMPLE history because the letters in the word "SAMPLE" stand for the elements of the history:

S = Symptoms

"What's wrong?" (known as the chief complaint)

A = Allergies

"Are you allergic to anything?"

M = Medications

"Are you taking any medications? What are they for?"

P = Past medical history

"Have you had this problem before? Do you have other medical problems?"

L = Last oral intake

"When did you last eat or drink anything? What was it?"

E = Events leading up to the illness or injury

Injury: "How did you get hurt?"
Illness: "What led to this problem?"

If the victim is unresponsive, you may be able to obtain the SAMPLE history information from family, friends, or bystanders.

Caution:

WHEN DOING A PHYSICAL EXAM

DO NOT aggravate injuries or contaminate wounds.

DO NOT move a victim with a possible spinal injury.

Physical Exam and SAMPLE History for Injured Victims

For an injured victim, start by reconsidering the cause (mechanism) of injury that you identified previously, during the scene survey ▶Table 1. This allows you to determine which procedures to use in checking an injured victim.

Table 1: Significant Mechanisms (Causes) of Injury

- Falls of more than 15 feet for adults, more than 10 feet for children, or more than three times the victim's height
- Vehicle collisions involving ejection, a rollover, high speeds, a pedestrian, a motorcycle, or a bicycle
- Unresponsive or altered mental status
- Penetrations of the head, chest, or abdomen (eg, stab or gunshot wounds) of the muscle between the neck and shoulder

Injured Victim With a Significant Mechanism of Injury For an injured victim with a significant mechanism of injury, stabilize the head (if the injury involves the head, neck, chest, or back) to keep it from moving, check ABC, perform a rapid physical examination from head to toe, and if possible, obtain a SAMPLE history.

Injured Victim with No Significant Mechanism of Injury The physical examination of a victim without a significant mechanism of injury should focus on the area(s) that the victim complains about. Determine the chief complaint—the problem as the victim describes it. For example, the victim might complain of "twisting" an ankle. Begin the physical examination at the location of the injury using the mnemonic **D-O-T-S.** Your assessment focuses on just the areas that the victim tells you are painful or that you suspect may be injured. After the physical exam, conduct a SAMPLE history.

Physical Exam and SAMPLE History for Ill Victims

With a responsive ill victim, first obtain the victim's SAMPLE history then conduct a physical examination focused on the victim's chief complaint (symptoms). With an unresponsive ill victim, perform a rapid physical examination first, followed by the victim's SAMPLE history (if possible from bystanders).

Medical Identification Tags Look for medical identification tags, which may be beneficial in identifying allergies, medications, allergies, or medical history ▶Figure 5. A medical-alert tag, worn as a necklace or as a bracelet, contains the wearer's medical problem(s) and a 24-hour telephone number that offers, in case of an emergency, access to the victim's medical history plus names of doctors

Victim Assessment Sequence

+ Determine responsiveness
↓
+ Perform initial assessment (ABCs)

Injured Victim

1. Significant Mechanism of Injury:
   a. Physical exam (head to toe)
   b. SAMPLE history
2. No Significant Mechanism of Injury:
   a. Physical exam (examine only complaint)
   b. SAMPLE history

Ill Victim

1. Responsive:
   a. SAMPLE history
   b. Physical exam (examine only complaint)
2. Unresponsive:
   a. Physical exam (head to toe)
   b. SAMPLE history (from bystanders)

Figure 5 Medic Alert® identification tag

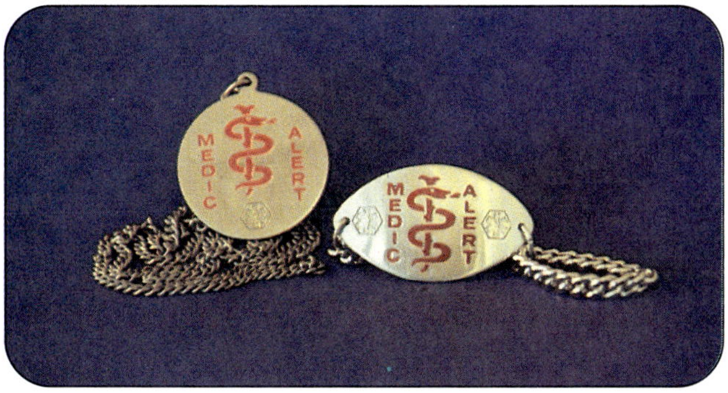

and close relatives. Necklaces and bracelets are durable, instantly recognizable, and less likely than cards to be separated from the victim in an emergency.

What to Do Until EMS Arrives

The initial assessment, physical examination, and SAMPLE history are done quickly so that injuries and illnesses can be identified and given first aid and, if necessary, transportation can be arranged. After the most serious problems have been cared for, regularly recheck the victim.

Recheck the victim's responsiveness, airway, breathing, circulation, and the effectiveness of first aid. Do this at least every 15 minutes for an alert victim, who has no serious injury or illness, and at least every five minutes for a victim who is unresponsive; has difficulties with airway, breathing, or circulation, including major blood loss; or has a significant mechanism of injury. Report your findings to EMS personnel when they arrive.

Learning Activities

Finding Out What's Wrong

Directions: Circle Yes if you agree with the statement, and circle No if you disagree.

Yes No **1.** An initial survey's purpose is to find life-threatening conditions.

Yes No **2.** Crying or screaming victims should be treated before quiet ones.

Yes No **3.** Most injured victims require a complete victim assessment.

Yes No **4.** In a physical exam, you usually begin at the head and work down the body.

Yes No **5.** Tapping a victim's shoulder helps in determining the victim's responsiveness.

Yes No **6.** The mnemonic D-O-T-S helps in remembering what to collect about the victim's history that may be useful.

Yes No **7.** For all injured and suddenly ill persons, look for medical-alert identification.

Yes No **8.** The mnemonic SAMPLE can remind you how to examine an area for signs of an injury.

Scenario: During a mid-morning break, a co-worker screams that somebody has collapsed in the hallway. As a company designated first aider, you push your way through a crowd of people gathered around the victim. You recognize Clyde, one of the older employees who is about to retire from the company, lying on the floor motionless. You notice that he wears a medical-alert identification bracelet.

____**9.** After confirming that the scene is safe, you next check Clyde for:

A. breathing **B.** signs of circulation **C.** broken bones **D.** responsiveness

____**10.** If he were unresponsive, you would:

A. open his airway and check for breathing
B. look for signs of circulation
C. look and feel for broken bones
D. look at his medical-alert ID tag

____**11.** If Clyde were responsive and breathing, what would you next check?

A. physical exam **B.** victim's history

____**12.** For injured victims, which usually comes first?

A. physical exam **B.** victim's history

____**13.** The physical exam on an adult should be started at the victim's:

A. head **B.** chest **C.** feet

____**14.** Which of these would the medical-alert identification bracelet help identify?

A. allergies **B.** medications **C.** medical history **D.** all of these

____**15.** When checking Clyde's eyes, you should look for:

A. color of the iris
B. reaction of pupils to light
C. equal or unequal size of the pupils
D. both B and C

Chapter 4

Bleeding and Shock

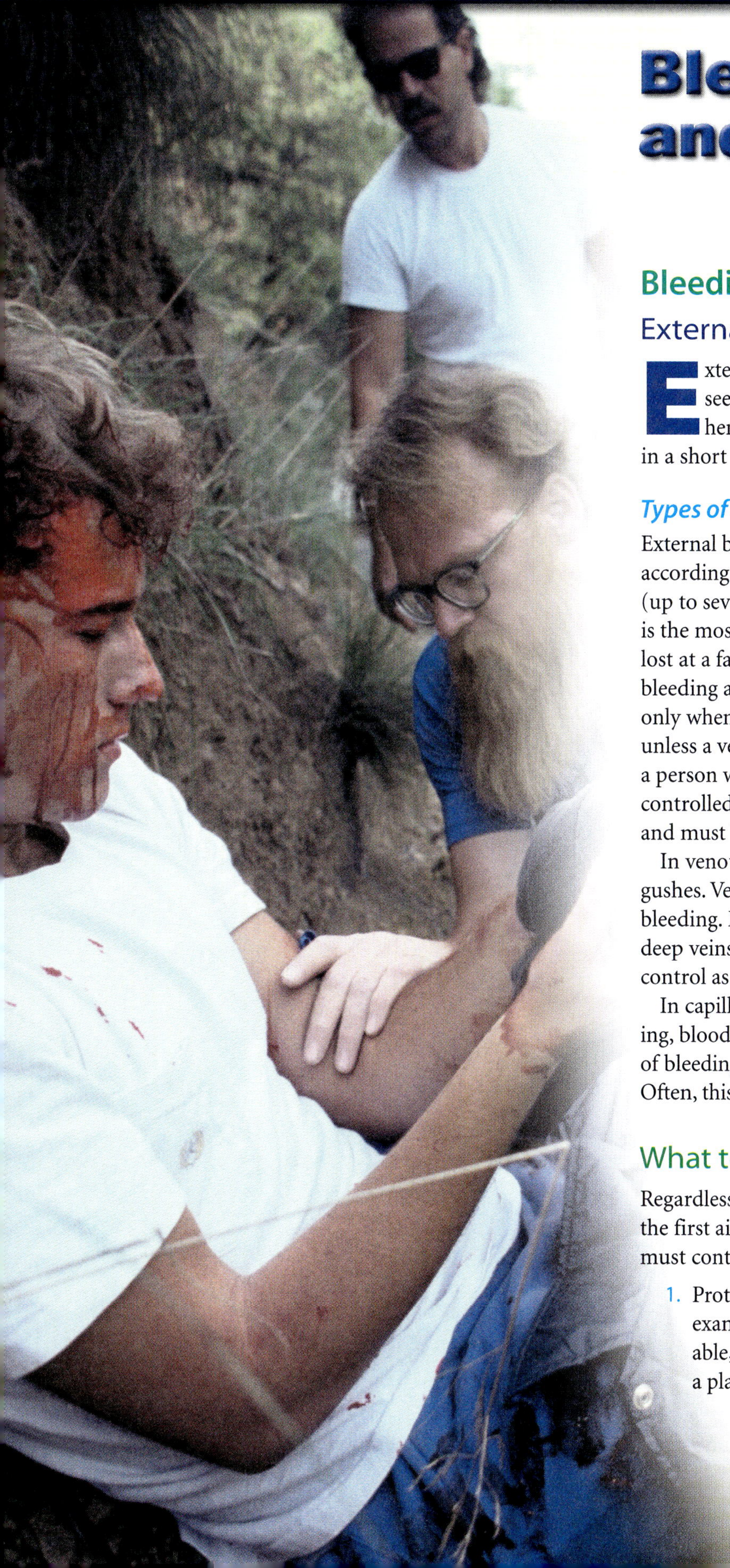

Bleeding

External Bleeding

External bleeding occurs when blood can be seen coming from an open wound. The term hemorrhage refers to a large amount of bleeding in a short time.

Types of External Bleeding

External bleeding can be classified into three types according to its source. In arterial bleeding, blood spurts (up to several feet) from the wound. Arterial bleeding is the most serious type of bleeding because blood is lost at a fast rate, leading to a large blood loss. Arterial bleeding also is less likely to clot because blood can clot only when it is flowing slowly or not at all. However, unless a very large artery has been cut, it is unlikely that a person will bleed to death before the flow can be controlled. Nevertheless, arterial bleeding is dangerous and must be controlled.

In venous bleeding, blood from a vein flows steadily or gushes. Venous bleeding is easier to control than arterial bleeding. Most veins collapse when cut. Bleeding from deep veins, however, can be as massive and as hard to control as arterial bleeding.

In capillary bleeding, the most common type of bleeding, blood oozes from capillaries—the most common type of bleeding. It usually is not serious and easily controlled. Often, this type of bleeding will clot and stop by itself.

What to Do

Regardless of the type of bleeding or the type of wound, the first aid is the same. First, and most important, you must control the bleeding (▶Skill Scan):

1. Protect yourself against disease by wearing medical exam gloves. If medical exam gloves are not available, use several layers of gauze pads, plastic wrap, a plastic bag, clean cloths or waterproof material.

Skill Scan Bleeding Control

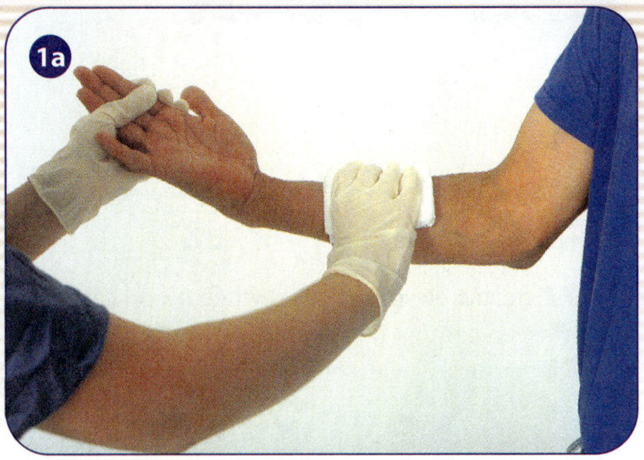

1a. Direct pressure stops most bleeding. Wear medical exam gloves, and place a sterile gauze pad or a clean cloth over wound.

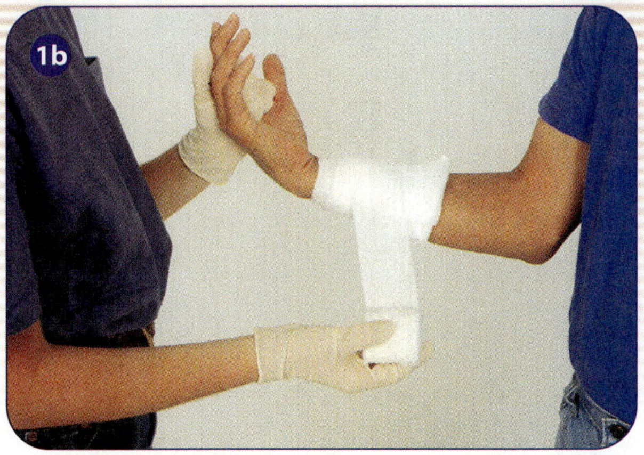

1b. A pressure bandage can free you to attend to other injuries or victims.

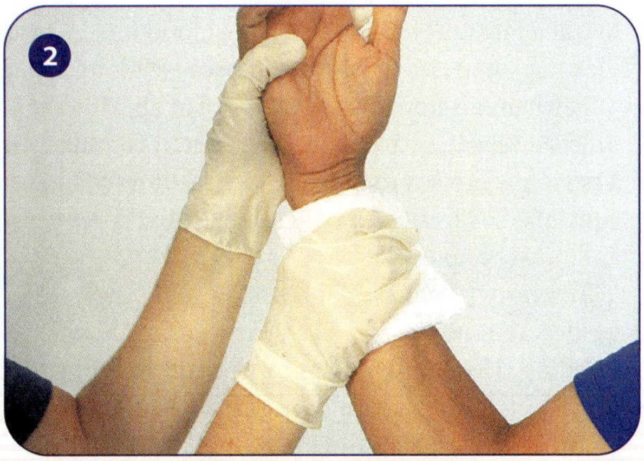

2. If bleeding continues, use elevation to help reduce blood flow. Combine with direct pressure over the wound.

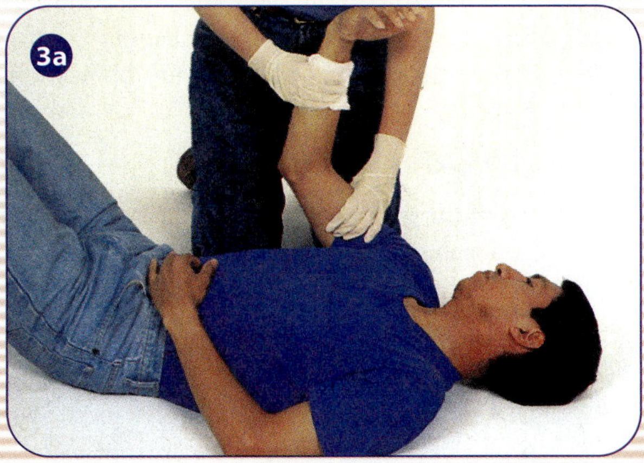

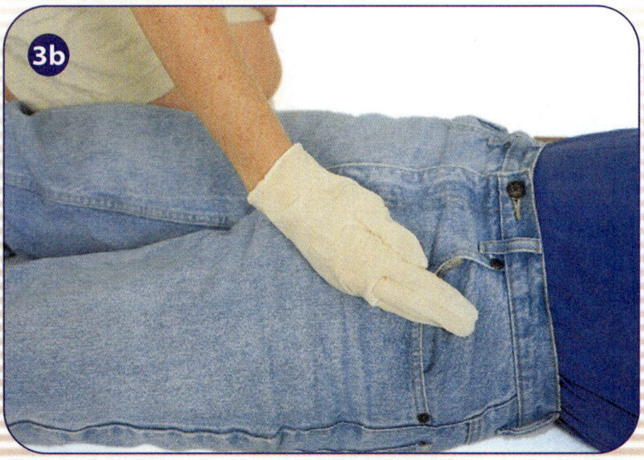

3. If bleeding continues, apply pressure at a pressure point to slow blood flow. Locations are: (**a**) brachial or (**b**) femoral. Combine with direct pressure over the wound.

You can even have the victim apply pressure on the wound with his or her own hand. After bleeding has stopped and the wound has been cared for, vigorously wash your hands with soap and water.

2. Expose the wound by removing or cutting the clothing to find the source of the blood.

Caution:

DO NOT touch a wound with your bare hands. If you must use your bare hands, do so only as a last resort. After the bleeding has stopped and the wound has been cared for, vigorously wash your hands with soap and water.

DO NOT use direct pressure on an eye injury, a wound with an embedded object, or a skull fracture.

DO NOT remove a blood-soaked dressing. Apply another dressing on top and keep pressing.

3. Place a sterile gauze pad or a clean cloth such as a handkerchief, washcloth, or towel over the entire wound and apply direct pressure with your fingers or the palm of your hand. The gauze or cloth allows you to apply even pressure.
4. If bleeding is from an arm or leg, elevate the injured area above heart level as you continue to apply pressure to reduce blood flow. Elevating the extremity means that gravity will make it difficult for the body to pump blood to the affected limb.
5. If the bleeding continues, keep applying direct pressure over the wound and apply pressure at a pressure point to slow the flow of blood. A pressure point is where an artery near the skin's surface passes close to a bone, against which it can be compressed. The most accessible pressure points on both sides of the body are the brachial point in the upper inside arm and the femoral point in the groin.
6. To free you to attend to other injuries or victims, use a pressure bandage to hold the dressing on the wound. Wrap a roller gauze bandage tightly over the dressing and above and below the wound site.
7. When you cannot apply direct pressure (eg, in the case of a protruding bone, skull fracture, or embedded object), use a doughnut-shaped (ring) pad to control bleeding. To make a ring pad, wrap one end of a narrow bandage (roller or cravat) several times around your four fingers to form a loop. Pass the other end of the bandage through the loop and wrap it around and around until the entire bandage is used and a ring has been made.
8. When bleeding stops, use procedures in Chapter 6 for wound care.

Caution:

Tourniquets are rarely needed and can damage nerves and blood vessels. Using a tourniquet may cause the loss of an arm or leg. If you do use one, apply wide, flat materials—never rope or wire—and do not loosen it.

Internal Bleeding

Internal bleeding occurs when the skin is not broken and blood is not seen. It can be difficult to detect but can be life threatening. Internal bleeding comes from injuries that do not break the skin or from nontraumatic disorders such as ulcers.

What to Look For

The signs of internal bleeding may take days to appear:

- bruises or contusions of the skin
- painful, tender, rigid, bruised abdomen
- vomiting or coughing up blood
- stools that are black or contain bright red blood

What to Do

For severe internal bleeding, follow these steps:

1. Monitor ABCs.
2. Expect vomiting. If vomiting occurs, keep the victim lying on his or her left side for so that the vomiting can drain. This will also prevent the victim from inhaling vomitus and will prevent expulsion of vomit from the stomach.
3. Treat for shock by raising the victim's legs 8 to 12 inches and covering the victim with a coat or blanket to keep him or her warm. See page 24 for when to use other body positions.
4. Seek immediate medical attention.

Bruises are a form of internal bleeding but are not life threatening. To treat bruises see page 31.

BLEEDING

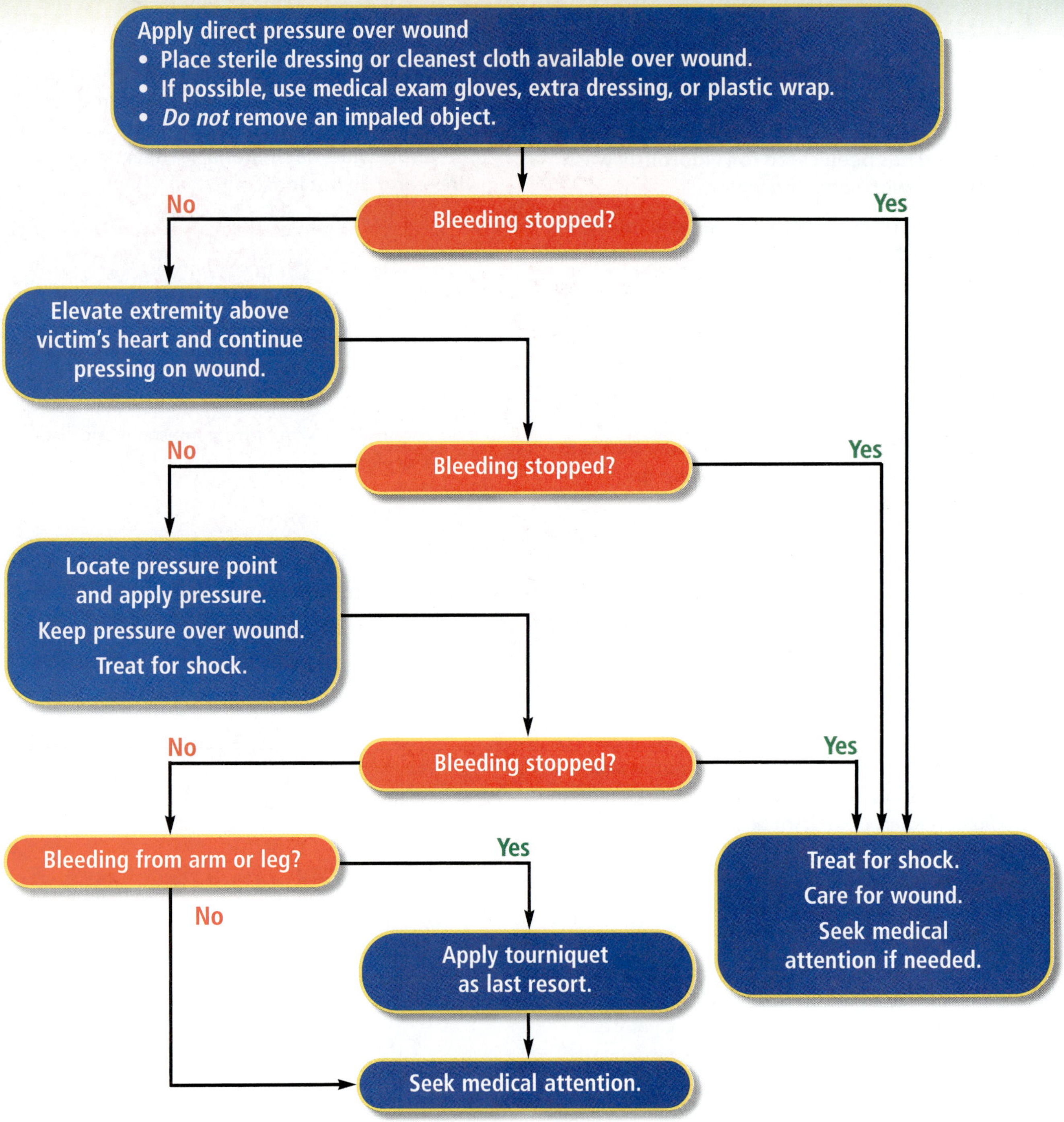
Apply direct pressure over wound
• Place sterile dressing or cleanest cloth available over wound.
• If possible, use medical exam gloves, extra dressing, or plastic wrap.
• *Do not* remove an impaled object.
No
Bleeding stopped?
Yes
Elevate extremity above victim's heart and continue pressing on wound.
No
Bleeding stopped?
Yes
Locate pressure point and apply pressure.
Keep pressure over wound.
Treat for shock.
No
Bleeding stopped?
Yes
Bleeding from arm or leg?
Yes
No
Apply tourniquet as last resort.
Seek medical attention.
Treat for shock.
Care for wound.
Seek medical attention if needed.

Caution:

DO NOT give a victim anything to eat or drink. It could cause nausea and vomiting, which could result in inhaling foreign material into the lungs (aspiration). Food or liquids could cause complications during surgery if it is needed.

Shock

Shock refers to circulatory system failure, which happens when insufficient amounts of oxygenated blood is provided for every body part. Because every injury affects the circulatory system to some degree, first aiders should automatically treat injured victims for shock.

To understand shock, think of the circulatory system as having three components: a working pump (the heart), a network of pipes (the blood vessels), and an adequate amount of fluid (the blood) pumped through the pipes. Damage to any of these components can deprive tissues of blood and produce the condition known as shock.

Shock can be classified as one of three types according to which component fails.

- *Pump failure:* the heart cannot pump sufficient blood. For example, a major heart attack can damage the heart muscle so the heart cannot squeeze and therefore cannot push blood through the blood vessels.
- *Fluid loss:* a significant amount of fluid, usually blood, is lost from the system.
- *Pipe failure:* blood vessels (pipes) enlarge and the blood supply is insufficient to fill them. This can result when the nervous system is damaged, such as with a spinal injury or drug overdose).

What to Look For

- altered mental status: anxiety and restlessness
- pale, cold, and clammy skin, lips, and nail beds
- nausea and vomiting
- rapid breathing and pulse
- unresponsiveness when shock is severe

What to Do

Even if an injured victim does not have signs or symptoms of shock, first aiders should treat for shock ►Skill Scan .

1. Treat life-threatening injuries and other severe injuries.
2. Lay the victim on his or her back.
3. Raise the victim's legs 8 to 12 inches. Raising the legs allows the blood to drain from the legs back to the heart ►Skill Scan .
4. Prevent body heat loss by putting blankets and coats under and over the victim.

Anaphylaxis

A powerful reaction to substances eaten or injected can occur within minutes or even seconds. This reaction, called **anaphylaxis,** can cause death if it is not treated immediately.

Common Causes of Anaphylaxis

Well-known causes of anaphylaxis include:

- medications (penicillin and related drugs, aspirin, sulfa drugs)
- food and food additives (shellfish, nuts, eggs, monosodium glutamate, nitrates, nitrites)
- insect stings (honeybee, yellow jacket, wasp, hornet, fire ant)
- plant pollen
- radiographic dyes

Caution:

DO NOT mistake anaphylaxis for other reactions such as hyperventilation, anxiety attacks, alcohol intoxication, or low blood sugar.

What to Look For

Anaphylaxis typically comes on within minutes of exposure to the offending substance, peaks in 15 to 30 minutes, and is over within hours.

Signs and symptoms of anaphylaxis include:

- sneezing, coughing, wheezing
- shortness of breath
- tightness and swelling in the throat
- tightness in the chest

Skill Scan Positioning the Shock Victim

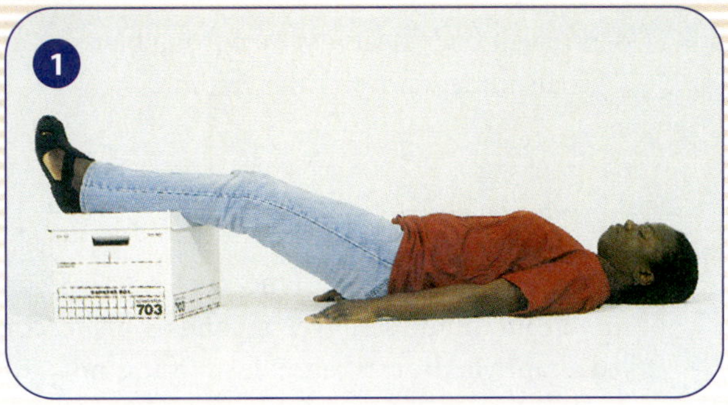

1. Usual shock position. Elevate the legs 8 to 12 inches (if spinal injury is not suspected).

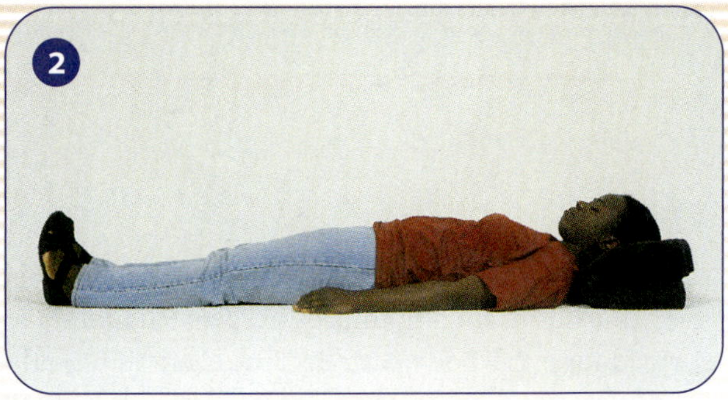

2. Elevate the head for head injury (if spinal injury not suspected).

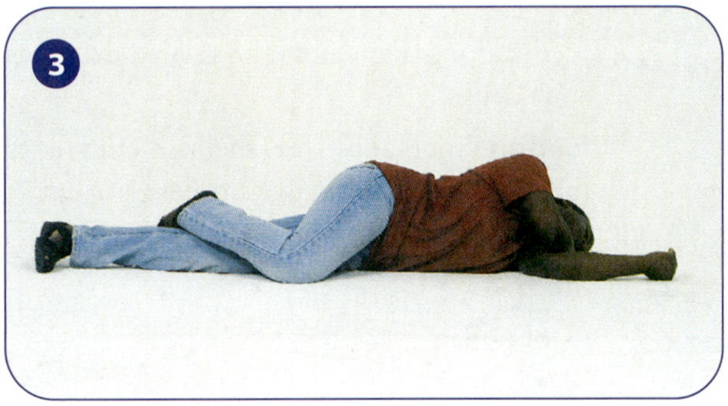

3. Lay an unresponsive, breathing victim on his or her side.

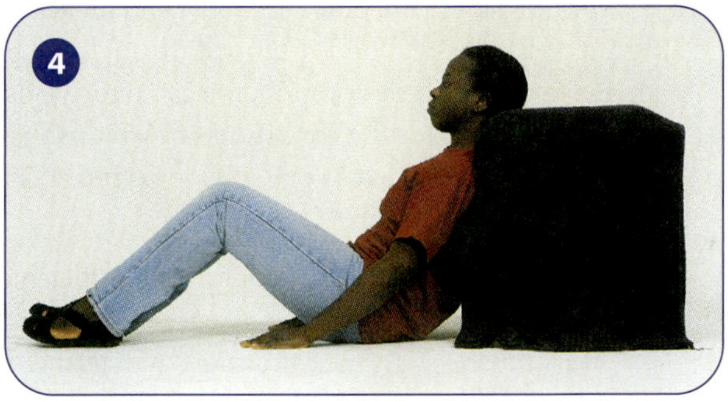

4. Use a half-sitting position for those with breathing difficulties, chest injuries, or a heart attack.

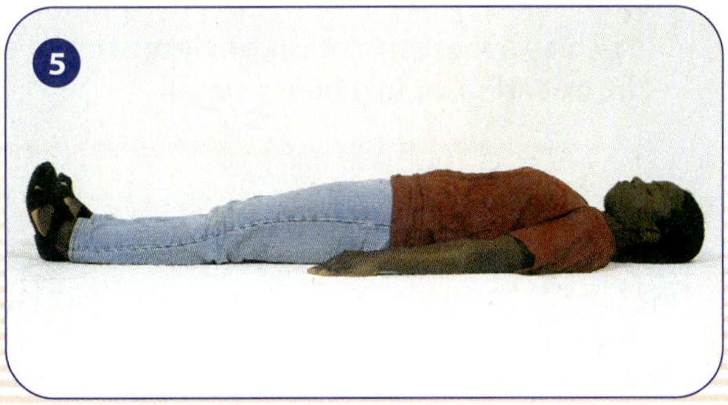

5. Keep victim flat if a spinal injury is suspected or victim has leg fractures.

- increased pulse rate
- swelling of the mucous membranes (tongue, mouth, nose)
- blueness around lips and mouth
- dizziness
- nausea and vomiting

What to Do

1. Check ABCs.
2. Seek immediate medical attention.
3. If the victim has his or her own physician-prescribed epinephrine, help the victim use it ▶Figure 1A–B.

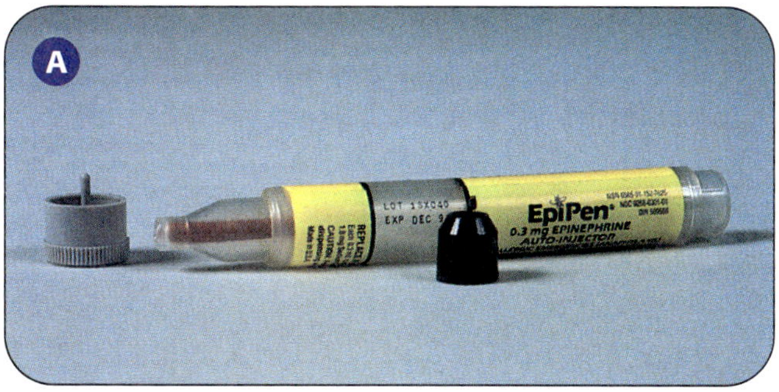

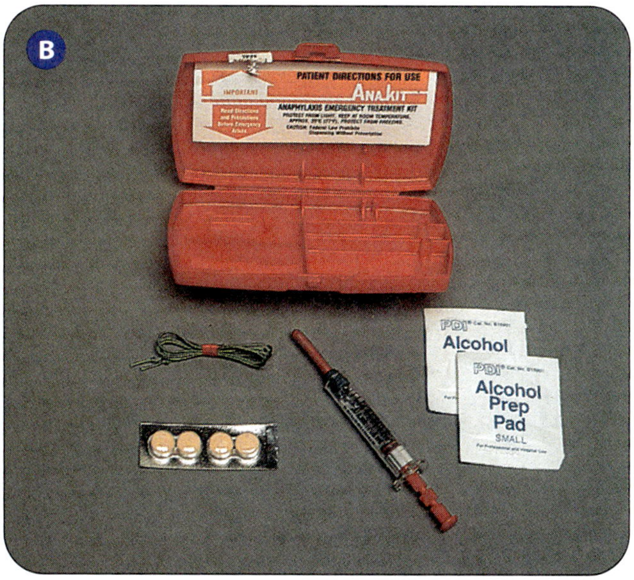

Figure 1 A–B **A.** Doctor-prescribed preloaded epinephrine autoinjector. **B.** Doctor-prescribed preloaded epinephrine with 2 shots.

Learning Activities

Bleeding

Directions: Circle Yes if you agree with the statement, and circle No if you disagree.

Yes No **1.** Most cases of bleeding require more than direct pressure to stop the bleeding.

Yes No **2.** Remove and replace blood-soaked dressings.

Yes No **3.** Elevating an arm or leg alone will not control bleeding and must be used in combination with direct pressure over the wound.

Yes No **4.** If direct pressure and elevation fail to control bleeding, the next step would be to use a tourniquet.

Yes No **5.** Tourniquets are often needed.

Scenario: Jim, a 25-year-old construction worker, has been badly cut on his thigh by a circular power saw. Blood is flowing heavily. The cut is about six to eight inches long. What should you do?

____

____

____

____

Shock

Yes No **1.** Most severely injured victims should have their legs raised.

Yes No **2.** Give the victim something to drink.

Yes No **3.** Prevent body heat loss by putting blankets under and over the victim.

Yes No **4.** A shock victim with head injuries should be placed on his or her side.

Yes No **5.** A shock victim with breathing difficulty or chest injury should be placed on his or her back with the legs raised.

Scenario: You have controlled the construction worker's bleeding. He appears to be pale and is anxious and restless. What should you do?

____

____

____

____

Anaphylaxis

Yes No **1.** Anaphylaxis is another form of fainting.

Yes No **2.** Anaphylaxis can kill.

Yes No **3.** Ask the victim if he or she has doctor-prescribed epinephrine.

Scenario: On a nice summer day, Susan is weeding in the front of the company's office building. Suddenly, she begins slapping her legs. She has disturbed a nest of yellow jackets, and is stung more than a dozen times. Susan complains that she feels hot, and has begun coughing, sneezing, and wheezing. You notice that her face seems to be getting puffy. What should you do?

____

____

____

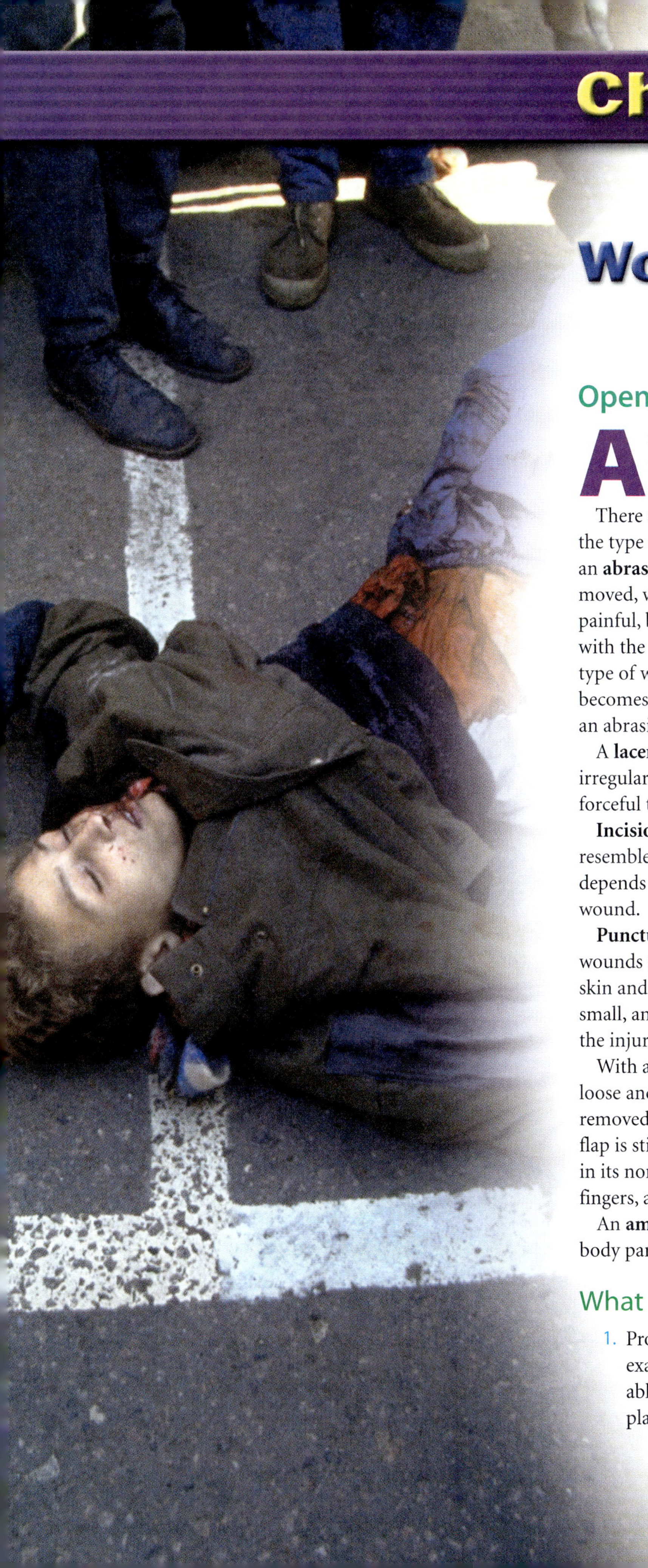

Chapter 5

Wounds

Open Wounds

An open wound is a break in the skin's surface that results in external bleeding and may allow bacteria to enter the body, causing infection.

There are several types of open wounds. Recognizing the type of wound helps in giving proper first aid. With an **abrasion** ▶Figure 1A, the top layer of skin is removed, with little or no blood loss. Abrasions tend to be painful, because the nerve endings often are torn along with the skin. Ground-in debris may be present. This type of wound can be serious if it covers a large area or becomes embedded with foreign matter. Other names for an abrasion are "scrape," "road rash," and "rug burn."

A **laceration** ▶Figure 1B is cut skin with jagged, irregular edges. This type of wound is usually caused by a forceful tearing away of skin tissue.

Incisions ▶Figure 1C tend to have smooth edges and resemble a surgical or paper cut. The amount of bleeding depends on the depth, the location, and the size of the wound.

Punctures ▶Figure 1D are usually deep, narrow wounds such as a stab wound from a nail or a knife in the skin and underlying organs. The entrance is usually small, and the risk of infection is high. The object causing the injury may remain impaled in the wound.

With an **avulsion** ▶Figure 1E, a piece of skin is torn loose and is either hanging from the body or completely removed. This type of wound can bleed heavily. If the flap is still attached and folded back, lay it flat and align it in its normal position. Avulsions most often involve ears, fingers, and hands.

An **amputation** involves the cutting or tearing off of a body part, such as a finger, toe, hand, foot, arm, or leg.

What to Do

1. Protect yourself against disease by wearing medical exam gloves. If medical exam gloves are not available, use several layers of gauze pads, clean cloths, plastic wrap or bags, or waterproof material. You

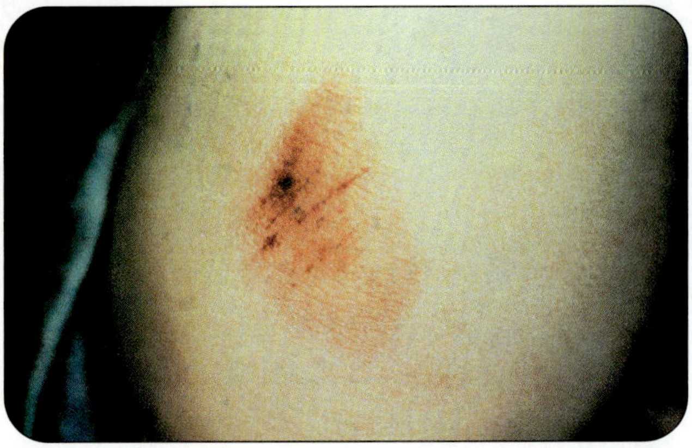

Figure 1A Abrasion

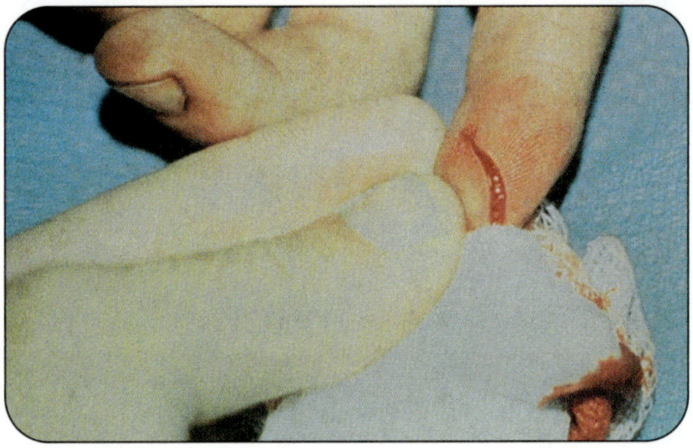

Figure 1B Laceration

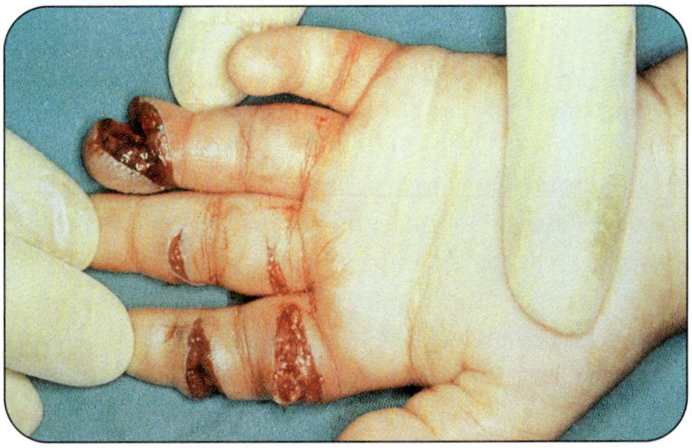

Figure 1C Incision

can even have the victim apply pressure with his or her own hand. Your bare hand should be used only as a last resort.

2. Expose the wound by removing or cutting clothing to see where the blood is coming from.
3. Control bleeding as described in Chapter 4.

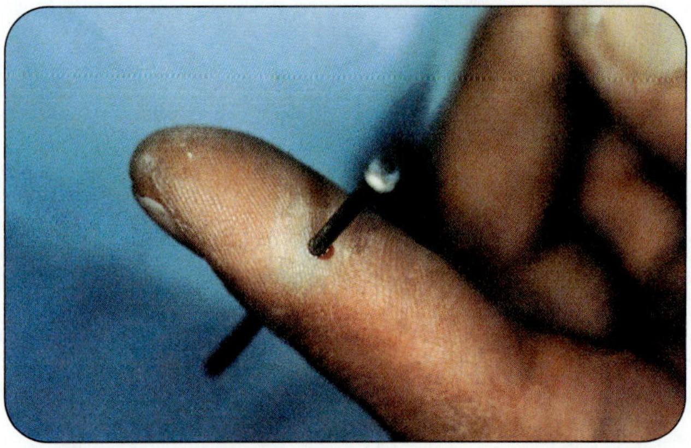

Figure 1D Puncture

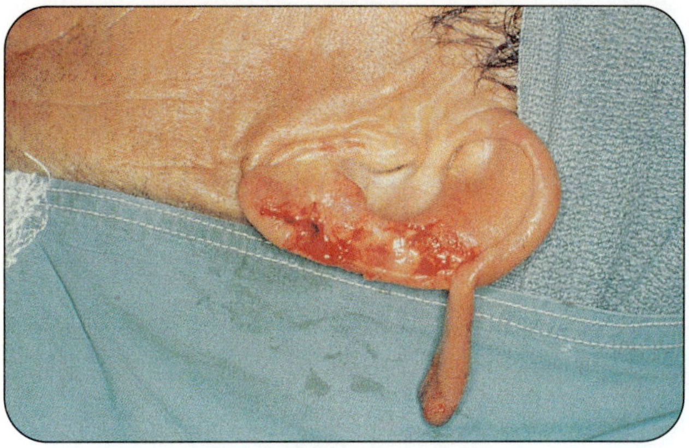

Figure 1E Avulsion

Caution:

DO NOT clean large, extremely dirty, or life-threatening wounds. Let hospital emergency department personnel do the cleaning.

DO NOT scrub a wound. Scrubbing a wound is debatable, and it can bruise the tissue.

Wound Care

A victim's wound should be cleaned to help prevent infection. Wound cleaning usually restarts bleeding by disturbing the clot, but it should be done anyway for shallow wounds. For severe bleeding, leave the pressure bandage in place until the victim can get medical attention.

To clean a shallow wound:

1. Wash inside the wound with soap and water.
2. Irrigate the wound with water from a faucet to provide sufficient quantity and pressure.

For a wound with a high risk for infection (eg, an animal bite, a very dirty or ragged wound, a puncture), seek medical attention for wound cleaning.

3. Remove small objects that don't flush out by irrigation with sterile tweezers.
4. If bleeding restarts, apply direct pressure.
5. Apply an antibiotic ointment such as Neosporin™. Cover the area with a sterile and, if possible, nonstick dressing. To keep the dressing in place on an arm or leg, use a self-adhering roller bandage or tape; on other parts of the body, use tape.
6. Change the dressing daily, or more often if it gets wet or dirty. If a wound bleeds after a dressing has been applied and the dressing becomes stuck, leave it on as long as the wound is healing. Pulling the scab loose to change the dressing retards healing and increases the chance of infection. If a sticking dressing must be removed, soak it in warm water to help soften the scab and make removal easier.

Caution:

DO NOT irrigate a wound with full-strength iodine preparations (eg, Betadine 10%) or isopropyl alcohol (70%). They kill body cells as well as bacteria and are painful. Also, some people are allergic to iodine.

DO NOT use hydrogen peroxide. It does not kill bacteria, it adversely affects capillary blood flow, and it extends wound healing.

DO NOT use antibiotic ointment on wounds that require sutures or on puncture wounds (the ointment may prevent drainage). Use an antibiotic ointment only on abrasions and shallow wounds.

Wound Infection

Any wound, large or small, can become infected ►Figure 2. Once an infection begins, damage can be extensive, so prevention is the best way to avoid the problem. A wound should be cleaned using the procedures described above.

It is important to know how to recognize and treat an infected wound. The signs and symptoms of infection include:

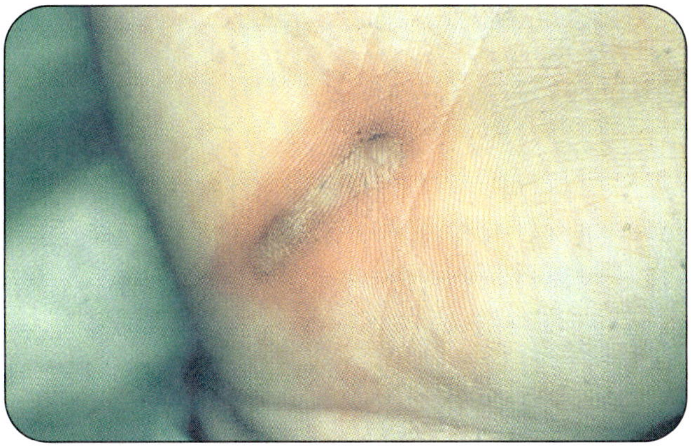

Figure 2 Infected wound

- swelling and redness around the wound
- a sensation of warmth
- throbbing pain
- pus discharge
- fever
- swelling of lymph nodes
- one or more red streaks leading from the wound toward the heart

The appearance of one or more red streaks leading from the wound toward the heart is a serious sign that the infection is spreading and could cause death. If chills and fever develop, the infection has reached the circulatory system (known as blood poisoning). Seek medical attention immediately.

Tetanus

The tetanus bacteria by itself does not cause tetanus. But when it enters a wound that contains little oxygen (eg, a puncture wound), the bacteria can produce a powerful poisonous toxin. The toxin travels through the nervous system to the brain and the spinal cord. It then causes contractions of certain muscle groups (particularly in the jaw). There is no known antidote to the toxin after it enters the nervous system.

A vaccination can completely prevent tetanus. Everyone needs an initial series of vaccinations to prepare the immune system to defend against the toxin. A booster shot once every 5 to 10 years is sufficient to jog the immune system's memory.

The guidelines for tetanus immunization boosters are as follows:

- Anyone with a wound who has never been immunized against tetanus should be given a tetanus vaccine and booster immediately.

- A victim who was once immunized but has not received a tetanus booster within the last 10 years should receive a booster.
- A victim with a dirty wound who has not had a booster for over five years should receive a booster.
- Tetanus immunization shots must be given within 72 hours of the injury to be effective.

Amputations ▼Figure 3

What to Do

1. Control the bleeding.
2. Treat the victim for shock.
3. Recover the amputated part and, whenever possible, take it with the victim.
4. To care for the amputated body part ►Figure 4:
    - The amputated part does not need to be cleaned.
    - Wrap the amputated part with a dry sterile gauze or other clean cloth.
    - Put the wrapped amputated part in a plastic bag or other waterproof container.
    - Keep the amputated part cool, but do not freeze. Place the bag or container with the wrapped part on a bed of ice.
5. Seek medical attention immediately.

Amputated body parts left uncooled for more than six hours have little chance of survival; 18 hours is probably the maximum time allowable for a part that has been cooled properly. Muscles without blood lose viability within four to six hours.

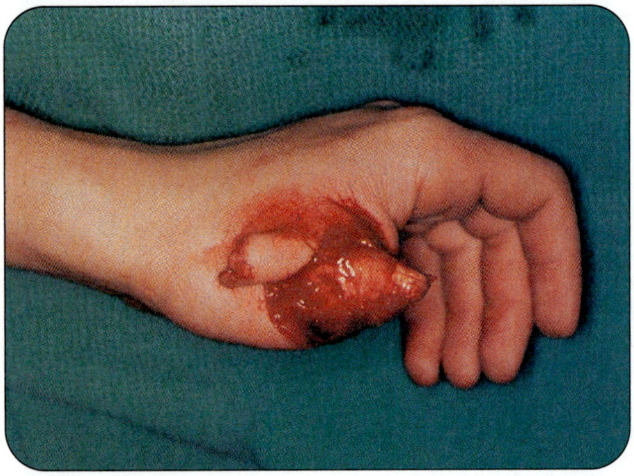

Figure 3 Amputation

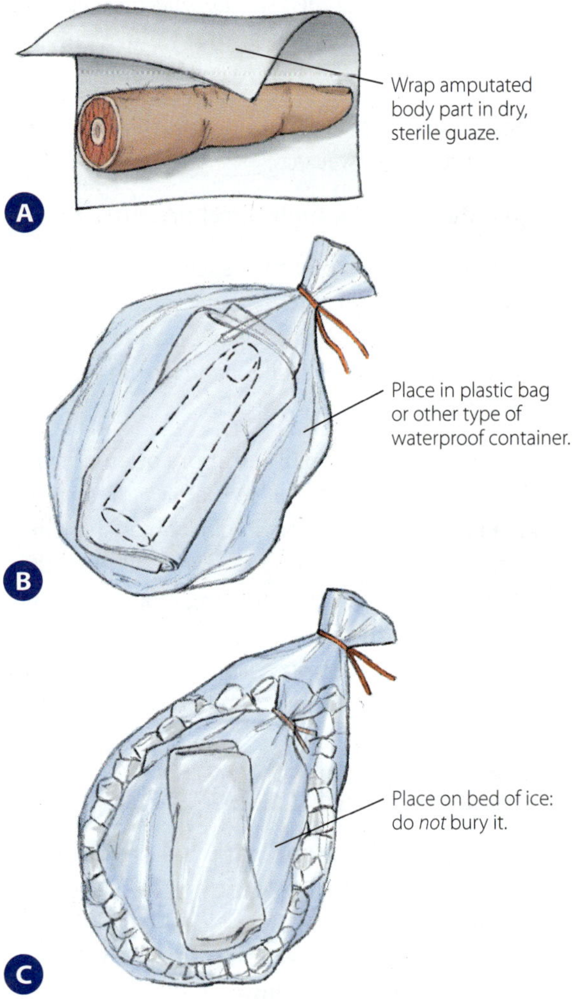

Figure 4 A–C Care of an amputated part

Caution:

DO NOT wrap an amputated part in a wet dressing or cloth. Using a wet wrap on the part can cause waterlogging and tissue softening, which will make reattachment more difficult.

DO NOT bury an amputated part in ice—place it on ice. Reattaching frostbitten parts is usually unsuccessful.

Impaled Objects

What to Do

1. Expose the area ►Figure 5. Remove or cut away clothing surrounding the injury.

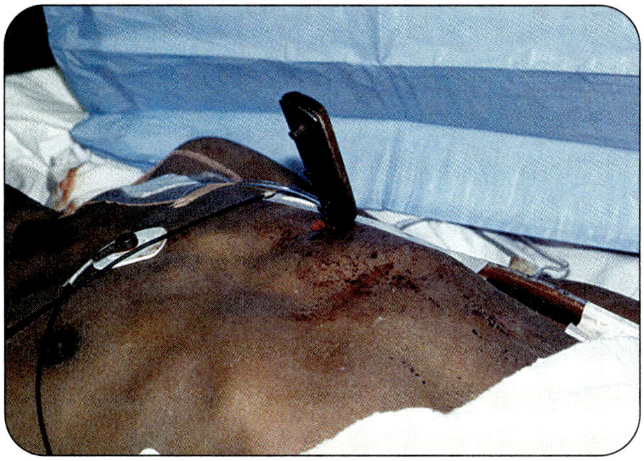

Figure 5

2. Do not remove or move an impaled object. Movement of any kind could produce additional bleeding and tissue damage.
3. Control any bleeding with pressure around the impaled object.
4. Stabilize the object with bulky dressings or clean cloths around the object.
5. Shorten the object only if necessary.

Closed Wounds

A closed wound happens when a blunt object strikes the body. The skin is not broken, but tissue and blood vessels beneath the skin's surface are crushed, causing bleeding within a confined area.

What to Do

1. Control bleeding by applying an ice pack for up to 20 minutes.
2. Apply an elastic bandage with a gauze pad between the bandage and the skin.
3. Check for a possible fracture.
4. Elevate an injured extremity above the victim's heart level to decrease pain and swelling.

Wounds That Require Medical Attention

As a guideline, seek medical attention for the following conditions:

- arterial bleeding
- uncontrolled bleeding
- a deep incision, laceration, or avulsion that
  - goes into the muscle or bone
  - is located on a body part that bends such as the elbow or knee
  - tends to gape widely
  - is located on the thumb or palm of the hand (nerves may be affected)
- a large or deep puncture wound
- a large embedded object or a deeply embedded object of any size
- foreign matter left in the wound
- human or animal bite
- possibility of a noticeable scar (sutured cuts usually heal with less scarring than unsutured ones)
- an eyelid cut (to prevent later drooping)
- a slit lip (easily scarred)
- internal bleeding
- any wound you are not certain how to treat
- tetanus immunization not up to date

Sutures (Stitches)

If sutures are needed, they should be made by a physician within six to eight hours of the injury. Suturing wounds allows faster healing, reduces infection, and lessens scarring.

Some wounds do not usually require sutures:

- wounds in which the skin's cut edges tend to fall together
- shallow cuts less than one inch long

Rather than close a gaping wound with butterfly bandages, cover the wound with sterile gauze. Closing the wound might trap bacteria inside, resulting in an infection. In most cases, a physician can be reached in time for sutures to be made.

Learning Activities

Wound Care

Directions: Circle Yes if you agree with the statement, and circle No if you disagree.

Yes No **1.** Wash shallow wounds with soapy water.

Yes No **2.** Irrigating a wound with water needs pressure.

Yes No **3.** Wounds with a high risk for infection (eg, animal bites, dirty wounds) require medical attention for proper wound cleaning.

Yes No **4.** Antibiotic ointment can be applied to any wound.

Yes No **5.** Hydrogen peroxide works well on wounds.

Scenario: Nancy used a knife to open a cardboard box, lost her grip on the knife, and received a shallow incision wound on her hand. What should you do?

____

____

____

Amputations

Yes No **1.** Recover any amputated part, regardless of size, and take it with the victim to the nearest hospital.

Yes No **2.** Cut off a partially attached part.

Yes No **3.** Wrap an amputated part in a dry, sterile gauze dressing, enclose it in something waterproof, and keep it cool.

Yes No **4.** Keep an amputated part packed (buried) in ice.

Yes No **5.** Do **NOT** let an amputated part become "water-logged" because reattaching it will be more difficult.

Scenario: Matt is mowing long wet grass, which begins to clog his mower's discharge opening. He reaches into the discharge chute to try to pull out the grass, and his fingers are struck by the mower's blade. Two fingers are cut off. You find him sitting on the ground firmly holding what remains of his fingers. What should you do?

____

____

____

Impaled Objects

Yes No **1.** Removing an impaled object could cause more bleeding.

Yes No **2.** Prevent an impaled object from moving by placing bulky padding around the object.

Scenario: At a construction site, a worker drove a large nail through his left hand with a nail gun. What should you do?

____

____

____

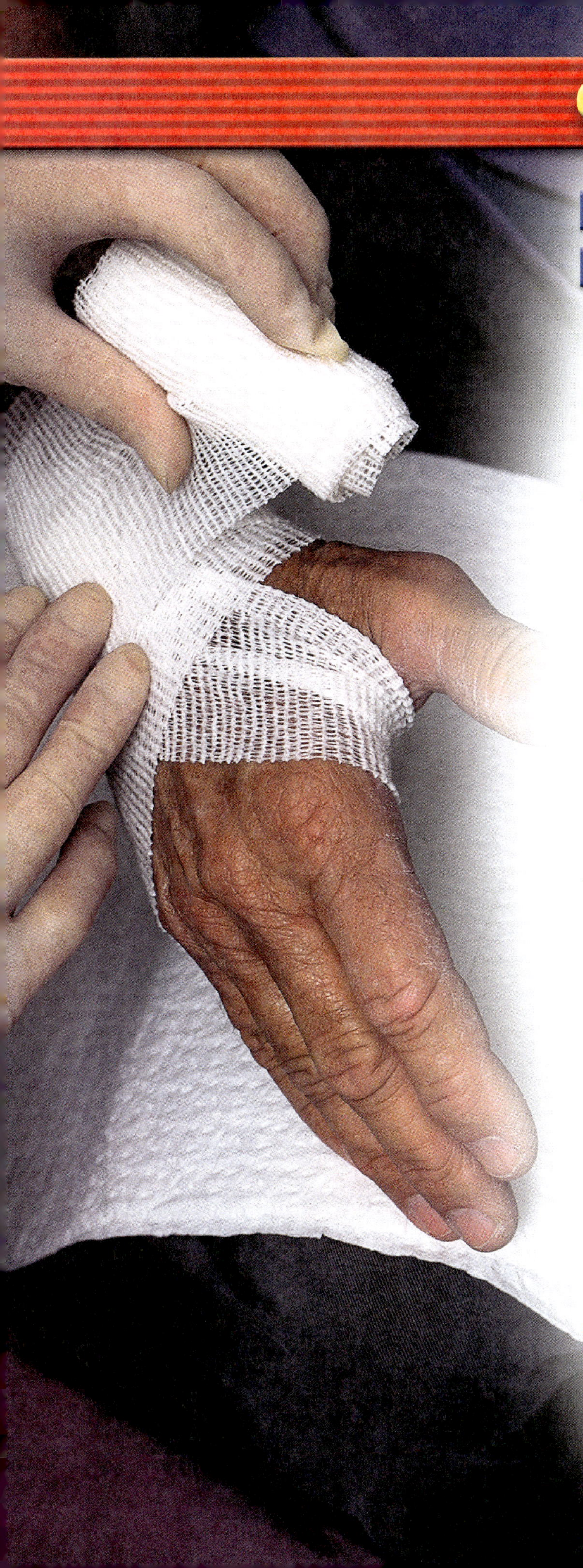

Chapter 6

Dressings and Bandages

Dressings

A dressing covers an open wound—it touches the wound. Whenever possible, a dressing should be:

- sterile. If a sterile dressing is not available, use a clean cloth (handkerchief, washcloth, towel).
- larger than the wound
- thick, soft, and compressible so pressure is evenly distributed over the wound
- lint-free

The purpose of a dressing is to:

- control bleeding
- prevent infection and contamination
- absorb blood and fluid drainage
- protect the wound from further injury

Types of Dressings

- ***Gauze pads*** are used for small wounds ▶Figure 1. They come in separately wrapped packages of various sizes (eg, 2 inches square; 4 inches square) and are sterile, unless the package is broken. Some gauze pads have a special coating to keep them from sticking to the wound and are especially helpful for burns or wounds secreting fluids.
- ***Adhesive strips*** (eg, Band-Aids™) are used for small cuts and abrasions and are a combination of both a sterile dressing and a bandage ▶Figure 2.
- ***Trauma dressings*** are made of large, thick, absorbent, sterile materials ▶Figure 3. Individually wrapped sanitary napkins can serve because of their bulk and absorbency, but they usually are not sterile.

Applying a Sterile Dressing

What to Do

1. Wear medical exam gloves whenever possible.
2. Use a dressing large enough to extend beyond the wound's edges. Hold the dressing by a corner. Place

the dressing directly over the wound. Do not slide it on.

3. Cover the dressing with one of the types of bandages referenced below.

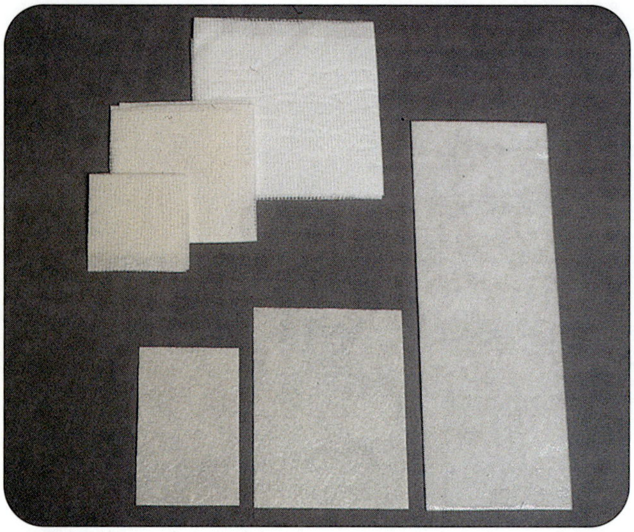

Figure 1 Gauze pads

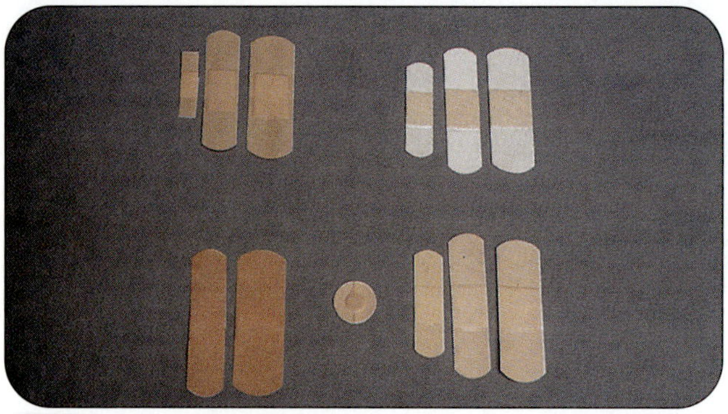

Figure 2 Adhesive strips

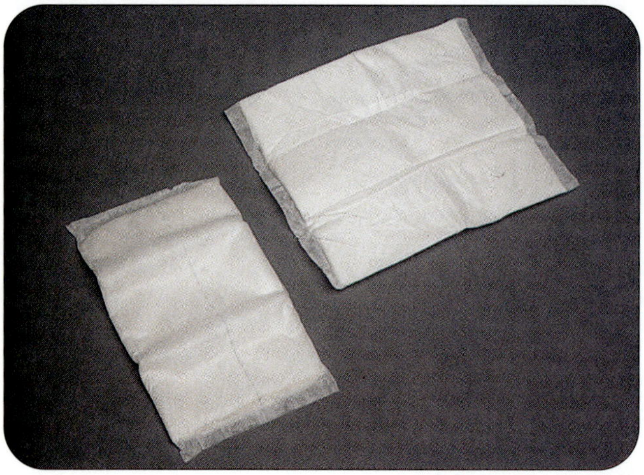

Figure 3 Trauma dressings

Caution:

DO NOT touch any part of the wound or any part of the dressings that will be in contact with the wound.

Bandages

A bandage can be used to:

- hold a dressing in place over an open wound
- apply direct pressure over a dressing to control bleeding
- prevent or reduce swelling
- provide support and stability for an extremity or joint

A bandage should be clean but need not be sterile.

Caution:

DO NOT bandage so tightly as to restrict blood circulation. Always check the extremity's pulse. If you cannot feel the pulse, loosen the bandage.

DO NOT bandage so loosely that the dressing will slip. This is the most common bandaging error. Bandages tend to stretch after a short time.

DO NOT cover fingers or toes unless they are injured. They need to be observed for color changes due to impaired circulation.

DO NOT use elastic bandages over a wound. First aiders have a tendency to apply them too tightly.

Signs that a bandage is too tight:

- blue tinge to the fingernails or toenails
- blue or pale skin color
- tingling or loss of sensation
- coldness of the extremity
- inability to move the fingers or toes

Types of Bandages

There are four basic types of bandages:

- ***Roller bandages*** come in various widths, lengths, and types of material. For best results, use different widths for different body areas (►Skill Scans):

- 1-inch width for fingers
- 2-inch width for wrists, hands, feet
- 3-inch width for elbows, arms
- 4- or 6-inch width for ankles, knees, legs

These can be *self-adhering, conforming bandages* ▼Figure 4 that come as rolls of slightly elastic, gauzelike material in various widths. They can also be *gauze rollers* made of cotton. These are rigid and nonelastic. Another type of roller bandage is an *elastic roller bandage* ►Figure 5 used for compression on sprains, strains, and contusions. Elastic bandages are not usually applied over dressings to cover a wound.

When commercial roller bandages are unavailable, you can *improvise bandages* from neckties or strips of cloth torn from a sheet or other similar material.

- ***Triangular bandages*** ►Figure 6 are available commercially or can be made from a 36- to 40-inch square of preshrunk cotton muslin material that is cut diagonally from corner to corner to produce two triangular pieces of cloth. The longest side is called the ***base***; the corner directly across from the base is the ***point***; the other two corners are called ***ends***. A triangular bandage may be applied two ways:
    - As a cravat (folded triangular bandage). The point is folded to the center of the base and folded in half again from the top to the base to form a cravat. It is to apply pressure evenly over a dressing, to hold splints in place, or used as a swathe (binder) around the victim's body to stabilize an injured arm in an arm sling.
    - Fully opened (not folded). Best used for an arm sling.
- ***Adhesive tape*** comes in rolls and in a variety of widths. It is often used to secure roller bandages and small dressings in place. Paper tape or special dermatologic tape should be used if the victim has an allergy to adhesive tape.
- ***Adhesive strips*** are used for small cuts and abrasions and are a combination of a dressing and a bandage.

Figure 4 Self-adhering conforming bandages of various sizes (3 on right) and gauze bandages (2 on left)

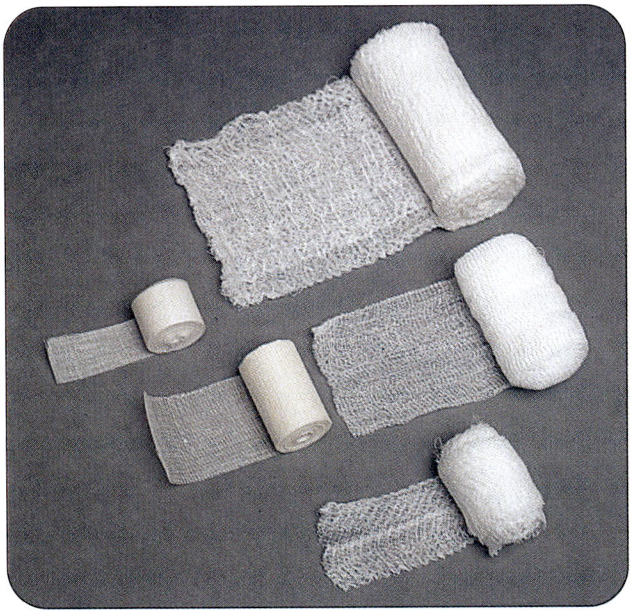

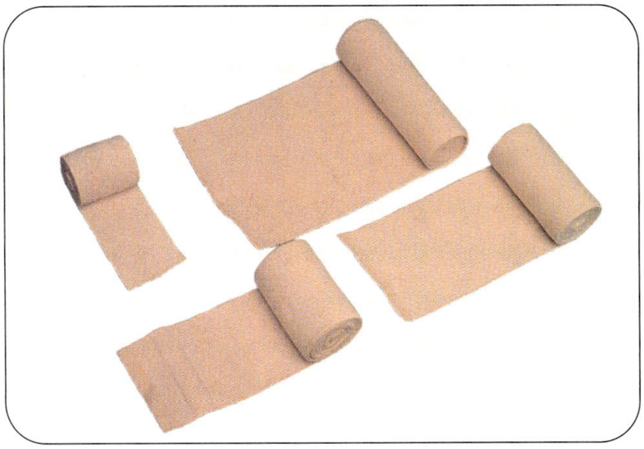

Figure 5 Elastic bandages of various sizes

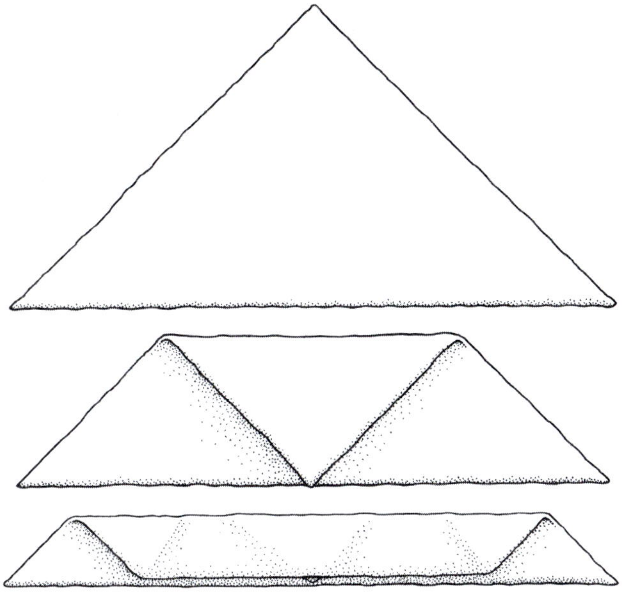

Figure 6 A triangular bandage folded into a cravat

Skill Scan Roller Bandage

Roller Bandage for Hand

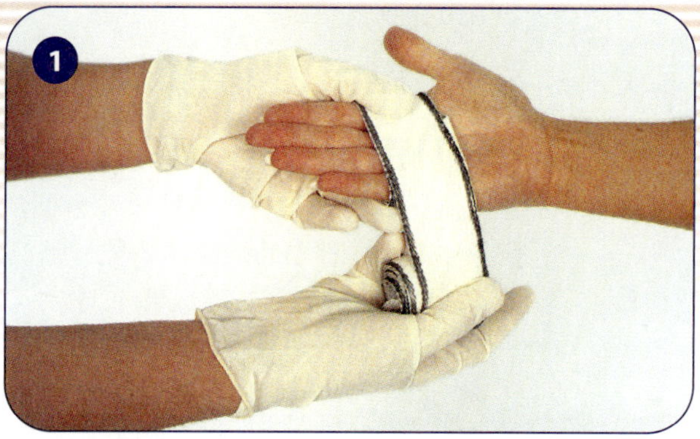

1. Anchor the bandage with one or two turns around the palm of the hand.

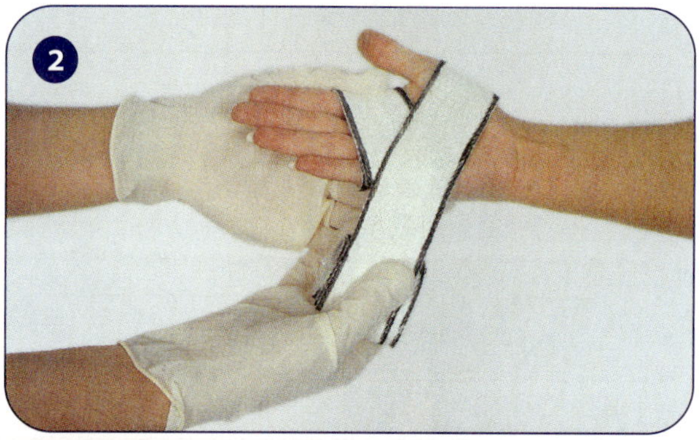

2. Carry it diagonally across the back of the hand and then around the wrist.

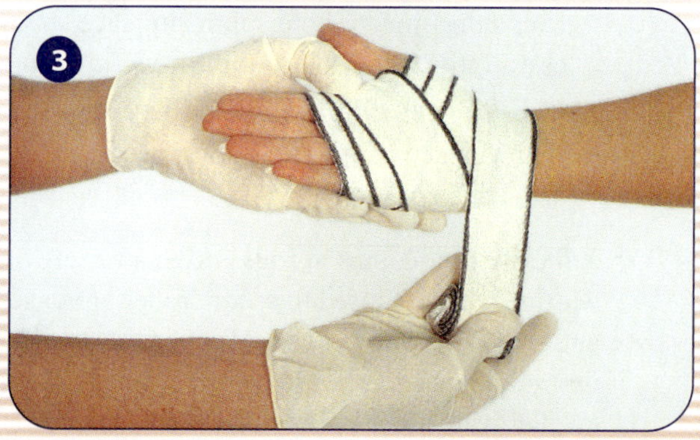

3. Repeat this figure-8 maneuver with overlapping wraps.

Roller Bandage for Elbow or Knee

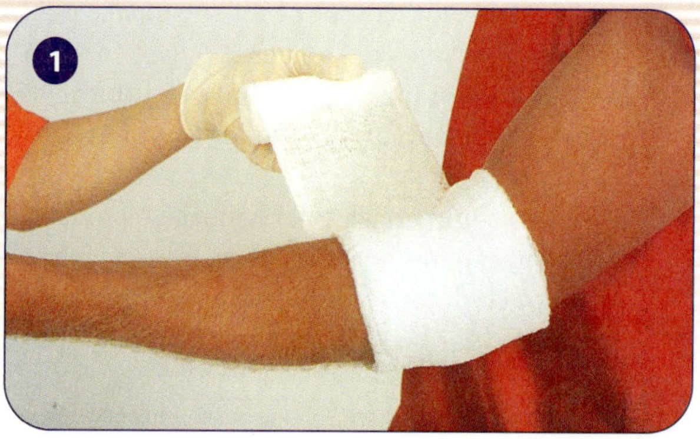

1. Bend arm. Wrap the bandage around the elbow several times.

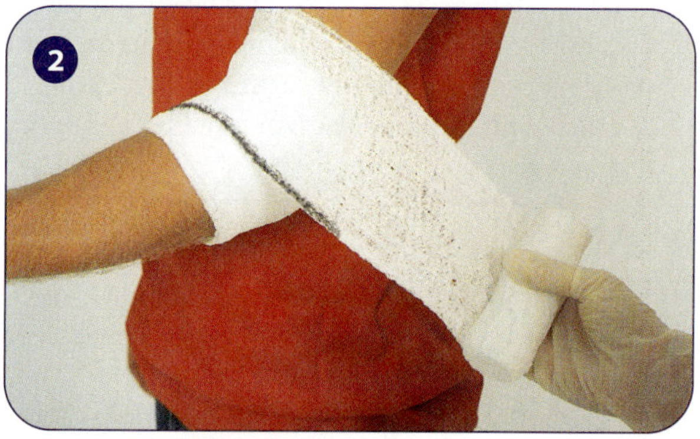

2. Make a diagonal turn to the upper arm.

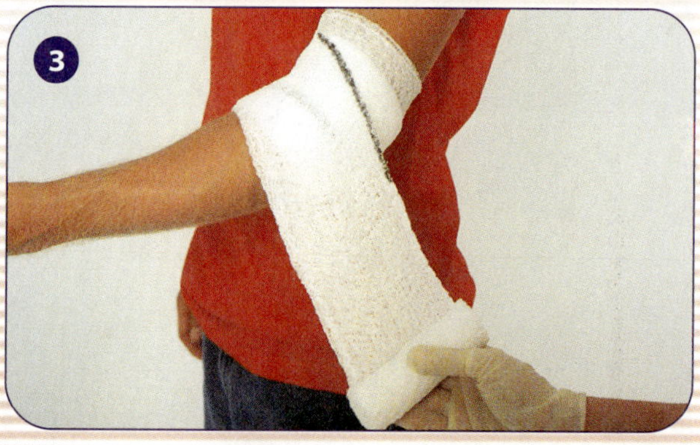

3. Make a diagonal turn around the forearm and continue this figure-8 maneuver.

Skill Scan Roller Bandage (Self-adhering), Figure 8

Roller Bandage for Ankle

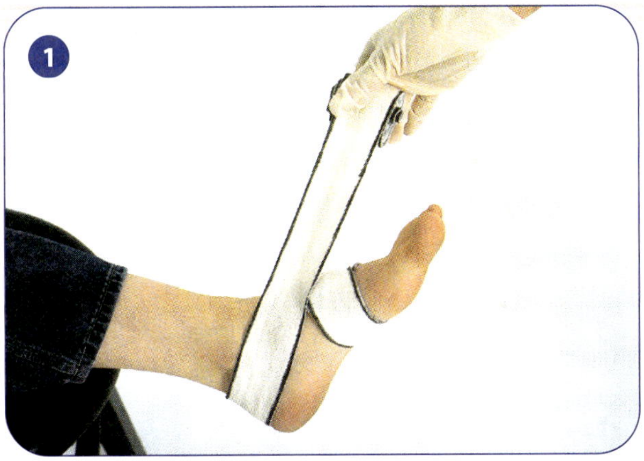

1. Anchor the bandage with one or two turns around the foot. Bring bandage diagonally across the top of the foot and around back of the ankle.

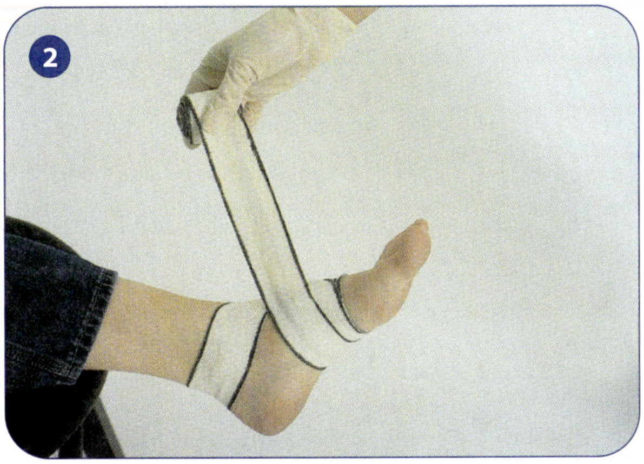

2. Continue bandage across the top of the foot and under the arch.

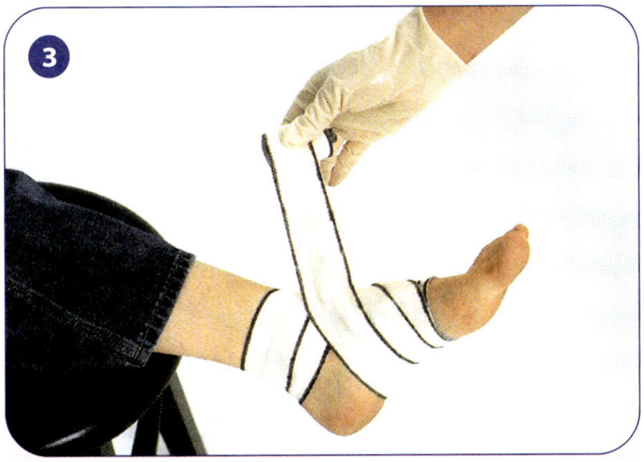

3. Continue figure-8 turns, with each turn overlapping the last turn.

Learning Activities

Dressings and Bandages

Directions: Circle Yes if you agree with the statement, and circle No if you disagree.

Yes No **1.** Bandages are used to secure dressings in place over a wound.

Yes No **2.** Dressings are used to control bleeding and prevent contamination.

Yes No **3.** Adhesive strips are types of bandages used for large wounds.

Yes No **4.** Fingers and toes should not be covered unless they are injured.

Yes No **5.** Triangular bandages can be used to control bleeding or to support splints for broken bones.

Scenario: A child "skinned" his knee when he fell off his bike. What should you do for this child?

____

____

____

____

Scenario: A worker has cut the palm of his hand on a sharp piece of metal. What should you do?

____

____

____

____

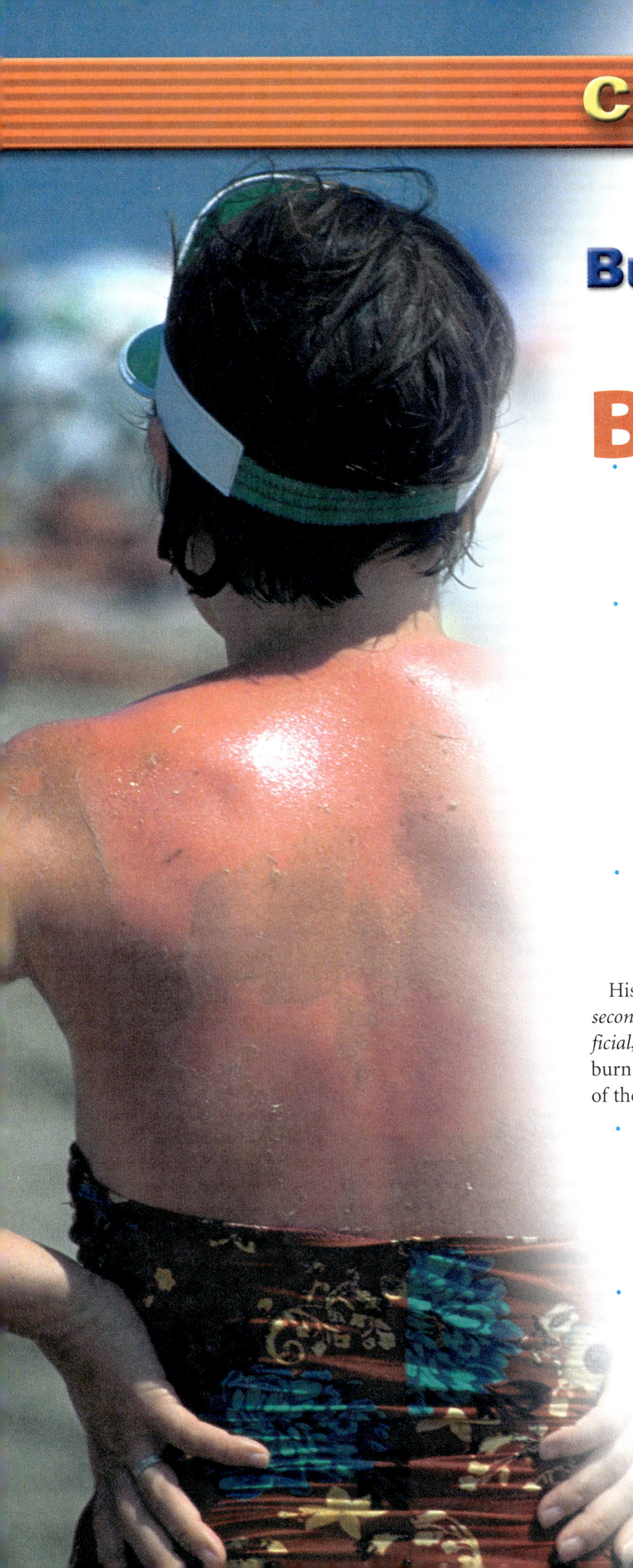

Chapter 7

Burns

Burn injuries can be classified as thermal (heat), chemical, or electrical.

- *Thermal (heat) burns.* Not all thermal burns are caused by flames. Contact with hot objects, flammable vapor that ignites and causes a flash or an explosion, and steam or hot liquid are other common causes of burns.
- *Chemical burns.* A wide range of chemical agents can cause tissue damage and death if they come in contact with the skin. As with thermal burns, the amount of tissue damage depends on the duration of contact, the skin thickness in the area of exposure, and the strength of the chemical agent. Chemicals will continue to cause tissue destruction until the chemical agent is removed. Three types of chemicals—acids, alkalis, and organic compounds—are responsible for most chemical burns.
- *Electrical burns.* The severity of an injury from contact with electrical current depends on the type of current (direct or alternating), the voltage, the area of the body exposed, and the duration of contact.

Historically, burns have been described as *first-degree*, *second-degree*, and *third-degree* injuries. The terms *superficial*, *partial thickness*, and *full thickness* are often used by burn-care professionals because they are more descriptive of the tissue damage.

- **First-degree (superficial) burns** affect the skin's outer layer (epidermis) ▶Figure 1. Characteristics include redness, mild swelling, tenderness, and pain. Healing occurs without scarring, usually within a week. The outer edges of deeper burns often are first-degree burns.
- **Second-degree (partial-thickness) burns** extend through the entire outer layer and into the inner skin layer ▶Figure 2. Blisters, swelling, weeping of fluids, and severe pain characterize these burns, because the capillary blood vessels in the dermis are damaged and give up fluid into surrounding tissues. Intact blisters provide a sterile, waterproof covering.

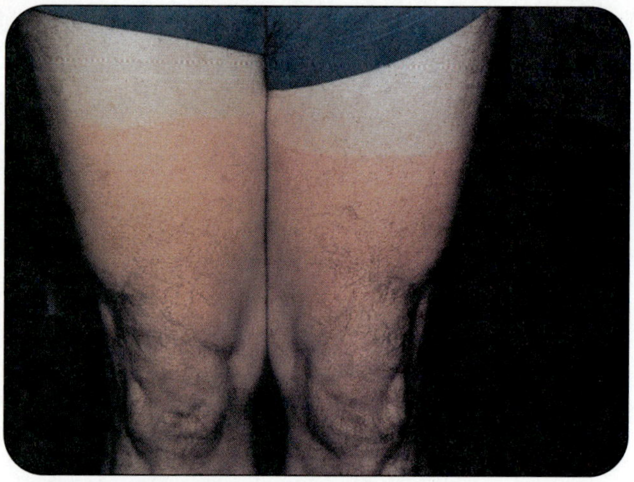

Figure 1 First-degree burn

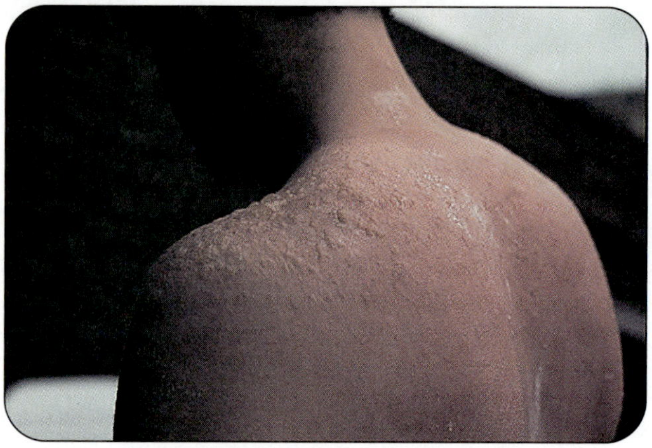

Figure 2 Second-degree burn blisters

Once a blister breaks, a weeping wound results and the risk of infection increases.

- **Third-degree (full-thickness) burns** are severe burns that penetrate all the skin layers, into the underlying fat and muscle ▶Figure 3. The skin looks leathery, waxy, or pearly gray and sometimes charred. There is a dry appearance, because capillary blood vessels have been destroyed and no more fluid is brought to the area. The skin does not blanch after being pressed because the area is dead. The victim feels no pain from a third-degree burn because the nerve endings have been damaged or destroyed. Any pain that is felt is from surrounding burns of lesser degrees. Medical care for a third-degree burn involves removing the dead tissue and often a skin graft to heal properly.

Respiratory damage may result from breathing heat or the products of combustion; from being burned by a

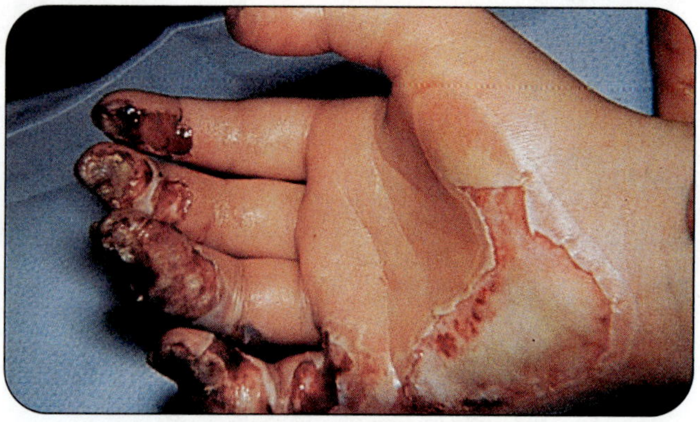

Figure 3 Second- and third-degree burns

flame while in a closed space; or from being in an explosion. Swelling occurs in 2 to 24 hours, restricting or even completely shutting off the airway so that air cannot reach the lungs. *All respiratory injuries must receive medical care.*

Thermal Burns

What to Do

1. Stop the burning! Burns can continue to injure tissue for a surprisingly long time. If clothing is burning, have the victim roll on the ground using the "stop, drop, and roll" method. Smother the flames with a blanket or douse the victim with water. Stop a person whose clothes are on fire from running, which only fans the flames. The victim should not remain standing, because he or she is more apt to inhale flames.
2. Check ABC.
3. Determine the depth (degree) of the burn. Making an assessment of burn depth will help you decide whether to seek medical care for the victim. You should be aware that it can be difficult to tell a burn's depth because the destruction varies within the same burn. Even experienced physicians may not know the true depth for several days after the burn.
4. Determine the extent of the burn. This means estimating how much body surface area the burn covers. A rough guide known as the Rule of Nines assigns a percentage value to each part of an adult's body ▶Figure 4. The entire head is 9%, one complete arm is 9%, the front torso is 18%, the complete back is 18%, and each leg is 18%. The rule of nines must be modified to take into account the different proportions of a small child. In small

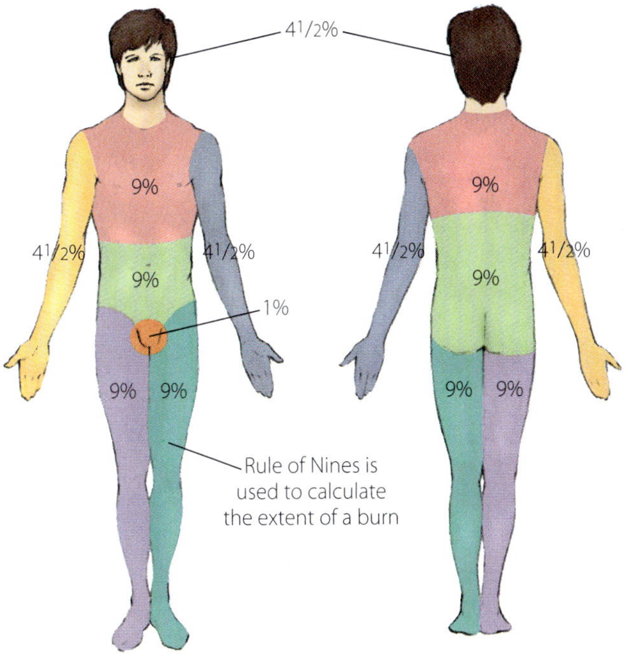

Figure 4 Rule of Nines

Caution:

DO NOT remove clothing stuck to the skin—pulling will further damage the skin.

DO NOT forget to remove jewelry as soon as possible—swelling could make jewelry difficult to remove later.

children and infants, the head accounts for 18% and each leg is 14%.

For small or scattered burns, use the rule of the palm. The victim's hand, excluding the fingers and the thumb, represents about 1% of his or her total body surface. Estimate the *unburned* area in number of hands.

5. Determine what parts of the body are burned. Burns on the face, hands, feet, and genitals are more severe than on other body parts. A circumferential burn (one that goes around a finger, toe, arm, leg, neck, or chest) is considered more severe than a noncircumferential one because it can have constriction and tourniquet effects on circulation and, in some cases, breathing. All these burns require medical care.
6. Determine if other injuries or preexisting medical problems exist or if the victim is elderly (over 55) or very young (under five). A medical problem or belonging to one of those age groups increases a burn's severity.
7. Determine the burn's severity ▼Table 1. This forms the basis for how to treat the burned victim. Most burns are minor, occur at home, and can be managed outside a medical setting. Seek medical attention for all moderate and severe burns, as classified by the ABA, or if any of the following conditions applies:

- The victim is under 5 or over 55 years of age.
- The victim has difficulty breathing.
- Other injuries exist.

Table 1: Burn Severity

Minor Burns
First-degree burn covering less than 50% BSA* in adults (face, hands, feet, or genitals not burned)
Second-degree burn covering less than 15% BSA in adults
Second-degree burn covering less than 10% BSA in children/elderly persons
Third-degree burn covering less than 2% BSA in adults (face, hands, feet, or genitals not burned)
Moderate Burns
First-degree burn covering more than 50% BSA in adults
Second-degree burn covering 15% to 30% BSA in adults
Second-degree burn covering 10% to 20% BSA in children/elderly persons
Third-degree burn covering 2% to 10% BSA in adults (face, hands, or feet not burned)
Critical Burns
First-degree burn covering more than 70% BSA
Second-degree burn covering more than 30% BSA in adults
Second-degree burn covering more than 20% BSA in children/elderly persons
Third-degree burn covering more than 10% BSA in adults
Third-degree burn covering more than 2% BSA in children/elderly persons or any part of the face, hands, feet or genitals
Also most inhalation injuries, electrical injuries, and burns accompanied by major trauma or significant preexisting conditions

*BSA = body surface area
Source: Adapted from the American Burn Association categorization

THERMAL BURNS

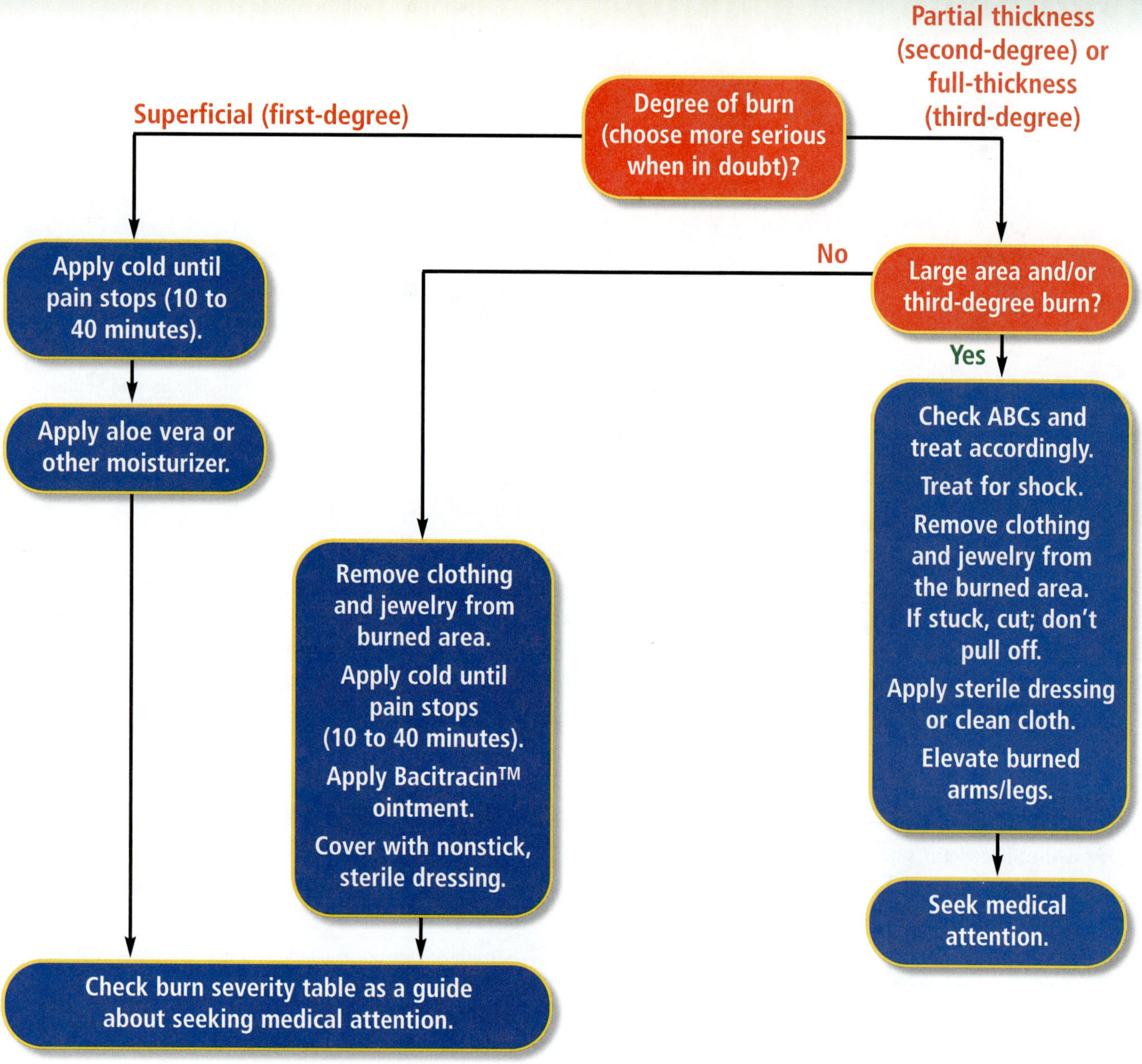

- An electrical injury exists.
- The face, hands, feet, or genitals are burned.
- Child abuse is suspected.
- The surface area of a second-degree burn is greater than 15% of the body surface area.
- The burn is third-degree.

Burn Care

Burn care aims to reduce pain, protect against infection, and prevent evaporation.

Care of First-Degree Burns

1. Immerse the burned area in cold water or apply a wet, cold cloth to reduce pain ▼Figure 5. Apply cold until the part is pain free both in and out of the water (usually in 10 minutes, but it may take up to 45 minutes). Cold also stops the burn from progressing into deeper tissue. If cold water is unavailable, use any cold drinkable liquid to reduce the temperature of the burned skin.
2. Give ibuprofen to relieve pain and inflammation. Give children acetaminophen.
3. After the burn cools, apply an aloe vera gel or an inexpensive skin moisturizer lotion to keep the skin moistened and to reduce itching and peeling. Aloe vera has antimicrobial properties and is an effective analgesic.
4. Keep a burned arm or leg elevated.

Figure 5 Immerse the burn in cold water.

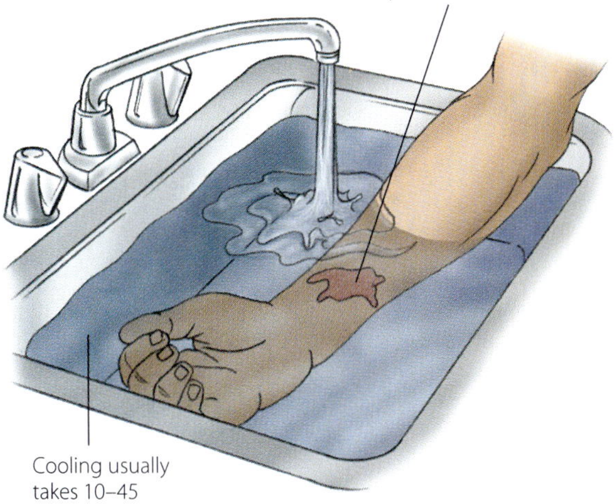

Caution:

DO NOT apply cold to more than 20% of an adult's body surface (10% for children); widespread cooling can cause hypothermia. Burn victims lose large amounts of heat and water.

DO NOT apply salve, ointment, grease, butter, cream, spray, home remedy, or any other coating on a burn until after it cools. Such coatings are unsterile and can lead to infection. They also can seal in heat, causing further damage.

Care of Small Second-Degree Burns (<20% BSA)

1. Follow steps 1 and 2 of First-Degree Burn care.
2. After the burn cools, apply a thin layer of bacitracin ointment. Topical antibiotic therapy like bacitracin does not sterilize a wound, but it does decrease the number of bacteria to a level that can be controlled by the body's defense mechanisms and prevents the entrance of bacteria.
3. Cover the burn with a dry, nonsticking, sterile dressing or a clean cloth. Covering the burn reduces the amount of pain by keeping air from the exposed nerve endings. The main purpose of a dressing over a burn is to keep the burn clean, prevent moisture loss through evaporation, and reduce pain. If toes or fingers have been burned, place dry dressings between them.
4. Have the victim drink as much water as possible without becoming nauseous.

Caution:

DO NOT cool more than 20% of an adult's body surface area (10% for a child) except to extinguish flames.

DO NOT break any blisters. Intact blisters serve as excellent burn dressings. Cover a ruptured blister with bacitracin ointment and a dry, sterile dressing.

CHEMICAL BURNS

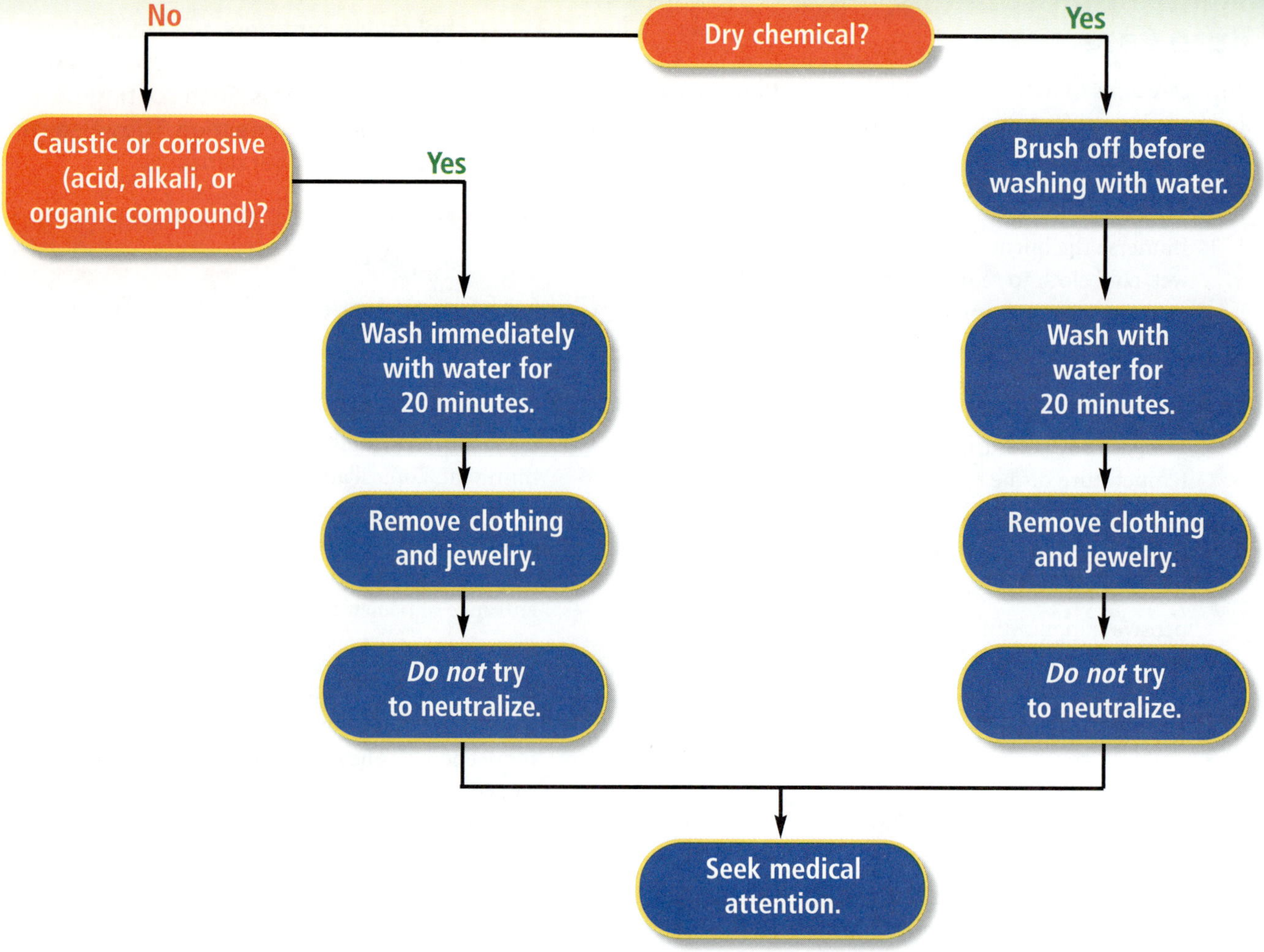

Care of Large Second-Degree Burns (>20% BSA)

Do not apply cold because it may cause hypothermia.

1. Follows steps 2 through 4 of Small Second-Degree Burn care (<20% BSA).
2. Seek medical attention.

Care of Third-Degree Burns

1. Cover the burn with a dry, nonsticking, sterile dressing or a clean cloth.
2. Treat the victim for shock by elevating the legs and keeping the victim warm with a clean sheet or blanket.
3. Seek medical attention.

Chemical Burns

A chemical burn is the result of a caustic or corrosive substance touching the skin (▼Figure 6). Because chemicals continue to "burn" as long as they are in contact with the skin, they should be removed from the victim as rapidly as possible.

First aid is the same for all chemical burns, except a few specific ones for which a chemical neutralizer has to be used. Alkalis such as drain cleaners cause more serious burns than acids such as battery acid because they penetrate deeper and remain active longer. Organic compounds such as petroleum products are also capable of burning.

Figure 6 Chemical burn from sulfuric acid

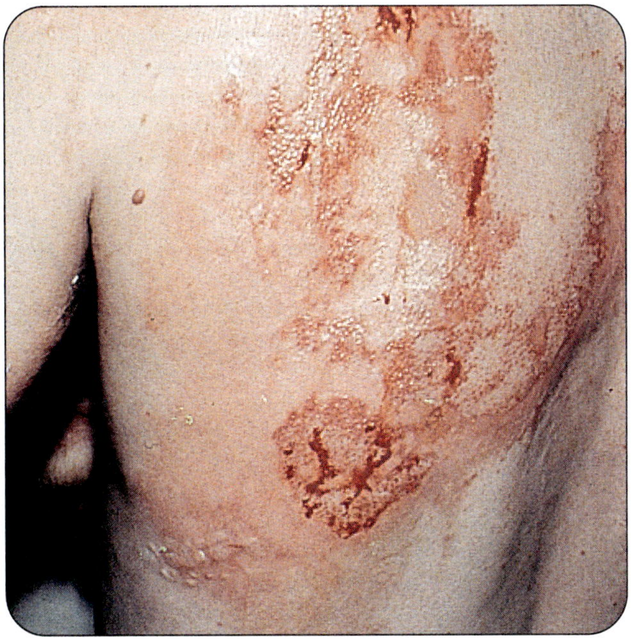

Caution:

DO NOT apply water under high pressure—it will drive the chemical deeper into the tissue.

DO NOT try to neutralize a chemical even if you know which chemical is involved—heat may be produced, resulting in more damage. Some product labels for neutralizing may be wrong. Save the container or the label for the chemical's name.

What to Do

1. Immediately remove the chemical by flushing the area with water (▼Figure 7). If available, use a hose or a shower. Brush dry powder chemicals from the skin *before* flushing, unless large amounts of water are immediately available. Water may activate a dry chemical and cause more damage to the skin. Take precautions to protect yourself from exposure to the chemical.
2. Remove the victim's contaminated clothing and jewelry while flushing with water. Clothing can hold chemicals, allowing them to continue to burn as long as they are in contact with the skin.
3. Flush for 20 minutes all chemical burns (skin, eyes). Washing with large amounts of water dilutes the chemical concentration and washes it away.
4. Cover the burned area with a dry, sterile dressing or, for large areas, a clean pillowcase.
5. Seek medical attention immediately for all chemical burns.

Figure 7 Flooding a chemical burn

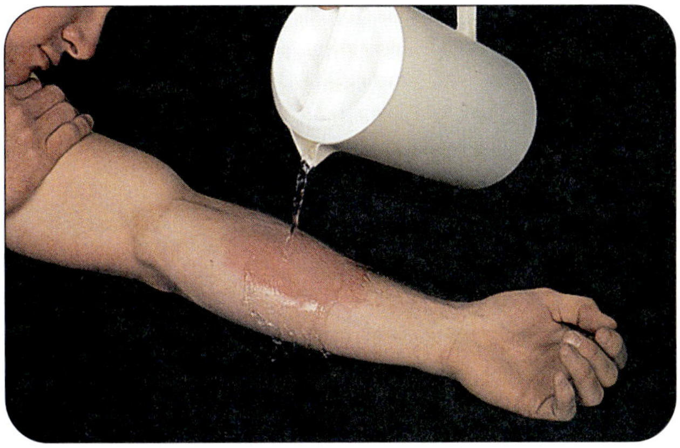

ELECTRICAL BURNS

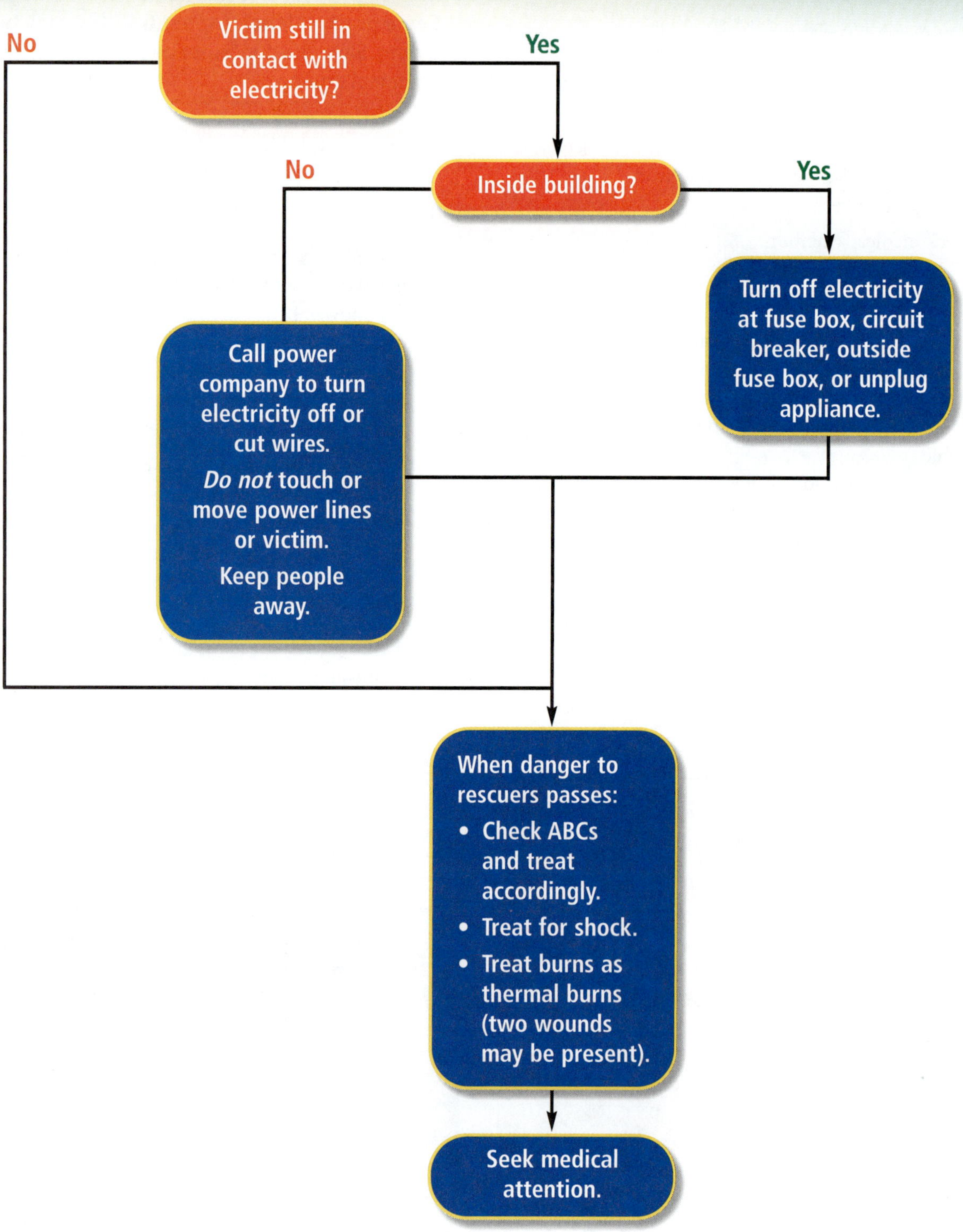

Electrical Burns

Even a mild electrical shock can cause serious internal injuries. A current of 1,000 volts or more is considered high voltage, but even the 110 volts found in ordinary household current can be deadly ▼Figures 8A and 8B.

There are three types of electrical injuries: thermal burn (flame), arc burn (flash), and true electrical injury (contact). A *thermal burn* (flame) results when clothing or objects in direct contact with the skin are ignited by an electrical current. These injuries are caused by the flames produced by the electrical current and not by the passage of the electrical current or arc.

An *arc burn* (flash) occurs when electricity jumps, or arcs, from one spot to another. The electrical current does not pass through the body. Although the duration of the flash may be brief, it usually causes extensive superficial injuries.

A *true electrical injury* (contact) happens when an electric current truly passes through the body. This type of injury is characterized by an entrance wound and an exit wound. The important factor in this type of injury is that the surface injury may be just the tip of the iceberg. High-voltage electrical currents passing through the body may disrupt the normal heart rhythm and cause cardiac arrest, burns, and other injuries.

During an electric shock, electricity enters the body at the point of contact and travels along the path of least resistance (nerves and blood vessels). The major damage occurs inside the body—the outside burn may appear small. Usually, the electricity exits where the body touches a surface or comes in contact with a ground (eg, a metal object). Sometimes, a victim has more than one exit site.

Figure 8A Electrical burn on toe

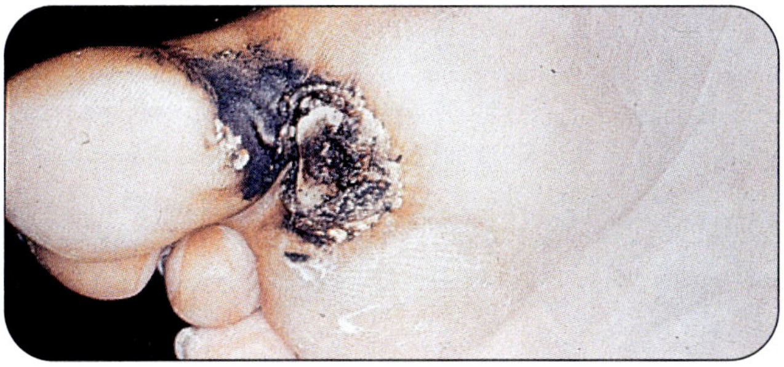

Figure 8B Electrical burn caused by chewing through electrical cord

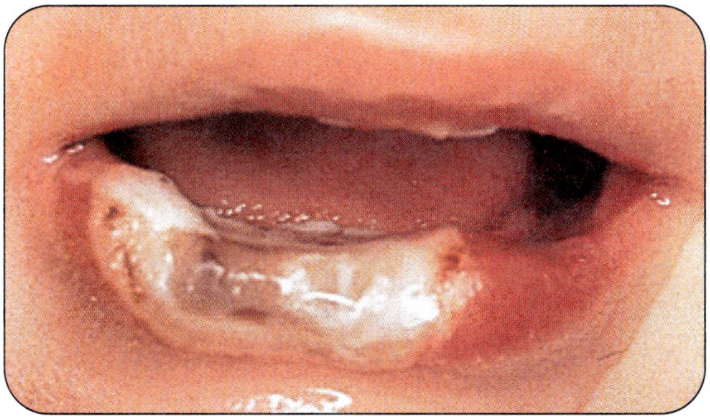

What to Do

1. Make sure the area is safe. Unplug, disconnect, or turn off the power. If that is impossible, call the power company or EMS for help.
2. Check ABCs.
3. If the victim fell, check for a spinal injury.
4. Treat the victim for shock by elevating the legs 8 to 12 inches if no spinal injury is suspected; prevent heat loss by covering the victim with a coat or blanket.
5. Seek medical attention immediately. Electrical injuries usually require burn center care.

Contact with a Power Line (Outdoors)

If the electric shock is from contact with a downed power line, the power *must* be turned off before a rescuer approaches anyone who may be in contact with the wire.

If you feel a tingling sensation in your legs and lower body as you approach a victim, stop. The sensation signals that you are on energized ground and that an electrical current is entering through one foot, passing through your lower body, and leaving through the other foot. Raise one foot off the ground, turn around, and hop to a safe place.

If you can safely reach the victim, do not attempt to move any wires, even with wooden poles, tools with wood handles, or tree branches. Do not use objects with a high moisture content and certainly not metal objects. You should not use wood-handled rakes, brooms, or shovels because if the voltage is high enough (you seldom will know how much voltage is involved), those objects can conduct electricity and you will be electrocuted. Do not attempt to move downed wires at all unless you are trained and are equipped with tools that can handle the high voltage.

Wait until trained personnel with the proper equipment can cut the wires or disconnect them. Prevent bystanders from entering the danger area.

Contact Inside Buildings

Most electrical burns that occur indoors are caused by faulty electrical equipment or careless use of electrical appliances. Turn off the electricity at the circuit breaker, fuse box, or outside switch box or unplug the appliance if the plug is undamaged. Do not touch the appliance or the victim until the current is off.

Once there is no danger to rescuers, first aid can begin.

Learning Activities

Thermal (Heat) Burns

Directions: Circle Yes if you agree with the statement, and circle No if you disagree.

Yes No **1.** Relieve pain and tissue damage from a burn by holding the part in a sink filled with running cold water.

Yes No **2.** Pain and inflammation can be relieved with aspirin or ibuprofen in those who can tolerate these over-the-counter medications.

Yes No **3.** Later, a layer of antibiotic ointment or aloe vera gel can be applied on first- and second-degree burns.

Yes No **4.** Butter can be effective on first- and second-degree burns.

Scenario: Tracy is boiling water to make hot chocolate in the office kitchen. She reaches across the stove for a cup. The sleeve of her blouse touches the flame of the gas burner and ignites, sending fire racing up her arm. Her screams bring you and others racing into the kitchen. She has second-degree burns on about 7% of her body. What should you do?

____

____

Chemical Burns

Yes No **1.** When washing chemicals off the body, flush with water for at least five minutes.

Yes No **2.** When washing chemicals off the body, use high pressure water.

Yes No **3.** Do not try to neutralize a chemical because more damage may result.

Yes No **4.** Brush dry powder chemicals from the skin before flushing unless large amounts of water are immediately available.

Scenario: Tim is a 28-year-old man using a caustic drain cleaner to unclog a bathroom sink. Fifteen minutes after applying the chemical, he runs water into the sink, but the drain remains clogged. He then ignores the instructions on the drain cleaner package and uses a plunger to clear the drain. The solution in the sink splashes on his arm. What should you do?

____

____

Electrical Burns

Yes No **1.** If a victim is in contact with an outdoor electrical wire, try to move it with a wooden pole or handle.

Yes No **2.** If the victim is inside a building, turn off the electricity at the fuse box, circuit-breaker, outside switch box, or unplug the appliance.

Scenario: Steve is trimming hedges using an old electric hedge trimmer, which is falling apart, but works. Because the three-pronged grounding plug is a little wobbly, Steve connects it to a two-pronged adapter, plugs the adapter into an outlet, and starts working on the hedges along a metal chain-link fence. Things are going well until Steve leans against the fence for support, and a powerful electric current shoots through his body, causing him to fall over. When you arrive, he is motionless. What do you do?

____

____

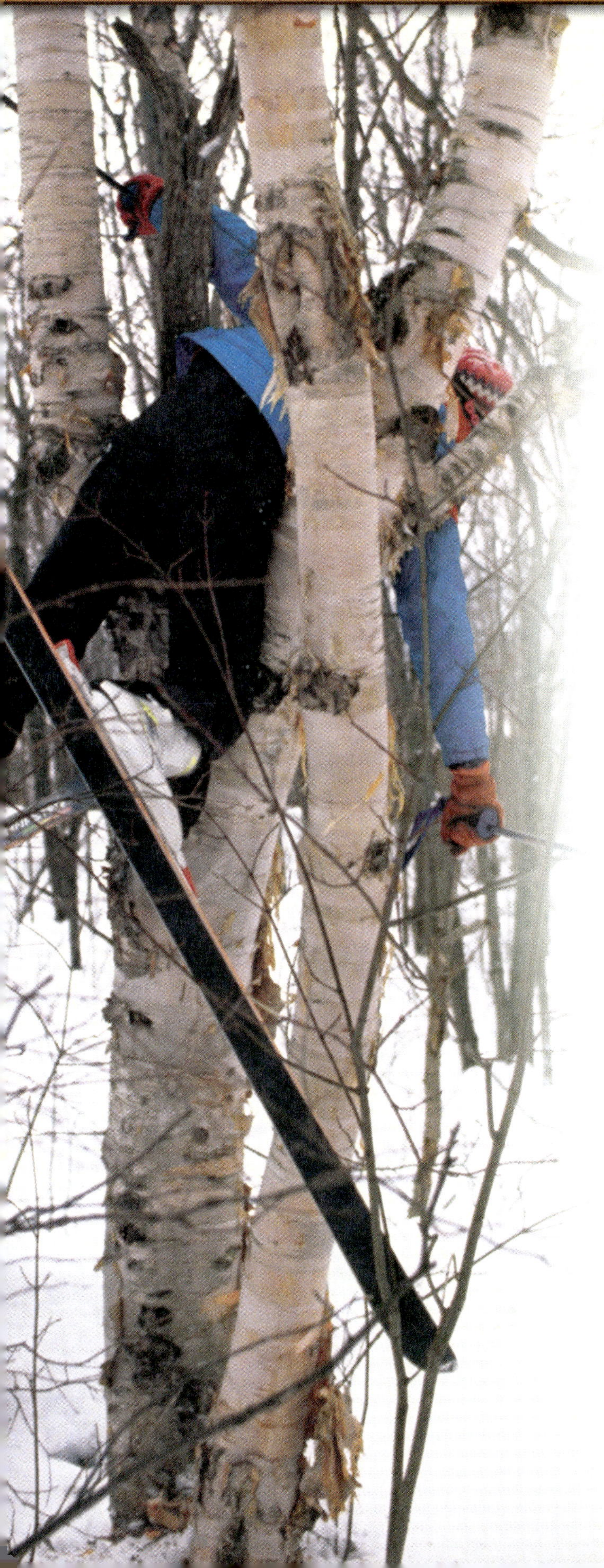

Chapter 8

Head and Spinal Injuries

Head Injuries

Head injury is a broadly used term. It is important to distinguish the various types of head injuries—scalp wounds, skull fractures, and brain injuries.

Scalp Wounds

A bleeding scalp wound does not affect the blood supply to the brain. The brain obtains its blood supply from arteries in the neck, not the scalp. A severe scalp wound may have an accompanying skull fracture, impaled object, or spinal injury.

What to Do

1. Wear medical exam gloves.
2. Control bleeding by gently applying direct pressure with a dry sterile dressing. If the dressing becomes blood-filled, do not remove it. Add another dressing on top of the first one.
3. If you suspect a skull fracture, apply pressure around the edges of the wound and over a broad area rather than on the center of the wound. Use a doughnut (ring) pad around the area.
4. Keep the head and shoulders slightly elevated to help control bleeding if you do not suspect a spinal injury.

Caution:

DO NOT remove an embedded object; instead stabilize it in place with bulky dressings. If you suspect a skull fracture, do not clean a scalp wound or irrigate it because the fluid can carry debris and bacteria into the brain.

HEAD INJURIES

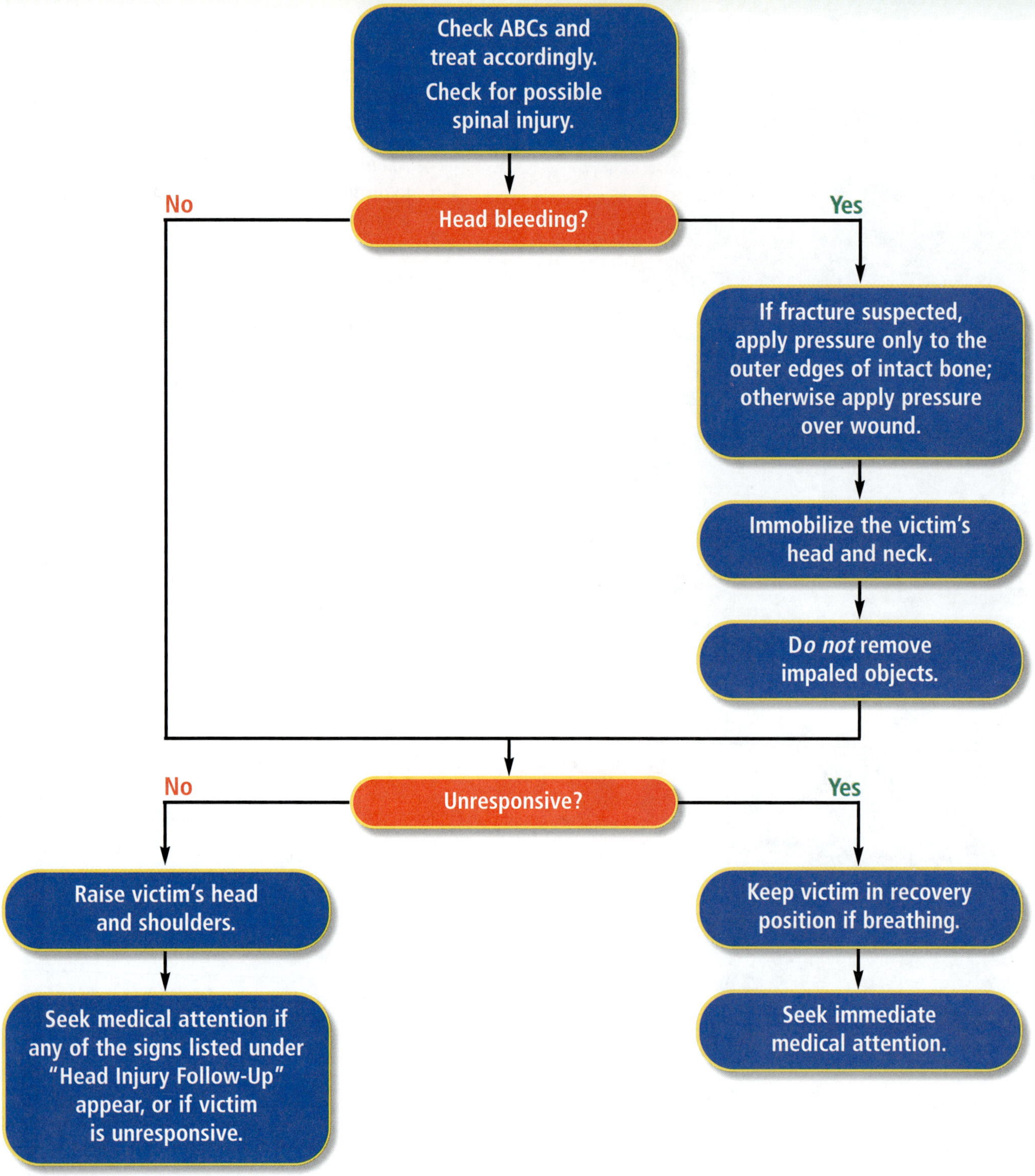

Head Injury Follow-Up

If any of the following signs appear within 48 hours of a head injury, seek medical attention:

- **Headache:** Expect a headache. But if it lasts more than one or two days or increases in severity, however, seek medical advice.
- **Nausea, vomiting:** If nausea lasts more than two hours, seek medical advice. Vomiting once or twice, especially in children, may be expected after a head injury. Vomiting does not tell anything about the severity of the injury. However, if vomiting begins again hours after the initial episodes have ceased, consult a physician.
- **Drowsiness:** Allow a victim to sleep, but wake the victim at least every two hours to check the state of consciousness and sense of orientation by asking his or her name and an information-processing question (eg, "Recite the months of the year backwards starting with December"). If the victim cannot respond or appears confused or disoriented, call a physician.
- **Vision problems:** If the victim "sees double," if the eyes fail to move together, or if one pupil appears to be larger than the other, seek medical advice.
- **Mobility:** If the victim cannot use his or her arms or legs as well as previously or is unsteady in walking, seek medical care.
- **Speech:** If the victim has slurred speech or is unable to talk, consult a doctor.
- **Seizures or convulsions:** If the victim has a violent involuntary contraction (spasm) or series of contractions of the skeletal muscles, seek medical assistance.

Skull Fracture

What to Look For

It is difficult to determine a skull fracture except by x-ray unless the skull deformity is severe. Signs and symptoms of a skull fracture include the following:

- Pain at the point of injury
- Deformity of the skull
- Bleeding coming from the ears or nose
- A clear, pink, watery fluid known as cerebrospinal fluid (CSF) leaking from an ear or the nose. A drop of CSF on a handkerchief, pillowcase, or other light-colored cloth will resemble a target, with a pink ring around a slightly blood-tinged center; this is called the "halo sign" or "ring sign."
- Discoloration around the eyes ("raccoon eyes") appearing several hours after the injury
- Discoloration behind an ear (known as "Battle's sign") appearing several hours after the injury
- Unequal sized pupils
- Profuse scalp bleeding if skin is broken. A scalp wound may expose the skull or brain tissue
- Penetrating wound (eg, from a bullet) or impaled object

What to Do

1. Monitor ABCs.
2. Cover wounds with a sterile dressing.
3. Stabilize the victim's neck against movement.
4. To control bleeding, apply pressure around the edges of the wound, not directly on it.

Brain Injuries

When the head is struck with sufficient force, the brain bounces against the inside of the skull.

The brain, like other body tissue, will swell from bleeding. Unlike other tissues, however, the brain is confined in the skull where there is little space for swelling. Therefore, swelling of brain tissue or accumulation of blood inside the skull compresses the brain and increases the pressure inside the skull, which interferes with brain functioning.

What to Look For

The following are frequently observed signs and symptoms of a concussion, according to the American Academy of Neurology and the Brain Injury Association:*

1. Confused facial expression
2. Slow to answer questions or follow instruction
3. Easily distracted and unable to follow through with normal activities
4. Walking in the wrong direction; unaware of time, date, and place
5. Making disjointed or incomprehensible statements
6. Stumbling, inability to walk straight line

---

* *Source:* Adapted from Management of Concussion in Sports, American Academy of Neurology and Brain Injury Association

7. Distraught, crying for no apparent reason
8. Asking the same question even though it has was already been answered, or unable to memorize and recall three words or three objects in sequence in five minutes
9. Coma, unresponsiveness

What to Do

1. Seek immediate medical attention for all brain-injury victims.
2. Suspect a spinal injury in an unresponsive victim until proved otherwise.
3. Monitor ABCs.
4. Control bleeding by covering wounds with sterile dressings as a barrier against infection. If you suspect a skull fracture, apply pressure around the wound edges, not directly on the wound.
5. Brain-injury victims tend to vomit. Rolling the victim onto his or her side while stabilizing the neck against movement will help drain vomit and keep the airway open.

Unfortunately, there is little a first aider can do for a brain injury. The victim must be transported to the care of a neurosurgeon.

Caution:

DO NOT stop the flow of blood or CSF from the ears or nose. Blocking either flow could increase pressure inside the skull.

DO NOT elevate the legs—that might increase pressure on the brain.

DO NOT clean an open skull injury—infection of the brain may result.

Eye Injuries

Eye injuries can involve minor conditions such as a foreign object such as dirt in the eye. But they can also involve more severe injuries that can compromise sight if not cared for immediately. Do not assume that any eye injury is innocent. When in doubt, seek medical attention immediately.

Penetrating Eye Injuries

Penetrating eye injuries are severe injuries that result when a sharp object such as a knife or a needle penetrates the eye and then is withdrawn or when pieces from a tool enter the eye and lodge there as foreign bodies.

What to Do

1. Seek immediate medical attention. Any penetrating eye injury should be managed in the hospital.
2. Stabilize any object. Stabilize a long protruding object with bulky dressings or clean cloths. You can place a protective paper cup or a piece of cardboard folded (►Figure 1) into a cone over the affected eye to prevent bumping of the object. For short objects, surround the eye without touching the object with a doughnut-shaped (ring) pad held on with a roller bandage.
3. Cover the undamaged eye. Most experts suggest that the undamaged eye should be covered to prevent sympathetic eye movement (ie, the injured eye moves when the undamaged one does) and aggravating the injury. Remember that the victim is unable to see when both eyes are covered and may be anxious. Make sure you explain everything you are doing.

Caution:

DO NOT wash out the eye with water.

DO NOT try to remove an object stuck in the eye.

DO NOT press on an injured eyeball or penetrating object.

Blows to the Eye

Blows to the eye can be minor to sight-threatening (►Figure 2).

What to Do

1. Apply an ice pack immediately for about 15 minutes to reduce pain and swelling. Do not exert any pressure on the eye.
2. Seek medical attention immediately if there is pain, reduced vision, or discoloration (a black eye).

Cuts of the Eye or Lid (►Figure 3)

What to Do

1. Bandage both eyes lightly.
2. Seek medical attention immediately.

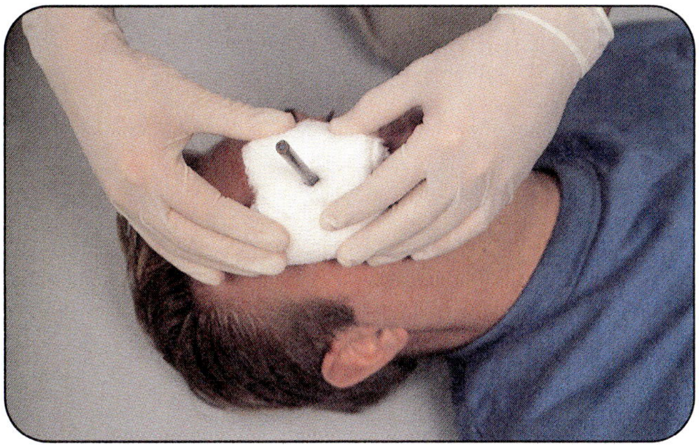

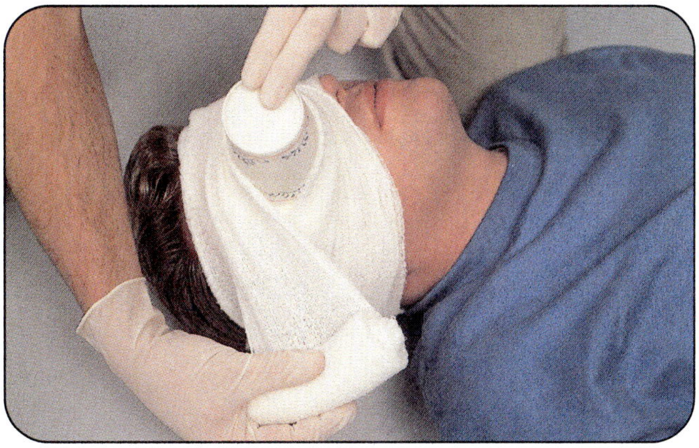

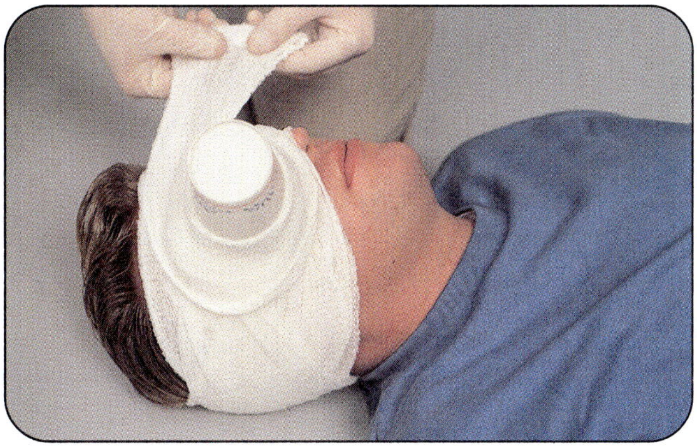

Figures 1A, 1B, and 1C Protecting a long penetrating object against movement (using paper cup)

Chemical Burns of the Eye

Chemical burns of the eyes are extremely sight-threatening. First aid may determine the fate of the eye and vision.

Alkalis cause greater damage than acids because they penetrate deeper and continue to burn longer. Common alkalis include drain cleaners, cleaning agents, ammonia, cement, plaster, and caustic soda. Common acids include hydrochloric acid, nitric acid, sulfuric (battery) acid, and acetic acid.

Because damage can happen in 1 to 5 minutes, the chemical must be removed immediately.

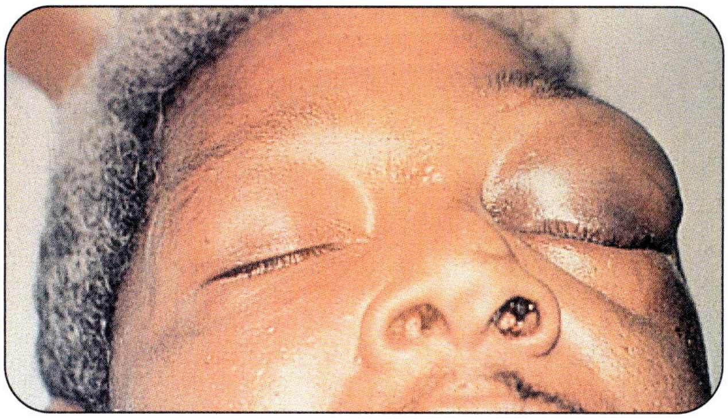

Figure 2 Blow to the eye

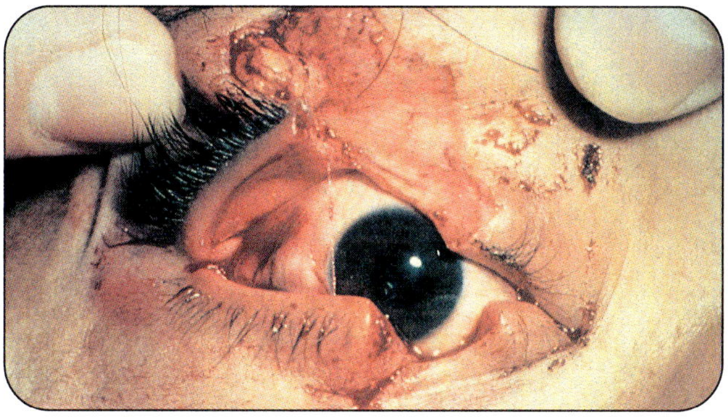

Figure 3 Lacerated eyelid

What to Do

1. Use your fingers to keep the eye open as wide as possible.
2. Flush the eye with water immediately ▼Figure 4. If possible, use warm water. If water is not available, use any nonirritating liquid.
   - Hold the victim's head under a faucet or pour water into the eye from any clean container for 20 minutes, continuously and gently. It is impossible to use too much water on these injuries.

Figure 4 Flushing eye for chemical burn

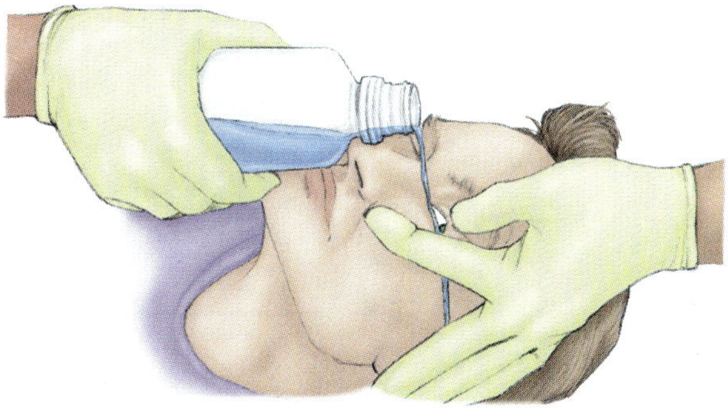

EYE INJURIES

Chemical in eye?

- **Yes** → Hold injured eye wide open; flush with warm water for 20 minutes. Loosely bandage both eyes. → Seek medical attention.
- **No** → **Object embedded in eye?**
  - **Yes** →
    1. *Do not* remove embedded object.

    2A. If object is long:
    - Place padding around object.
    - Place paper cup or cardboard folded in a cone over eye.

    2B. If object is short:
    - Place doughnut-shaped pad around eye.

    3. Cover uninjured eye with a dressing.
    4. Keep victim flat on back.

    → Seek medical attention.
  - **No** → **Loose object in eye?**
    - **Yes** → Attempt, in order, each procedure until one is effective.
      1. Pull upper eyelid down and over lower lid.
      2. Pull lower lid down and look at inner surface while victim looks up. If object is seen, remove with wet gauze.
      3. Lift upper eyelid over Q-tip. If object is seen, remove with wet gauze.

      If successful, medical attention is usually not needed.
    - **No** → **Cut on eye?**
      - **Yes** → *Do not* apply pressure. Cover both eyes with gauze pads. Position victim with head elevated. → Seek medical attention.
      - **No** → **Blow to eye?** → Keep victim flat on back with eyes closed. Place ice pack for 15 minutes. → Seek medical attention.

Seek medical attention.

- Irrigate from the nose side of the eye toward the outside, to avoid flushing material into the other eye.
- Tell the victim to roll the eyeball as much as possible to help wash out the eye.

3. Loosely bandage both eyes with cold, wet dressings.
4. Seek immediate medical attention.

Caution:

DO NOT try to neutralize the chemical. Water usually is readily available and better for eye irrigation.

DO NOT bandage eye tightly.

Eye Knocked Out

A blow to the eye can knock it from its socket.

What to Do

1. Cover the eye loosely with a sterile dressing that has been moistened with clean water. Do not try to push the eyeball back into the socket.
2. Protect the injured eye with a paper cup, a piece of cardboard folded into a cone, or a doughnut-shaped pad made from a roller gauze bandage or a cravat bandage.
3. Cover the undamaged eye.
4. Seek medical attention immediately.

Foreign Objects in Eye

Try one or more of the following techniques, beginning with the first step ▶Figure 5.

What to Do

1. Lift the upper lid over the lower lid, allowing the lashes to brush the object off the inside of the upper lid. Have the victim blink a few times and let the eye move the object out. If the object remains, keep the eye closed.
2. Try flushing the object out by rinsing the eye gently with warm water. Hold the eyelid open and tell the victim to move the eye as it is rinsed.
3. Examine the lower lid by pulling it down gently. If you can see the object, remove it with a moistened sterile gauze or clean cloth.

Figure 5 Removing foreign object from the eye

a. If tears or gentle flushing do not remove object, gently pull lower lid down. Remove an object by gently flushing with lukewarm water or a wet sterile gauze.

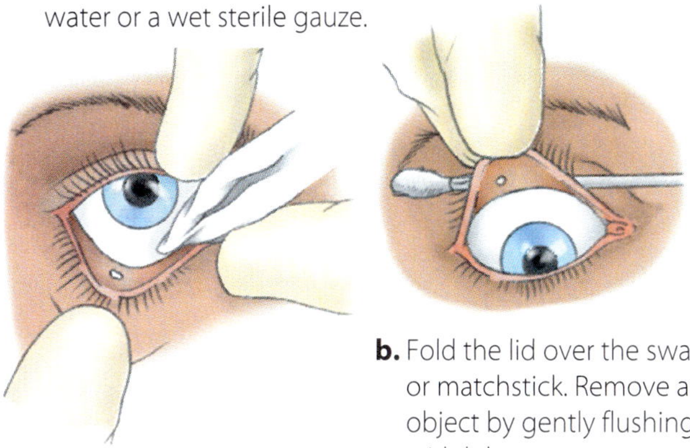

b. Fold the lid over the swab or matchstick. Remove an object by gently flushing with lukewarm water or a wet sterile gauze.

4. Examine the upper lid by grasping the lashes of the upper lid, placing a match stick or cotton-tipped swab across the upper lid and rolling the lid upward over the stick or swab. If you can see the object, remove it with a moistened sterile gauze or clean cloth or flush it out.

Caution:

DO NOT allow the victim to rub the eye.

DO NOT try to remove an embedded foreign object.

DO NOT use dry cotton (cotton balls or cotton-tipped swabs) or instruments (eg, tweezers) on an eye.

Eye Burns from Light

Burns can result if a person looks at a source of ultraviolet light (eg, sunlight, arc welding, bright snow, tanning lamps). Severe pain begins 1 to 6 hours after exposure.

What to Do

1. Cover both eyes with cold, wet packs. Tell the victim not to rub the eyes.
2. Have the victim rest in a darkened room. Do not allow light to reach the victim's eyes.
3. Give pain medication if needed.
4. Call an ophthalmologist for medical advice.

DENTAL INJURIES

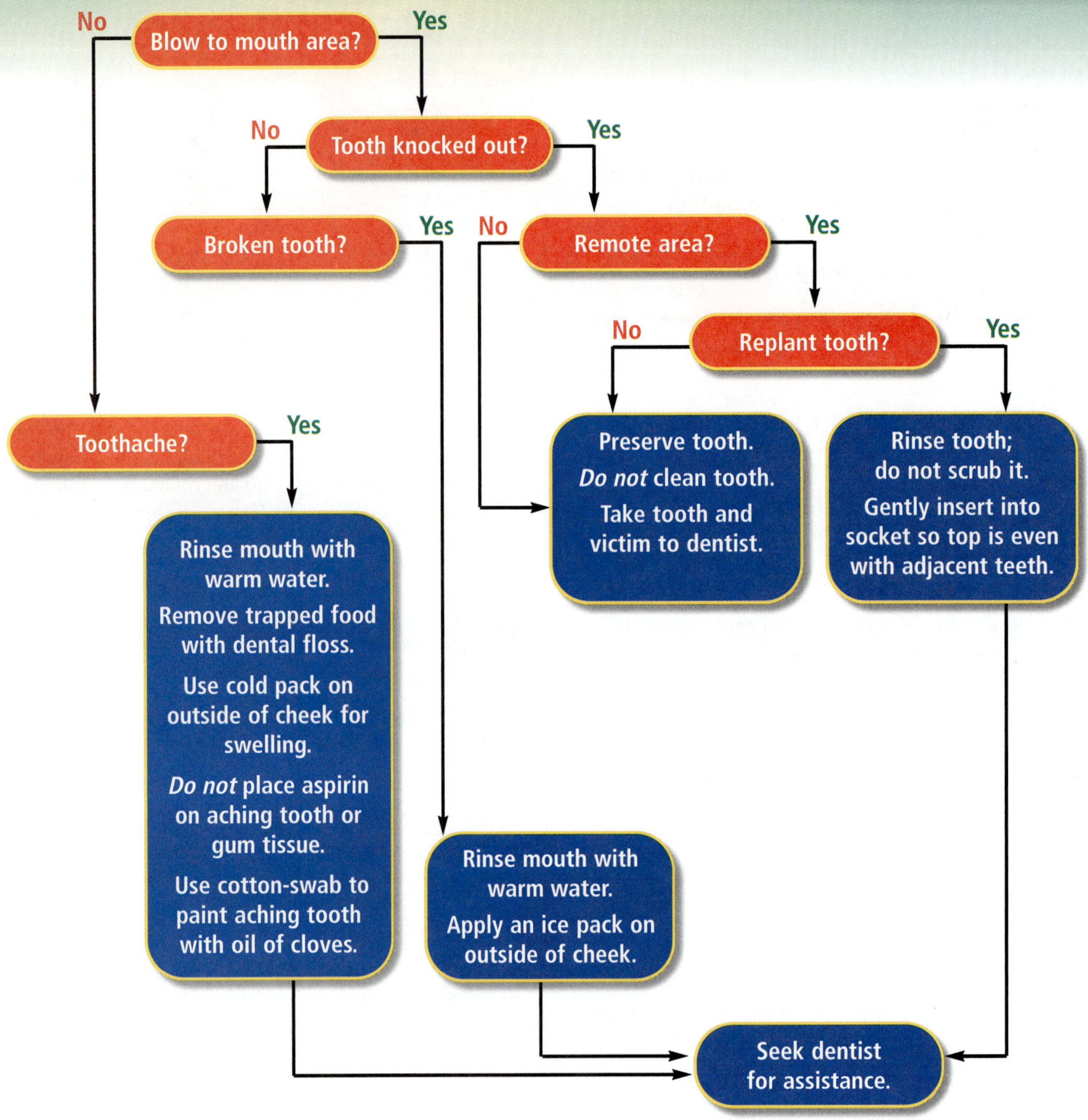

Nose Injuries

Nosebleeds

There are two types of nosebleeds:

- *Anterior (front of nose)* is the most common type (90%). Blood comes out of the nose through one nostril.
- *Posterior (back of nose)* type involves massive bleeding backward into the mouth or down the back of the throat. A posterior nosebleed is serious and requires medical attention.

Caution:

DO NOT allow the victim to tilt the head backward.

DO NOT probe the nose with a cotton-tipped swab.

DO NOT move the victim's head and neck if a spinal injury is suspected.

What to Do

1. Place the victim in a seated position.
2. Keep the victim's head tilted slightly forward so blood can run out the front of the nose, not down the back of the throat, which can cause choking, nausea, or vomiting.
3. Pinch (or have the victim pinch) all the soft parts of the nose together between the thumb and two fingers with steady pressure for five minutes. While pinching the nostrils, push the pinched parts against the bones of the face.
4. If bleeding persists, have the victim gently blow the nose to remove any irregular clots and excess blood and to minimize sneezing. This allows new clots to form. If available, spray the nose four times on each side with a decongestant spray (Afrin™, Neo-Synephrin™), then pinch the nostrils again for five minutes.
5. Apply an ice pack over the nose and cheeks to help control bleeding—especially if caused by a blow to the nose.
6. Seek medical attention if any of the following applies:
   - The nostril pinching and other methods do not stop the bleeding.
   - You suspect a posterior nosebleed.
   - The victim has high blood pressure or is taking anticoagulants (blood thinners) or large doses of aspirin.
   - Bleeding happens after a blow to the nose, and you suspect a broken nose.

Broken Nose

1. Seek medical attention.
2. Treat a nosebleed as described above.
3. Apply an ice pack to the nose for 15 minutes. Do not try to straighten a crooked nose.

Dental Injuries

Because dental emergencies generally cause considerable pain and anxiety, managing them promptly can provide great relief to the victim.

Knocked-Out Tooth

A knocked-out tooth is a common dental emergency ▼Figure 6. More than 90% of the two million teeth knocked out each year in the United States could be saved with proper treatment.

Emergency care for knocked-out teeth has changed dramatically in recent years. The first question you want to ask in this situation is, "Where is the tooth?" Time is crucial for successful reimplantation. After a tooth is knocked out, ligament fiber fragments remain attached to the tooth and to the bone in the socket. However, the ligament fibers begin to die soon after the injury. Therefore, it is important to prevent the tooth from drying. Moisture alone is not sufficient to preserve the tooth's ligament fibers. Steps must be taken both to prevent the tooth from becoming dehydrated and to protect the ligament fibers from damage.

Figure 6 Tooth knocked out

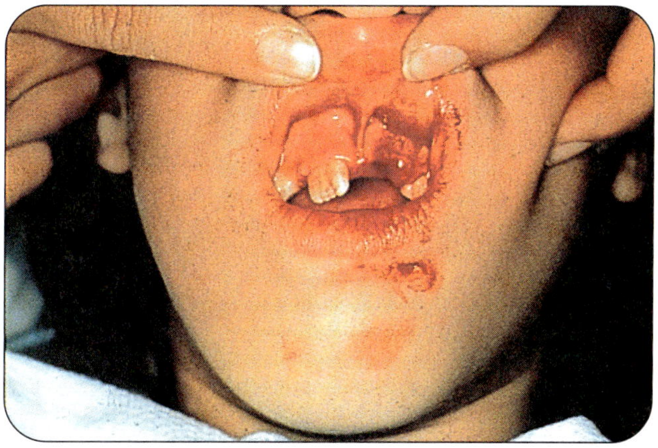

1. Have the victim rinse his or her month, and put a rolled gauze pad in the socket to control bleeding.
2. Find the tooth and handle it by the crown, not the root, to minimize damage to the ligament fibers.
3. The best place for a knocked-out tooth is its socket. A tooth can often be successfully reimplanted if it is replaced in its socket within 30 minutes after the injury; the odds of successful reimplantation decrease about 1% for every minute the tooth is absent from the socket. If you feel you can do this without causing more injury to the victim, gently rinse any debris from the tooth and try to place the tooth into the socket, using adjacent teeth as a guide. Apply pressure on the tooth so the top is even with the adjacent teeth.

   Immediate reinsertion is not always possible, however. The victim may be reluctant to put the knocked-out tooth back into its socket, especially if it has fallen on the ground and is covered with debris. Or the tooth may repeatedly fall out, putting the victim at risk of inhaling or swallowing it. In victims with multiple trauma, the presence of more serious injuries may prevent reinsertion.

   When immediate reinsertion is not possible, the tooth should be transported in a moist environment. The best transport medium is the Save-a-Tooth Kit™. Its use extends the viability of the ligament fibers for 6 to 12 hours. If this is not available, cool milk can be used.

   Some experts recommend that the tooth be placed in the victim's mouth to keep it moist until dental treatment is available. This method, although convenient, presents the risk of the tooth's being accidentally swallowed, especially by children.
4. Take the victim and the tooth to a dentist immediately even if it has been reinserted.

Dental Emergency Procedures

Toothache	Rinse the mouth vigorously with warm water to clean out debris. Use dental floss to remove any food that might be trapped between the teeth. ***(Do not place aspirin on the aching tooth or gum tissues.)*** See your dentist as soon as possible.
Orthodontic Problems (braces and retainers)	If a wire is causing irritation, cover the end of the wire with a small cotton ball, beeswax, or a piece of gauze until you can get to the dentist. If a wire is embedded in the cheek, tongue, or gum tissue, do not attempt to remove it. Go to your dentist immediately. If an appliance becomes loose or a piece of it breaks off, take the appliance and the piece and go to the dentist.
Knocked-Out Tooth	If the tooth is dirty, rinse it gently in running water. ***Do not scrub it*** or remove any attached tissue fragments. Gently insert and hold the tooth in its socket. If this is not possible, place the tooth in a container of milk or a special tooth-preserving solution. Go immediately to your dentist (within 30 minutes, if possible). Don't forget to bring the tooth.
Broken Tooth	Gently clean dirt or debris from the injured area by rinsing the mouth with warm water. Place cold compresses on the face, in the area of the injured tooth, to minimize swelling. Go to the dentist immediately.
Bitten Tongue or Lip	Apply direct pressure to the bleeding area with a clean cloth. If swelling is present, apply cold compresses. If bleeding does not stop, go to a hospital emergency room.
Object Wedged between Teeth	Try to gently remove the object with dental floss. Guide the floss and avoid cutting the gums. If not successful in removing the object, go to the dentist. Do not try to remove the object with a sharp or pointed instrument.
Possible Fractured Jaw	Immobilize the jaw by any means (necktie, dish towel). If swelling is present, apply cold compresses. Call your dentist or go immediately to a hospital emergency room.

Source: Copyright by the American Dental Association; reprinted with permission.

Broken Tooth ▼Figure 7

What to Do

1. Gently clean dirt and blood from the injured area with a sterile gauze pad or a clean cloth and warm water.
2. Apply an ice pack to the face in the area of the injured tooth to decrease swelling.
3. If you suspect a jaw fracture, stabilize the jaw by wrapping a bandage under the chin and over the top of the head.
4. Seek a dentist immediately.

Toothache

The tooth will be sensitive to heat and cold. Identify the diseased tooth by tapping the area with a spoon handle or similar object. A diseased tooth will hurt.

What to Do

1. Rinse the mouth with warm water to clean it out.
2. Use dental floss to remove any food that might be trapped between the teeth.
3. Give the victim pain medication such as ibuprofen.
4. Seek a dentist immediately.

Spinal Injuries

Head injuries serve as a clue to possible spinal injuries because the head may have been moved suddenly in one or more directions, damaging the spine.

What to Look For ►Skill Scan

- Painful movement of the arms or legs
- Numbness, tingling, weakness, or burning sensation in the arms or legs

Figure 7 Broken teeth

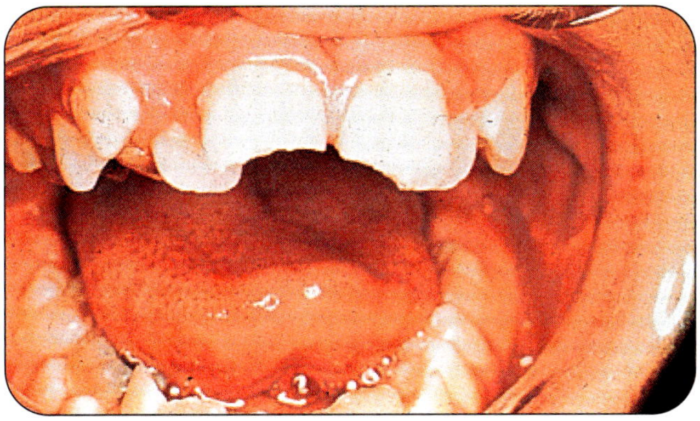

- Loss of bowel or bladder control
- Paralysis of the arms or legs
- Deformity (odd-looking angle of the victim's head and neck)
- Check a responsive victim by using techniques shown in the Skill Scan: *Checking for Spinal Injuries* of this chapter.

If the victim is unresponsive, do the following:

- Look for cuts, bruises, and deformities.
- Test responses by pinching the victim's hand (either palm or back of the hand) and bare foot (sole or top of the foot). No reaction could mean spinal damage.
- Ask bystanders what happened. If you still are not sure about a possible spinal injury, assume the victim has one until it is proved otherwise.

What to Do

1. Stabilize the victim against any movement ▼Figure 8, A–B.
2. Check ABC.

Figure 8, A–B **A.** Stabilize head against movement. **B.** To free yourself to help others, place heavy objects on each side of the head

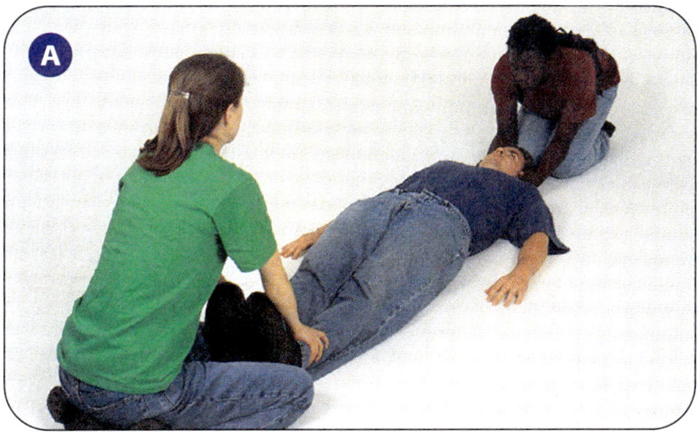

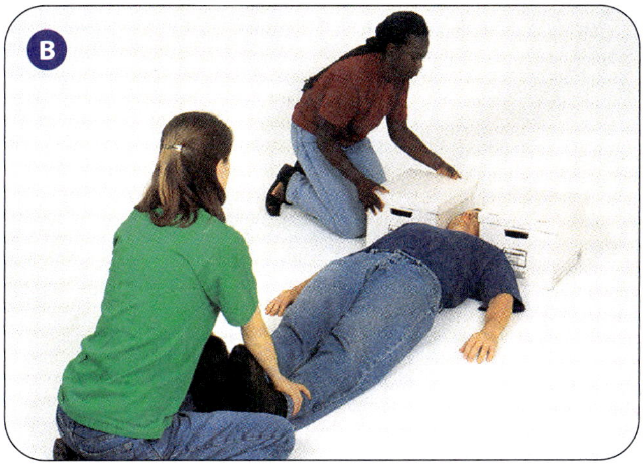

SPINAL INJURIES

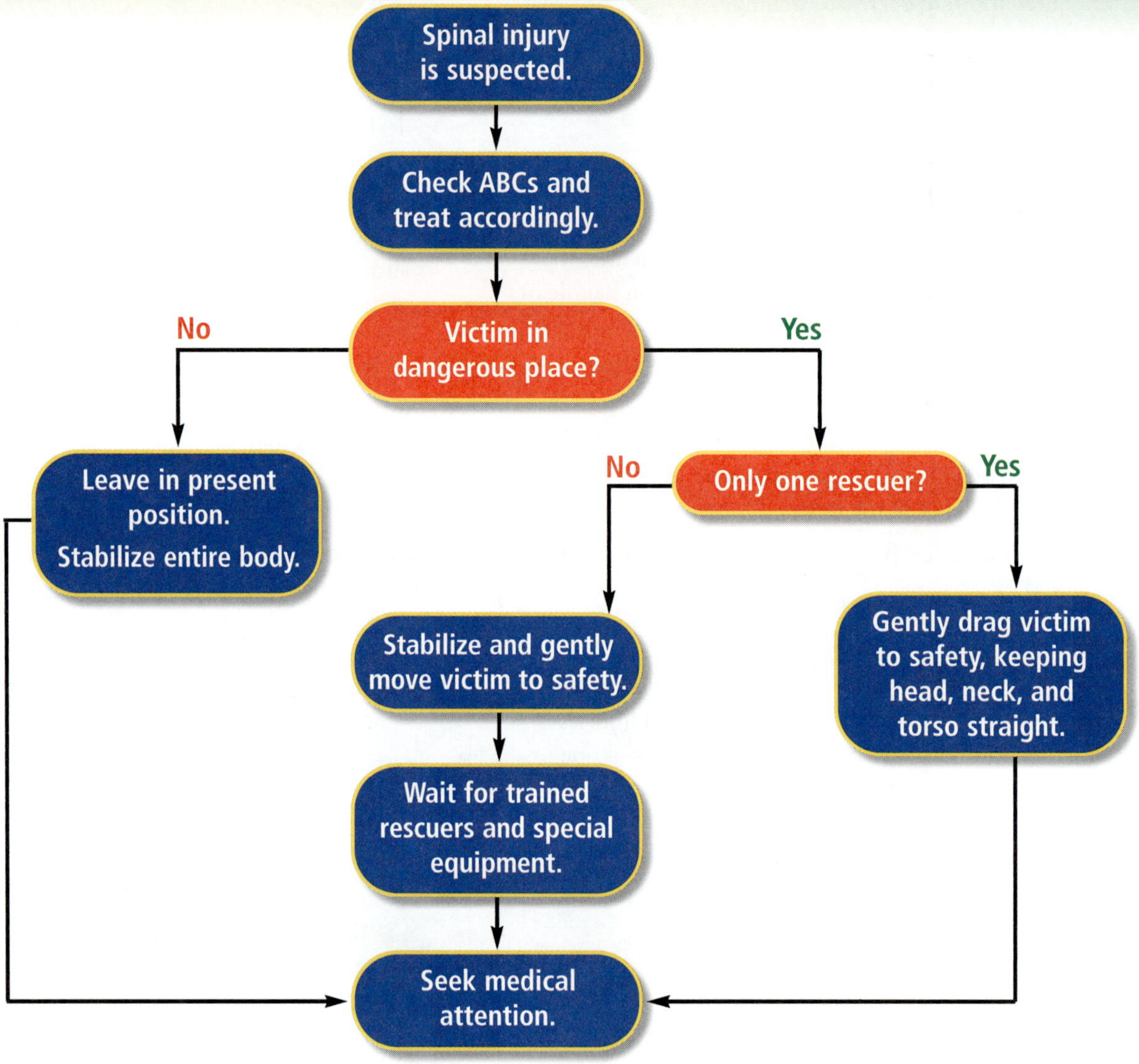

Skill Scan Checking for Spinal Injuries

Responsive Victim—Upper Extremity Checks

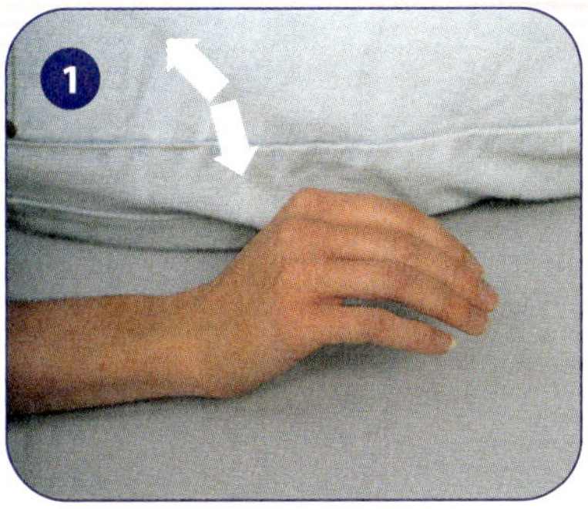

1. Victim wiggles fingers.

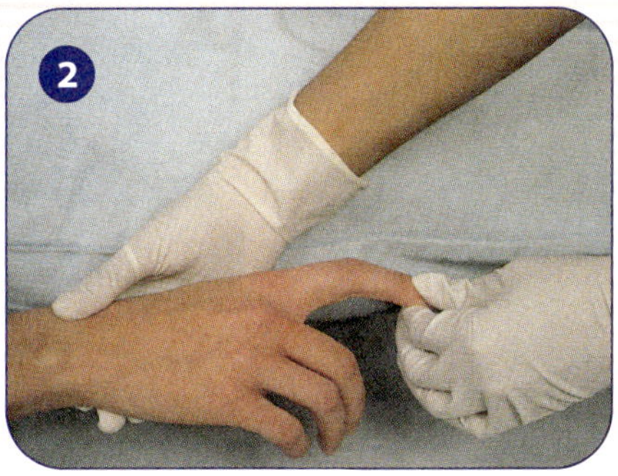

2. Victim feels rescuer squeeze fingers.

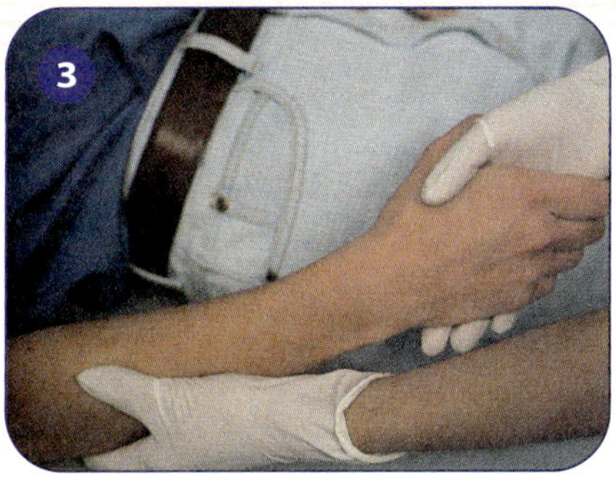

3. Victim squeezes rescuer's hand.

Responsive Victim—Lower-Extremity Checks

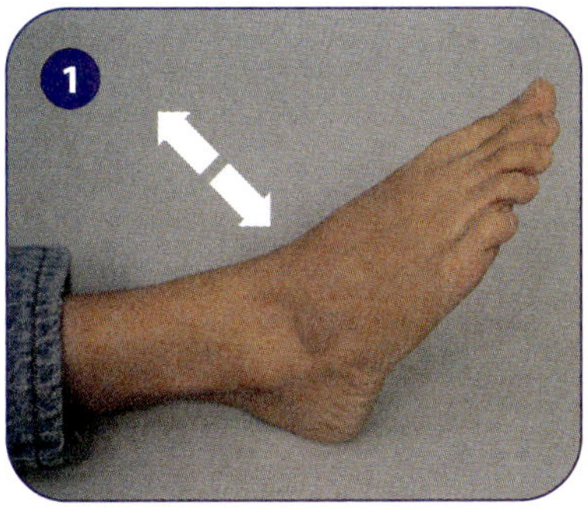

1. Victim wiggles toes.

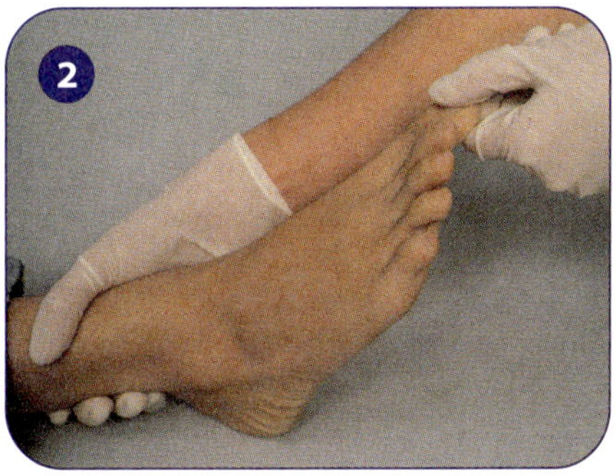

2. Victim feels rescuer squeezes toes.

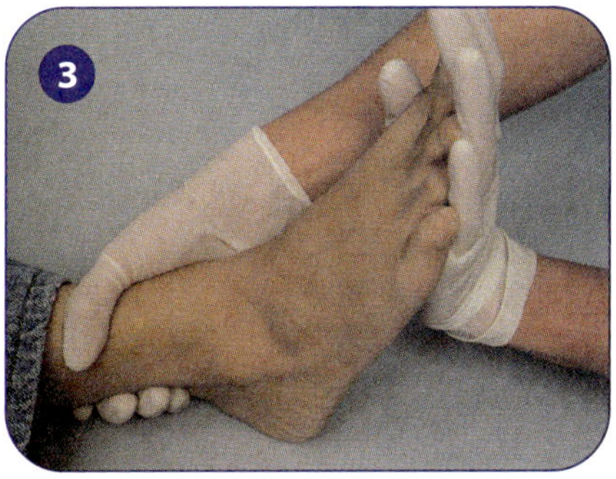

3. Victim pushes foot against rescuer's hand.

Learning Activities

Head Injuries

Directions: Circle Yes if you agree with the statement, and circle No if you disagree.

Yes No 1. Press around the edges of a suspected skull fracture and not directly on the wound.

Yes No 2. Do NOT remove impaled (embedded) objects.

Yes No 3. Head injured victims should be checked for a possible spinal injury.

Scenario: At work, you are called to help a carpenter who fell from a ladder. A bystander says that, though responsive now, the victim was previously motionless for a couple of minutes. The victim complains about a severe headache and dizziness. There is swelling on the back of his head. What should you do?

____

____

Eye Injuries

Yes No 1. After a blow to an eye, apply a cold pack for about 15 minutes.

Yes No 2. Tears are sufficient to flush a chemical from the eye.

Yes No 3. Use a clean, damp cloth to remove an object from the eyelid's surface.

Scenario: As Sam is attempting to jump-start the company car, a spark from the jump-cables ignites hydrogen gas accumulated in the battery. This causes the battery to explode. The battery cap flies off, and battery acid splashes into Sam's eyes. What should you do?

____

____

Dental Injuries

Yes No 1. Preserve a knocked-out tooth in mouthwash or rubbing alcohol.

Yes No 2. Scrub a knocked-out tooth before taking the victim to a dentist.

Yes No 3. Sometimes a knocked-out tooth should be reinserted by a first aider.

Scenario: Mike, age 20, was struck in the mouth by a pipe loosely suspended from a cable. He has spit out two of his front teeth, which are lying on the ground. What should you do?

____

____

Spinal Injuries

Yes No 1. Do NOT move a victim with a suspected spinal injury.

Yes No 2. Inability to move fingers and/or feet may indicate a spinal injury.

Yes No 3. A head injury may be a reason to suspect a spinal injury.

Scenario: You heard a loud crash when a car hit a concrete median. You have done a scene survey. The driver complains of numbness and loss of feeling in both legs. What should you do?

____

____

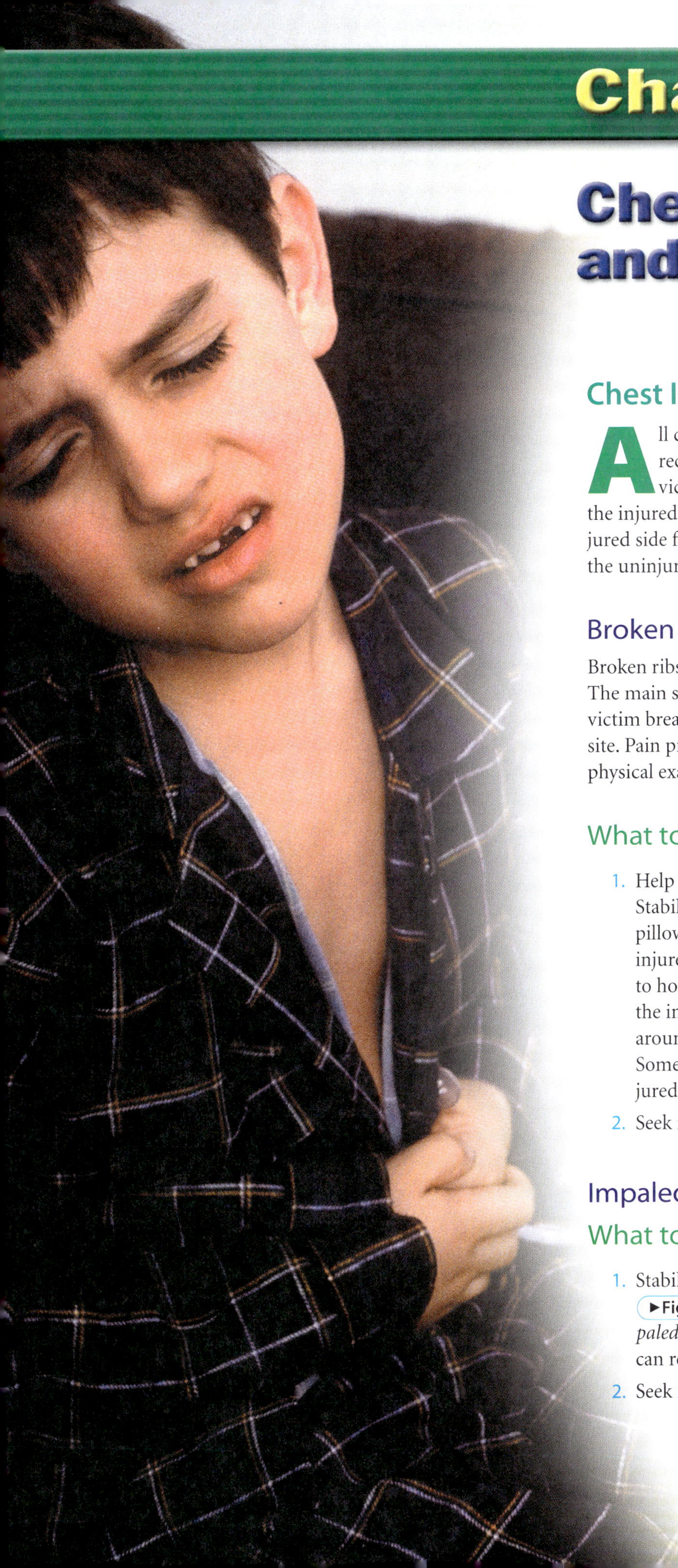

Chapter 9

Chest, Abdominal, and Pelvic Injuries

Chest Injuries

All chest injury victims should be checked and rechecked for ABCs. A responsive chest injury victim should usually sit up or be placed with the injured side down. This position protects the uninjured side from blood inside the chest cavity and allows the uninjured side to expand.

Broken Ribs

Broken ribs usually occur along the side of the chest. The main symptom of a broken rib is pain when the victim breathes, coughs, or moves and pain at the injured site. Pain produced when squeezing the chest during the physical exam is another indication of a broken rib.

What to Do

1. Help the victim find a comfortable position. Stabilize the ribs by having the victim hold a pillow or other similar soft object against the injured area ►Figure 1A and 1B. Or use bandages to hold the pillow in place or tie an arm over the injured area. Do not apply tight bandages around the chest because they restrict breathing. Some victims find comfort by lying on the injured side.
2. Seek medical attention.

Impaled Object in Chest

What to Do

1. Stabilize the object in place with bulky dressings ►Figure 2A and 2B. *Do not try to remove an impaled object*—bleeding and air in the chest cavity can result.
2. Seek medical attention.

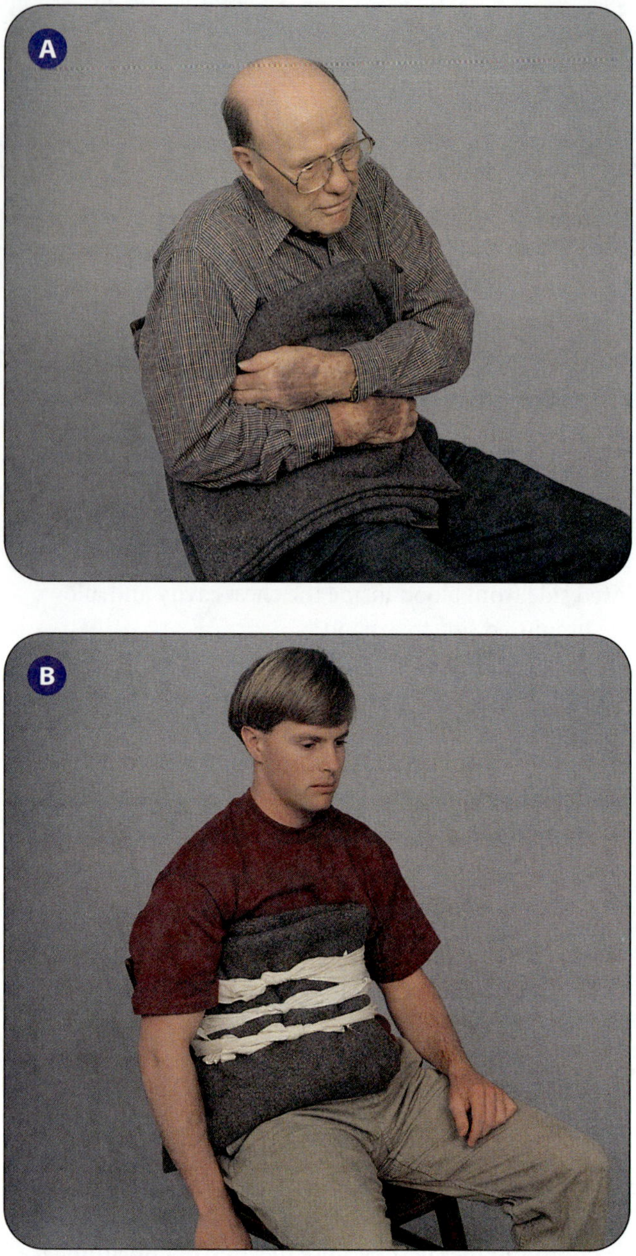

Figure 1, A–B Stabilize chest with soft object such as pillow, coat, or blanket (hold or tie).

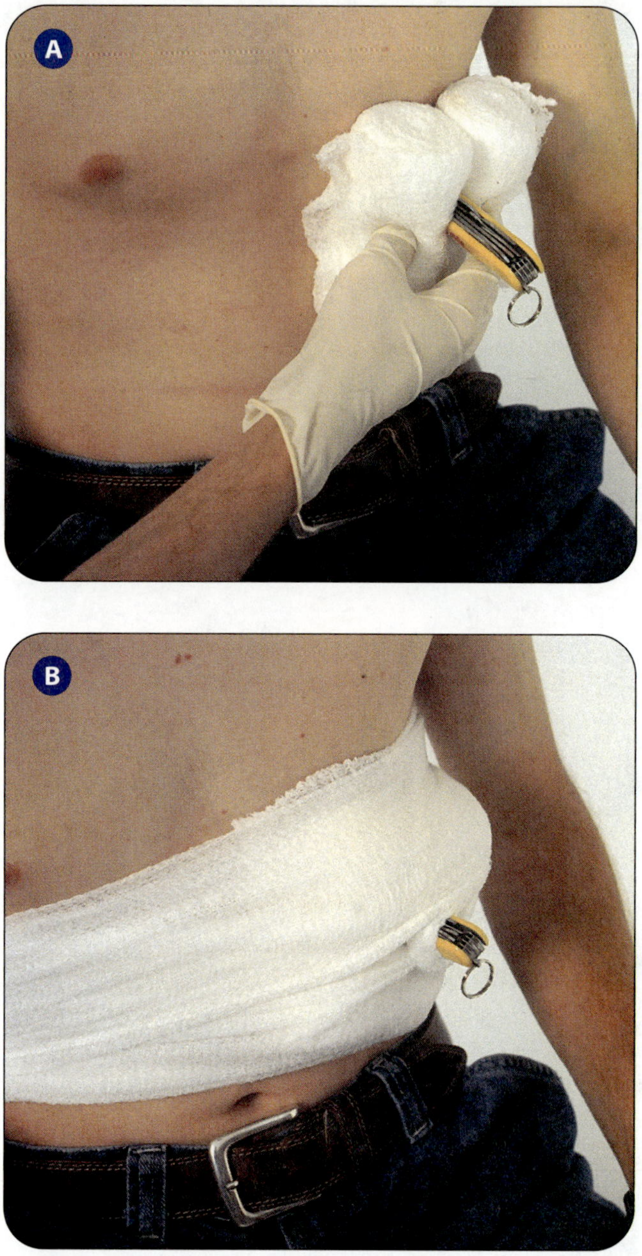

Figure 2, A–B **A.** Stabilize penetrating object with bulky padding. **B.** Secure padding and object.

Sucking Chest Wound

A sucking chest wound results when a chest wound allows air to pass into and out of the chest cavity with each breath.

What to Do

1. Have the victim take a breath and let it out; then seal the wound with anything available to stop air from entering the chest cavity. Plastic wrap or a plastic bag works well. Tape it in place but leave one corner untaped. This creates a flutter valve to prevent air from being trapped in the chest cavity. If plastic wrap is not available, you can use your gloved hand.
2. If the victim has trouble breathing or seems to be getting worse, remove the plastic cover (or your hand) to let air escape, then reapply.
3. Seek medical attention.

CHEST INJURIES

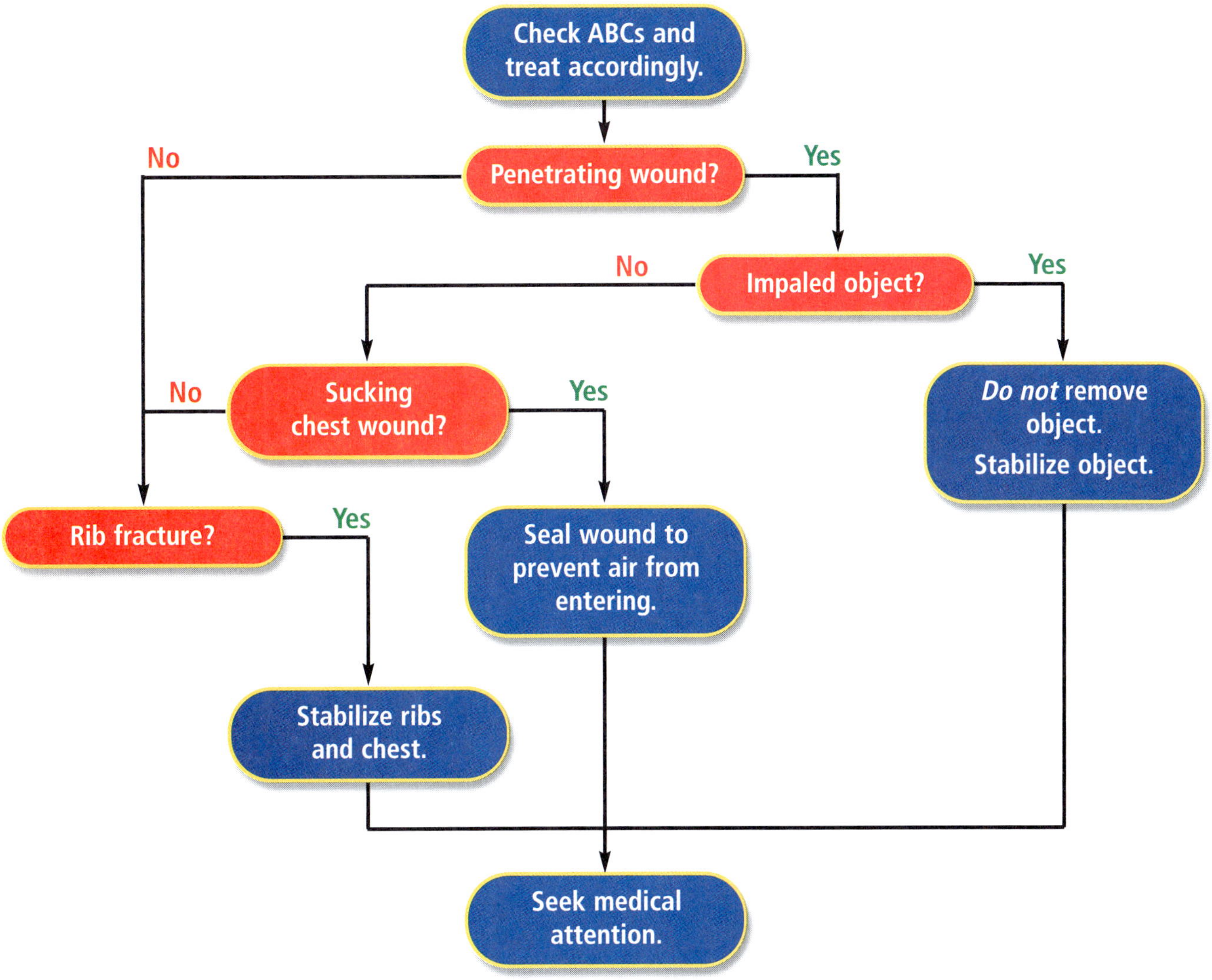

Abdominal Injuries

Blow to the Abdomen

Examine the abdomen by gently pressing different areas of the abdomen with your fingertips. Observe for pain, tenderness, muscle tightness, or rigidity. A normal abdomen is soft and not tender when pressed.

What to Do

1. Place the victim in a comfortable position and expect vomiting. Do not give the victim any food or drink. If you are hours from a medical facility, allow the victim to suck on a clean cloth soaked in water to relieve a dry mouth.
2. Seek medical attention.

Penetrating Wound

Expect internal organs to be damaged.

What to Do

1. If the penetrating object is still in place, stabilize the object and control bleeding by using bulky dressings around it. *Do not try to remove the object.*
2. Seek medical attention.

Protruding Organs

What to Do

Position the victim with head and shoulders slightly raised, and knees bent and raised.

1. Cover protruding organs with a moistened sterile dressing or clean cloth (▶Figure 3).
2. Place a towel lightly over the dressing to help maintain warmth
3. Seek medical attention.

Caution:

DO NOT try to reinsert protruding organs into the abdomen—you could introduce infection or damage the intestines.

DO NOT cover the organs tightly.

DO NOT cover the organs with any material that clings or disintegrates when wet.

DO NOT give anything to eat or drink.

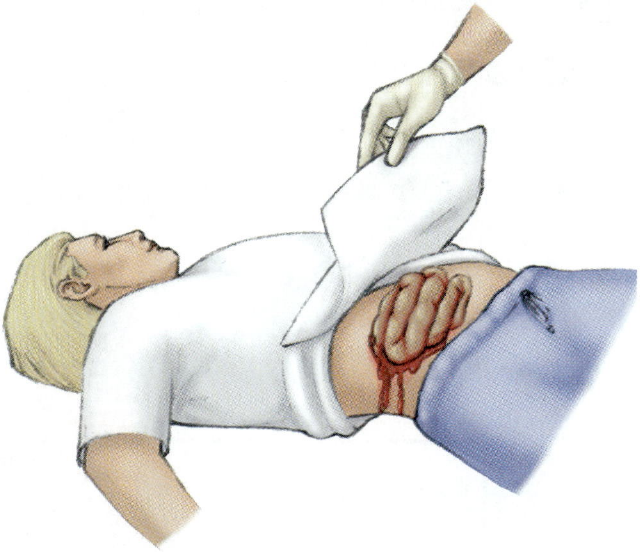

Figure 3 Do not reinsert protruding organs. Cover them with a moist, sterile dressing.

Pelvic Injuries

If you must move the victim, and you suspect a broken pelvis, gently press the sides of the pelvis downward and squeeze them inward at the iliac crests (upper points of the hips). A broken pelvis will be painful. Just like other injuries, if the victim is already complaining about pain, do not apply pressure.

What to Do

1. Treat the victim for shock.
2. Place padding between the victim's thighs, then tie the victim's knees and ankles together. If the knees are bent, place padding under them for support.
3. Keep the victim on a firm surface.
4. Seek medical attention.

Caution:

DO NOT roll the victim—additional internal damage could result.

DO NOT move the victim. Whenever possible, wait for the EMS ambulance, with its trained personnel and a backboard.

ABDOMINAL INJURIES

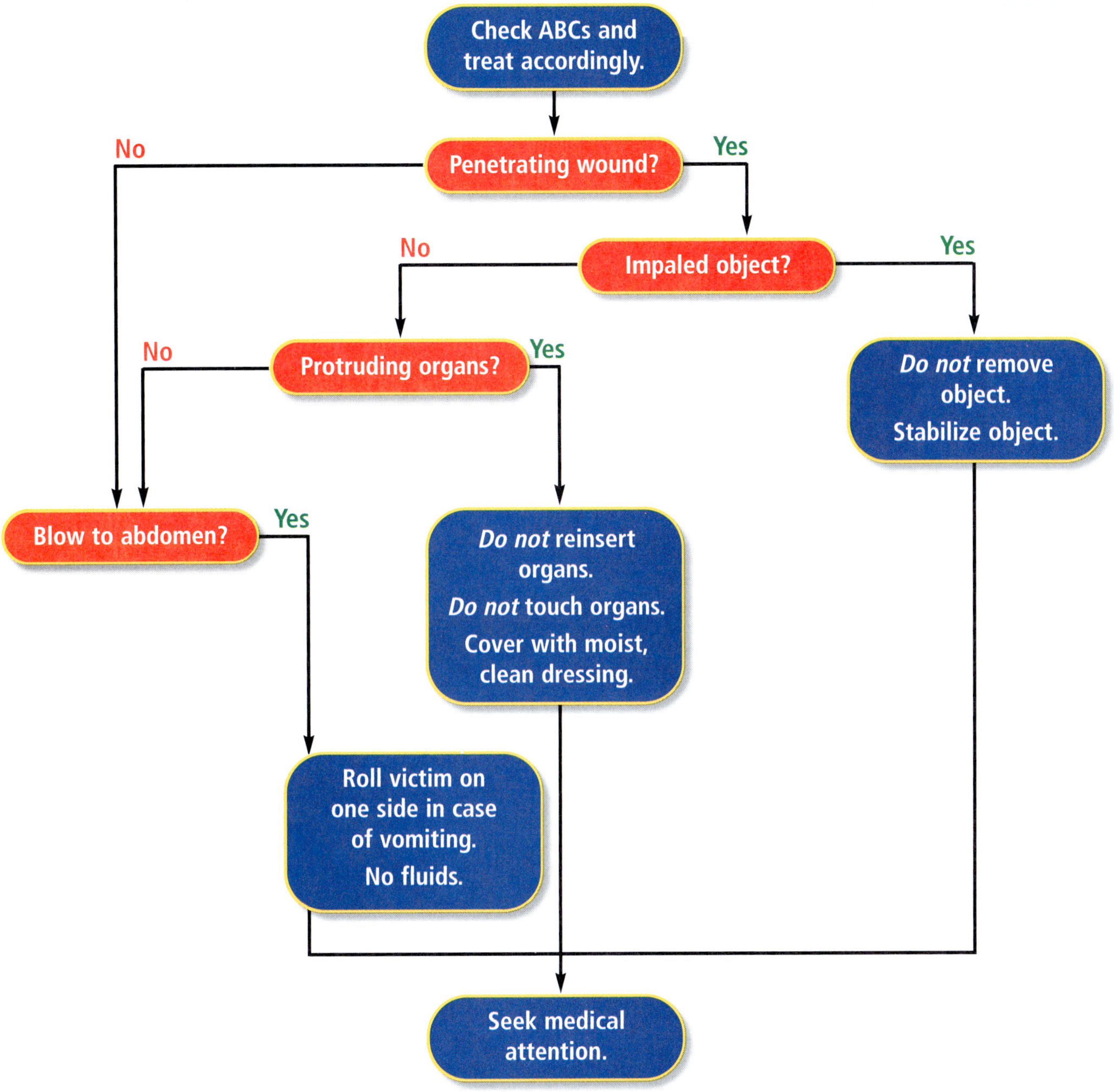

Learning Activities

Chest Injuries

Directions: Circle Yes if you agree with the statement, and circle No if you disagree.

Yes No **1.** Stabilize a broken rib by strapping (taping) a victim's chest as tightly as possible.

Yes No **2.** Stabilize an impaled (embedded) object in the chest with bulky padding to prevent it from moving.

Yes No **3.** Seal a chest wound that has air passing in and out of the chest.

Scenario: An iron rod broke and stuck into a construction worker's chest as he tied the rods for a concrete foundation. You are called over to help with the injured worker and you find that the iron rod has been removed. Air is passing into and out of the victim's chest with each breath he takes. What should you do?

____

____

____

Abdominal Injuries

Yes No **1.** Gently push protruding organs back through the abdominal wound.

Yes No **2.** The dressing covering exposed intestines should be kept dry.

Yes No **3.** Remove any penetrating object from the abdomen.

Yes No **4.** For a blow to the abdomen with suspected internal injuries, place the victim on his or her side.

Scenario: A 45-year-old repairman fell while carrying a replacement glass for a broken window. The new glass broke in several jagged pieces. You find him lying on his back with a blood-soaked shirt. You see a lacerated abdomen with several loops of bowel protruding through the laceration. What should you do?

____

____

____

Pelvic Injuries

Yes No **1.** Keep the victim on a firm surface.

Yes No **2.** Keep the victim's knees bent and place padding between the legs.

Scenario: An older secretary slipped while on stairs and fell down five steps. She is at the bottom of the stairs lying on her side. You suspect a pelvic fracture because she is complaining about severe pain in the pelvic area. What should you do?

____

____

____

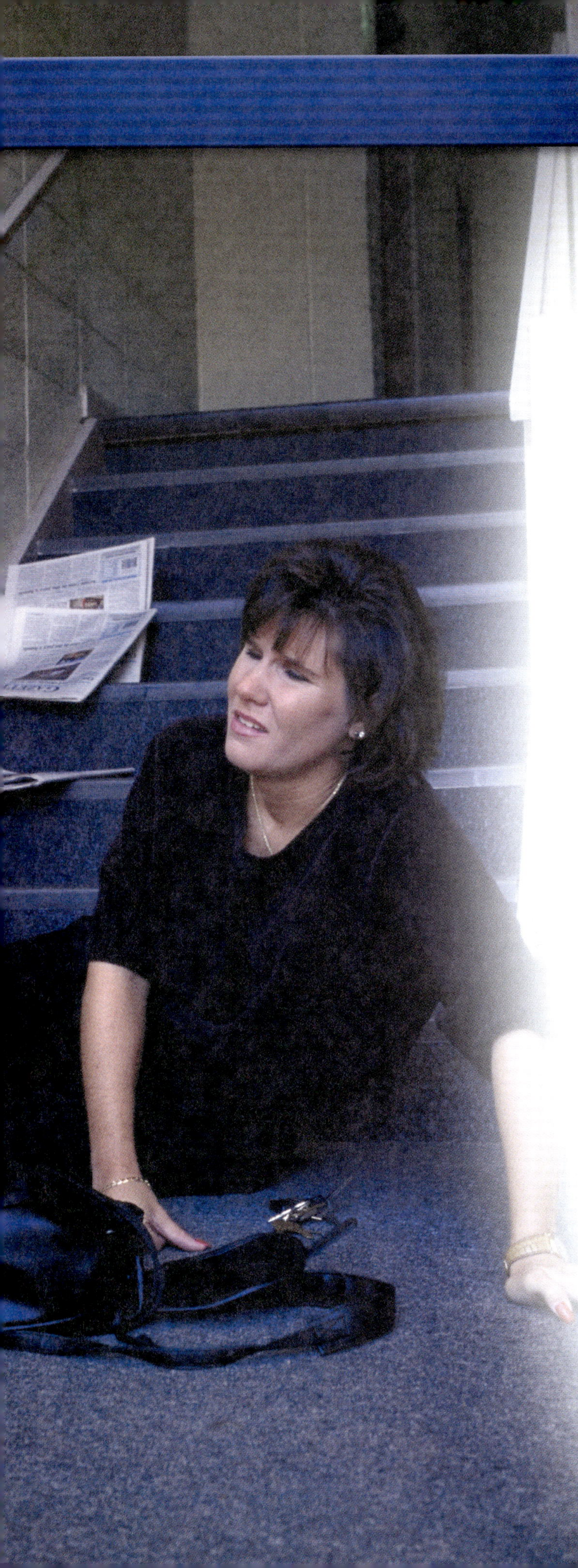

Chapter 10

Bone, Joint, and Muscle Injuries

Fractures

The terms "fracture" and "broken bone" have the same meaning: a break or crack in a bone. There are two categories of fractures ►Figure 1:

- Closed (simple) fracture ►Figures 2A and 2B. The skin is intact and no wound exists anywhere near the fracture site.
- Open (compound) fracture. The skin over the fracture has been damaged or broken ►Figure 3. The wound may result from bone protruding through the skin or by a direct blow that cuts the skin at the time of the fracture. The bone may not always be visible in the wound.

The real problems is not the broken bones themselves but the potential injury to the vital organs next to them.

What to Look For

It may be difficult to tell if a bone is fractured. When in doubt, treat the injury as a fracture. Use the mnemonic **D-O-T-S** (deformity, open wound, tenderness, swelling) found on page 15:

- *Deformity* might not be obvious. Compare the injured part with the uninjured part on the other side.
- *Open wound* may indicate an underlying fracture.
- *Tenderness* and pain are commonly found only at the injury site. Usually, the victim will be able to point to the site of the pain. A useful procedure for detecting a fracture is to gently feel along the bone; a victim's complaint about pain or tenderness serve as a reliable sign of a fracture.
- *Swelling* caused by bleeding happens rapidly after a fracture.

Additional signs and symptoms include:

- *Loss of use* may or may not occur. The victim may refuse to use the injured part if motion produces

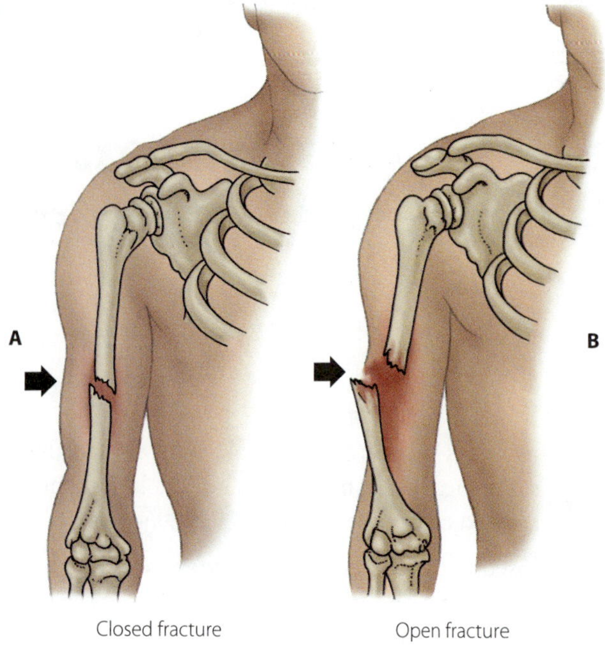

Figure 1 Fractures

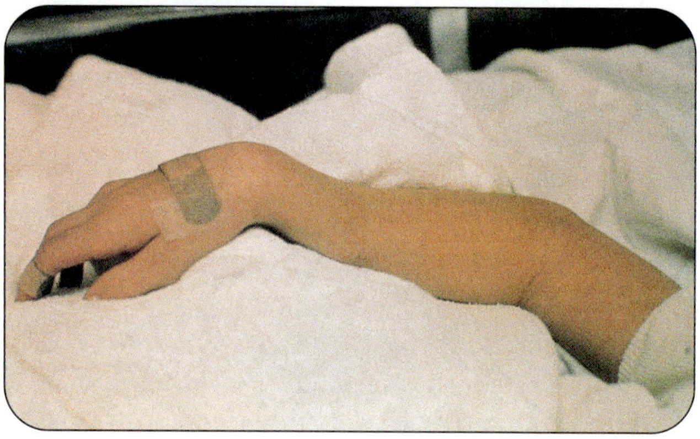

Figure 2A Forearm fracture

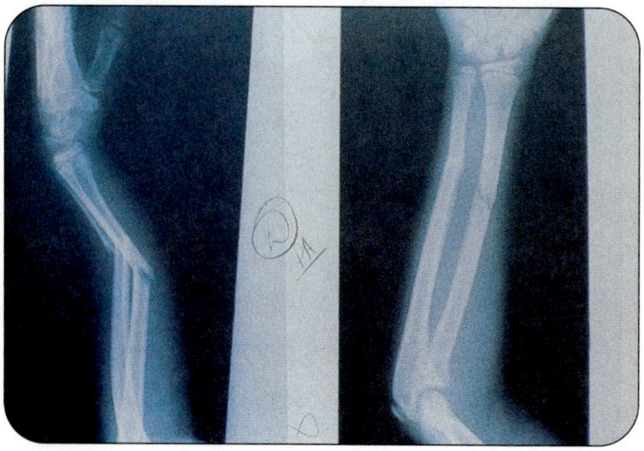

Figure 2B X-rays of victim with forearm fracture before and after setting

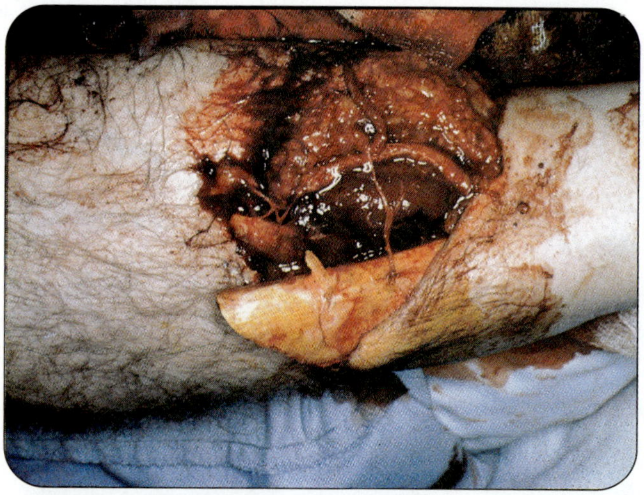

Figure 3 Open tibia, fibula fracture

pain. This is called "guarding." Sometimes, however, the victim is able to move a fractured limb with little or no pain.

- *A grating sensation* can be felt and sometimes even heard when the ends of the broken bone rub together. Do not move the injured limb in an attempt to detect it.
- *The history of the injury* can lead you to suspect a fracture whenever a serious accident has happened. The victim may have heard or felt the bone snap.

What to Do

1. Determine what happened and the location of the injury.
2. Gently remove clothing covering the injured area. Cut clothing at the seams if necessary.
3. Examine the area by looking and feeling for D-O-T-S).
   - Look at the injury site. Swelling and black-and-blue marks, which indicate that blood is escaping into the tissues, may come from either the bone end or associated muscular and blood vessel damage. Shortening or severe deformity (angulation) between the joints, deformity around the joints, shortening of the extremity, and rotation of the extremity when compared with the opposite extremity indicate a bone injury. Lacerations or even small puncture wounds near the site of a bone fracture are considered open fractures.
   - Feel the injured area. If a fracture is not obvious, gently press, touch, or feel along the length of the bone for deformities, tenderness, and swelling.

BONE INJURIES

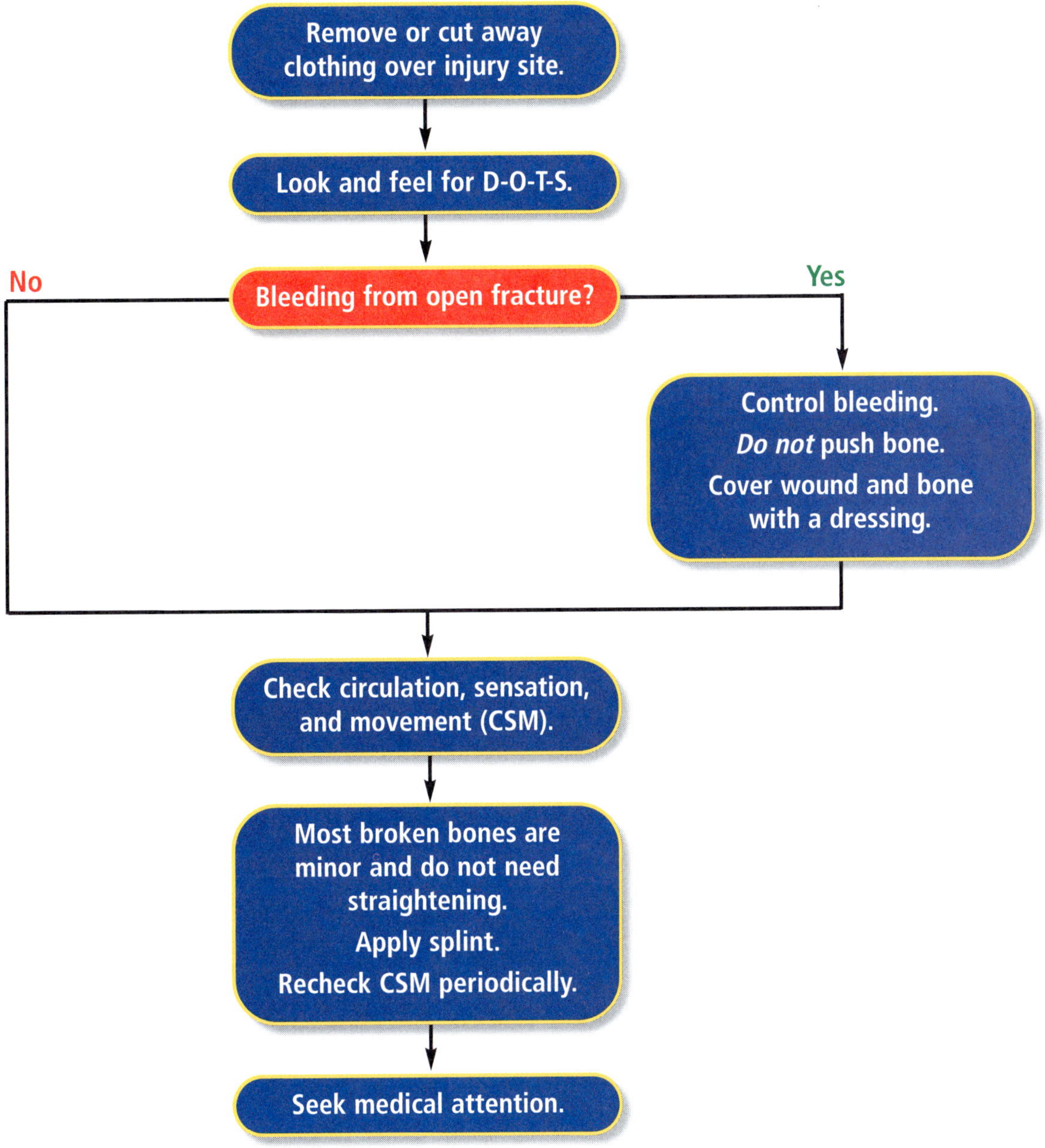

5. Check blood flow and nerves. Use the mnemonic CSM (circulation, sensation, movement) as a way of remembering what to do ▶Skill Scan.
    - *Circulation.* Feel for the radial pulse (located on the thumb side of the wrist) for an arm injury and the posterior tibial pulse (located between the inside ankle bone and the Achilles tendon) for a leg injury. A pulseless arm or leg is a significant emergency that requires immediate surgical care.
    - *Sensation.* This is the most useful sign. Lightly touch or squeeze the victim's toes or fingers and ask the victim what he or she feels. Loss of sensation is an early sign of nerve damage or spinal damage.
    - *Movement.* Inability to move develops later. Check for nerve damage by asking the victim to wiggle his or her toes or fingers. If the toes or fingers are injured, do not have the victim attempt to move them.

The major blood vessels of an extremity tend to run close to the bone. Any time a bone is broken, the adjacent blood vessels are at risk of being torn by bone fragments or pinched off between the ends of the broken bone. The tissues of the arms and legs cannot survive without a continuing blood supply for more than two or three hours. In that case seek immediate medical attention.

6. Use the RICE (rest-ice-compression-elevation) procedures (see page 75).
7. Use a splint to stabilize the fracture (see Chapter 11).
8. Seek medical attention.

Joint Injuries

Dislocations

A dislocation occurs when a joint comes apart and stays apart with the bone ends no longer in contact. The shoulders, elbows, fingers, hips, kneecaps, and ankles are the joints most frequently affected. Dislocations cause signs and symptoms similar to those of a fracture: deformity, severe pain, swelling, and the inability of the victim to move the injured joint. The main sign of a dislocation is deformity. A dislocated joint will definitely look different from an uninjured joint.

What to Do

1. Check the CSM (circulation, sensation, movement). If the end of the dislocated bone is pressing on nerves or blood vessels, numbness or paralysis may exist below the dislocation. Always check the pulses. If there is no pulse in the injured extremity, transport the victim to a medical facility immediately.
2. Use the RICE (rest, ice, compression, elevation) procedures.
3. Use a splint to stabilize the joint in the position in which it was found (see Chapter 11).
4. Do not try to reduce the joint (put the displaced parts back into their normal positions), because nerve and blood vessel damage could result.
5. Seek medical attention to reduce the dislocation.

Sprains

A sprain is an injury to a joint in which the ligaments and other tissues are damaged by violent stretching or twisting. Attempts to move or use the joint increase the pain. The skin around the joint may be discolored because of bleeding from torn tissues. It often is difficult to distinguish between a severe sprain and a fracture, because their signs and symptoms are similar.

Treatment consists of rest, ice, compression, and elevation (RICE). It is vitally important to keep a joint from swelling by applying cold promptly; it is even more important to make the swelling recede as quickly as possible with a compression (elastic) bandage.

Muscle Injuries

Strains

A muscle strain, also known as a "pulled muscle," occurs when a muscle is stretched beyond its normal range of motion, and tears.

What to Look For

Any of the following signs and symptoms may indicate a muscle strain:

- sharp pain
- extreme tenderness when the area is touched
- cavity, indentation, or bump that can be felt or seen
- severe weakness and loss of function of the injured part
- stiffness and pain when the victim moves the muscle

What to Do

Use the RICE procedures.

Skill Scan Checking an Extremity's CSM

Check an Upper Extremity For:

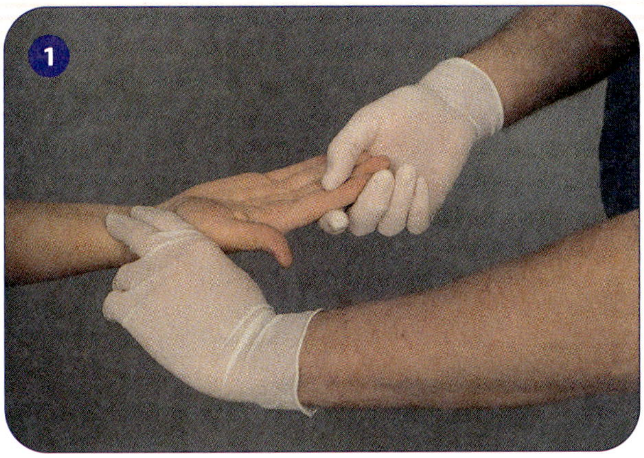

1. **C**irculation—radial pulse.

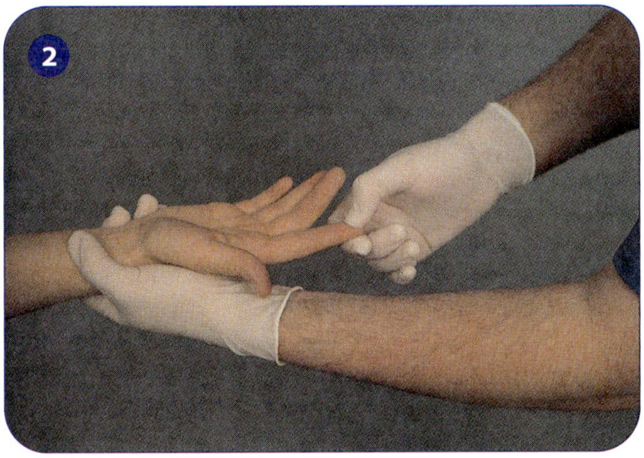

2. **S**ensation—squeeze fingers.

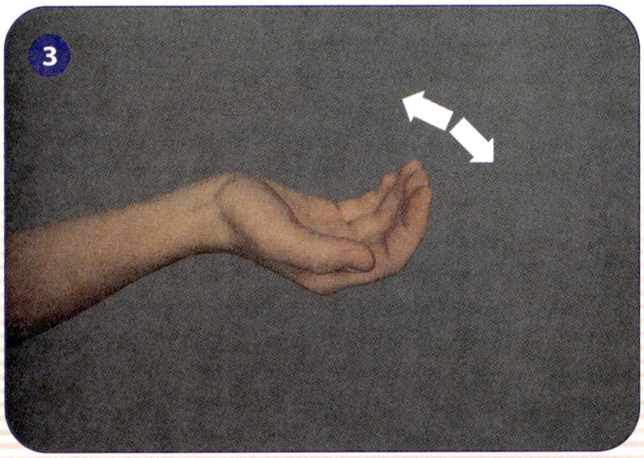

3. **M**ovement—wiggle fingers.

Check a Lower Extremity For:

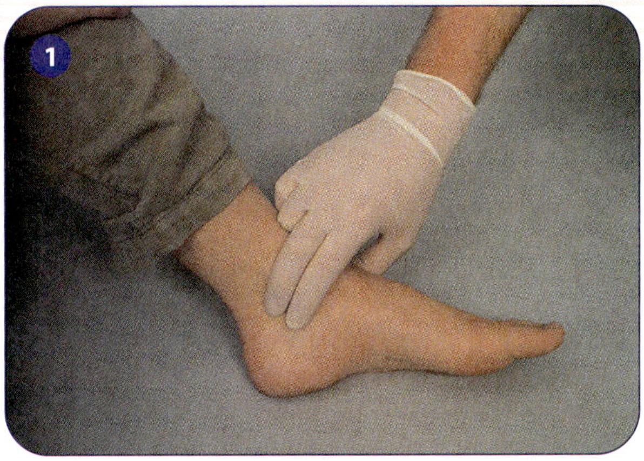

1. **C**irculation—posterial tibial pulse.

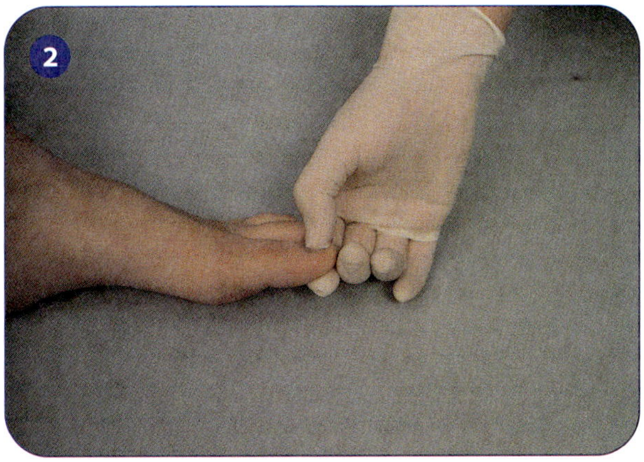

2. **S**ensation—squeeze toe.

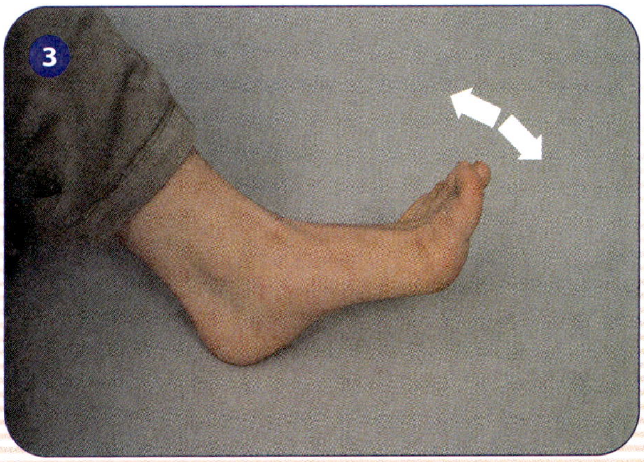

3. **M**ovement—wiggle toes.

SPRAINS, STRAINS, CONTUSIONS, DISLOCATIONS

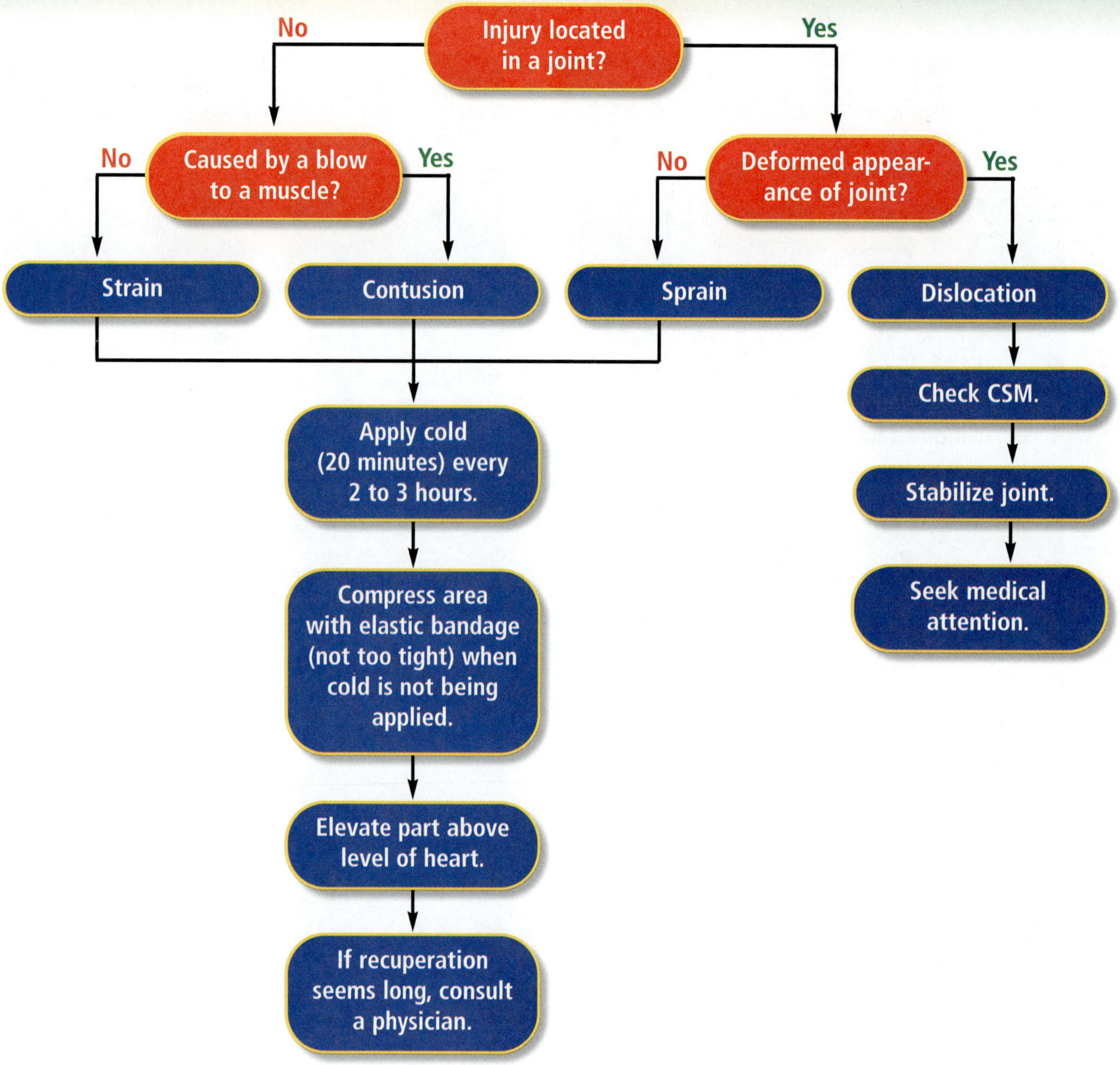

Contusions

A muscle contusion or bruise results from a blow to the muscle.

What to Look For

Any of the following signs and symptoms may occur in a muscle contusion:

- swelling
- pain and tenderness
- black-and-blue mark appearing hours later

What to Do

Use the RICE procedures.

Cramps

A cramp occurs when a muscle goes into an uncontrolled spasm and contraction, resulting in severe pain and restriction or loss of movement.

What to Do

There are many treatments for cramps. Try one or more of the following:

1. Have the victim gently stretch the affected muscle. Because a muscle cramp is an uncontrolled muscle contraction or spasm, a gradual lengthening of the muscle may help lengthen the muscle fibers and relieve the cramp.
2. Relax the muscle by applying pressure to it.
3. Apply ice to the cramped muscle to make it relax, unless you are in a cold environment.
4. Pinch the upper lip hard (an acupressure technique) to reduce calf-muscle cramping.
5. Drink lightly salted cool water (dissolve $\frac{1}{4}$ teaspoon salt in a quart of water) or a commercial sports drink.

Caution:

DO NOT give salt tablets to a person with muscle cramps. They can cause stomach irritation, nausea, and vomiting.

DO NOT massage or rub the affected muscle. This only causes more pain and does not relieve the cramping.

RICE Procedure for Bone, Joint, and Muscle Injuries

RICE is the acronym for the first aid procedures—rest, ice, compression, elevation—for bone, joint, and muscle injuries. The steps you take in the first 48 to 72 hours after such an injury can help to relieve, and even prevent, aches and pains. **Treat all extremity bone, joint, and muscle injuries with the RICE procedures. In addition to RICE, fractures and dislocations should be splinted to stabilize the injured area. (See Chapter 12 for splinting techniques.)**

R = Rest

Injuries heal faster if rested. Rest means the victim stays off the injured part. Using any part of the body increases the blood circulation to that area, which can cause more swelling of an injured part. Crutches may be used to rest leg injuries.

I = Ice

An ice pack should be applied to the injured area for 20 to 30 minutes every two or three hours during the first 24 to 48 hours. Skin treated with cold passes through four stages: cold, burning, aching, and numbness. When the skin becomes numb, usually in 20 to 30 minutes, remove the ice pack. After removing the ice pack, compress the injured part with an elastic bandage and keep it elevated (the "C" and "E" of RICE).

Cold constricts the blood vessels to and in the injured area, which helps reduce the swelling and inflammation as it dulls the pain and relieves muscle spasms. Cold should be applied as soon as possible after the injury—healing time often is directly related to the amount of swelling that occurs. Heat has the opposite effect when applied to fresh injuries: it increases circulation to the area and greatly increases both the swelling and the pain.

Use either of the following methods to apply cold to an injury:

- Put crushed ice (or cubes) into a double plastic bag, hot water bottle. Place the ice pack on the skin and then use an elastic bandage to hold the ice pack in place. Ice bags can conform to the body's contours.
- Use a chemical cold pack, a sealed pouch that contains two chemical envelopes. Squeezing the pack mixes the chemicals, producing a chemical reaction

Skill Scan RICE Procedures for an Ankle

1

R = Rest

Stop using the injured part. Continued use could cause further injury, delay healing, increase pain, and stimulate bleeding. Get the victim into a comfortable position, either sitting or lying down. This slows blood flow to the injured area.

1. R = Rest

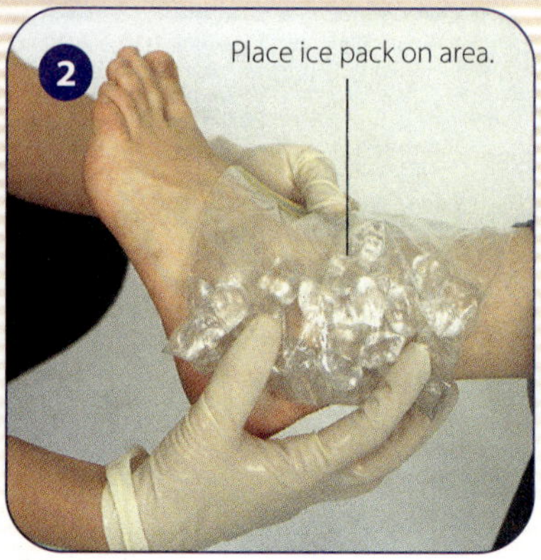

2. I = Ice

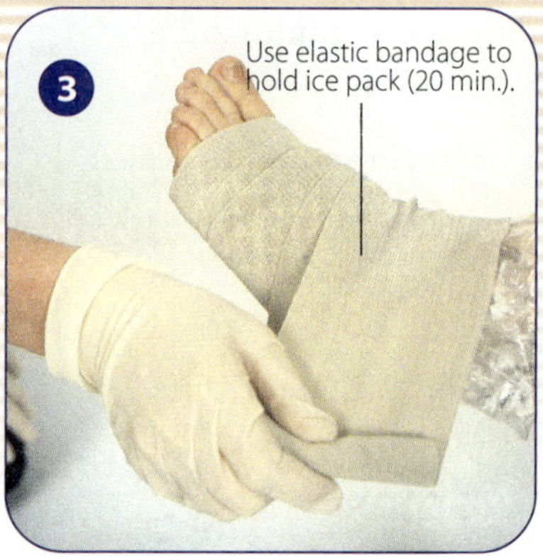

3. I = Ice

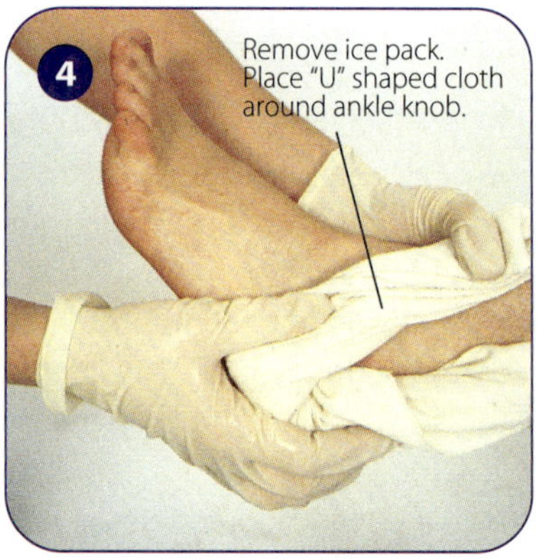

4. C = Compression

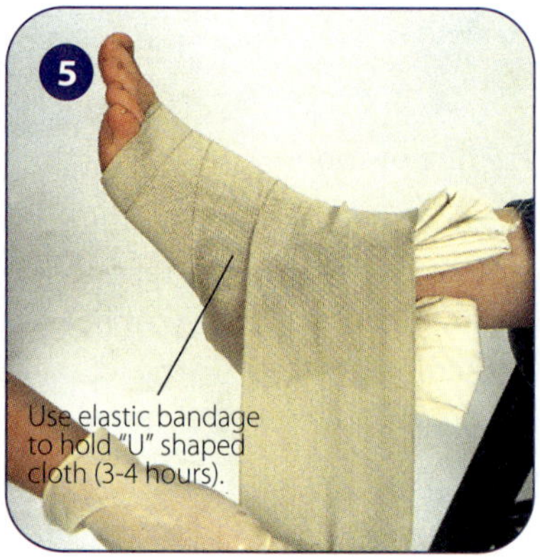

5. C = Compression

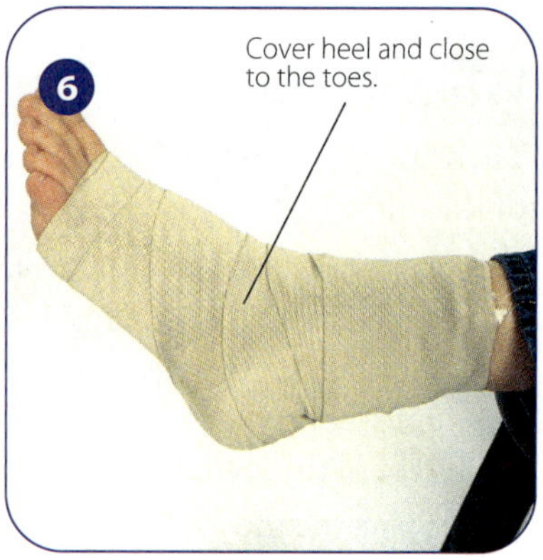

6. C = Compression

7

E = Elevation

Elevating the injured part is another way to decrease swelling and pain. As you apply ice or compression, elevate the part in a convenient manner. The aim of this step is to get the injured part higher than the heart, if possible.

7. E = Elevation

Repeat cycles of:

- ice pack for 20 minutes followed by
- compression for 3–4 hours for 24 to 48 hours (if severe, 72 hours)

that has a cooling effect. Although they do not cool as well as other methods, they are convenient to use when ice is not readily available. They lose their cooling power quickly, however, and can be used only once. Also, they may be impractical because they are expensive and can break.

Caution:

DO NOT apply an ice pack for more than 20 to 30 minutes at a time. Frostbite or nerve damage can result.

DO NOT apply cold if the victim has a history of circulatory disease, Raynaud's syndrome (spasms in the arteries of the extremities that reduce circulation), abnormal sensitivity to cold, or if the injured part has been frostbitten previously.

DO NOT stop using an ice pack too soon. A common mistake is the early use of heat, which will result in swelling and pain. Use an ice pack three to four times a day for the first 24 hours, preferably up to 48 hours, before applying any heat. For severe injuries, using ice for up to 72 hours is recommended.

C = Compression

Compressing the injured area may squeeze some fluid and debris out of the injury site. Compression limits the ability of the skin and of other tissues to expand and reduces internal bleeding. Apply an elastic bandage to the injured area, especially the foot, ankle, knee, thigh, hand, or elbow. Fill the hollow areas with padding such as a sock or washcloth before applying the elastic bandage.

Elastic bandages come in various sizes, for different body areas:

- 2-inch width, used for the wrist and hand
- 3-inch width, used for the ankle, elbow and arm
- 4- or 6-inch width, used for the ankle, knee, and leg

Start the elastic bandage several inches below the injury and wrap in an upward, overlapping (about one-half the bandage's width) spiral, starting with an even, slightly tight pressure. Gradually wrap more loosely above the injury. Stretch a new elastic bandage to about one third its maximum length for adequate compression. Leave fingers and toes exposed so possible color change can be easily observed. Compare the toes or fingers of the injured extremity with the uninjured one. Pale skin, pain, numbness, and tingling are signs that the bandage is too tight. If any of these symptoms appears, immediately remove the elastic bandage. Leave the elastic bandage off until all the symptoms disappear, then rewrap the area, less tightly. Always wrap from below the injury and move toward the heart.

Applying compression may be the most important step in preventing swelling. The victim should wear the elastic bandage continuously for the first 18 to 24 hours (except when cold is being applied). At night, have the victim loosen but not remove the elastic bandage.

For an ankle injury, place a horseshoe-shaped pad around the ankle knob and secure with the elastic bandage. The pad will help compress the soft tissues rather than just the bones. Wrap the bandage tightest nearest the toes and loosest above the ankle. It should be tight enough to decrease swelling but not tight enough to inhibit blood flow.

For a contusion or a strain, place a pad between the injury and the elastic bandage.

E = Elevation

Gravity slows the return of blood to the heart from the lower parts of the body. Once fluids get to the hands or feet, they have nowhere else to go and those parts of the body swell. Elevating the injured area, in combination with ice and compression, limits circulation to that area, helps limit internal bleeding, and minimize swelling.

It is simple to prop up an injured leg or arm to limit bleeding. Whenever possible, elevate the injured part above the level of the heart for the first 24 hours after an injury. If a fracture is suspected, do not elevate an extremity until it has been stabilized with a splint. Even then, some fractures should not be elevated.

Along with RICE, fractures and dislocations should be splinted. Chapter 11 describes splinting techniques for various parts of the body.

Caution:

DO NOT apply an elastic bandage too tightly. If applied too tightly, elastic bandages will restrict circulation.

ANKLE INJURIES

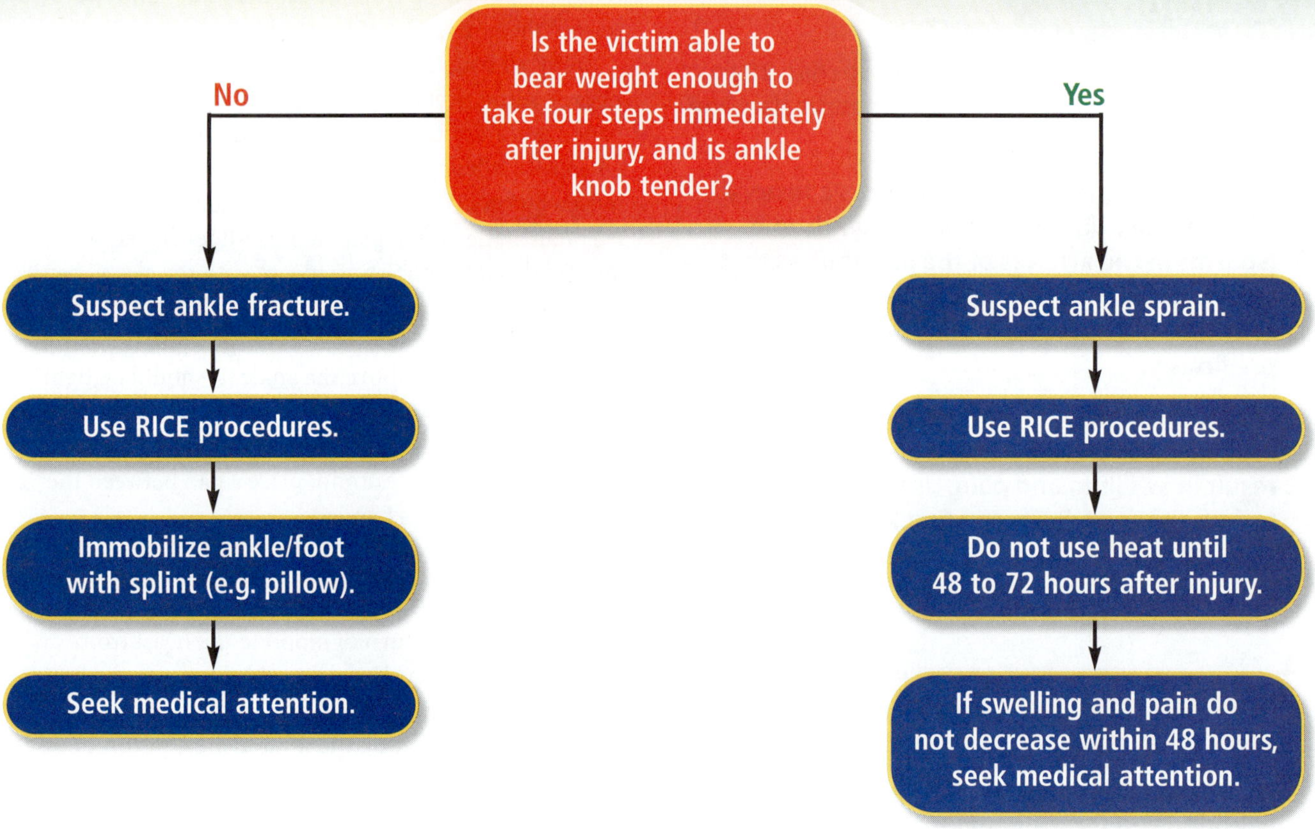

Blood under a Nail

When a fingernail has been crushed, blood collects under the nail. This condition usually is very painful because of the pressure of the blood pressing against the nail ▼Figure 4.

What to Do

1. Immerse the finger in ice water or apply an ice pack with the hand elevated.
2. By using one of the following methods, relieve the pressure under the injured nail:
   - Straighten the end of a metal (noncoated) paper clip or use the blunt (eye) end of a sewing needle. Hold the paper clip or needle with pliers and use a match or cigarette lighter to heat it until the metal is red hot. Press the glowing end of the paper clip or needle against the nail until it melts through. Little pressure is needed. The nail has no nerves, so this is a painless procedure ▶Figure 5.
   - Using a rotary action, drill through the nail with the sharp point of a knife.

Figure 4 Relieve pain by releasing blood under a nail.

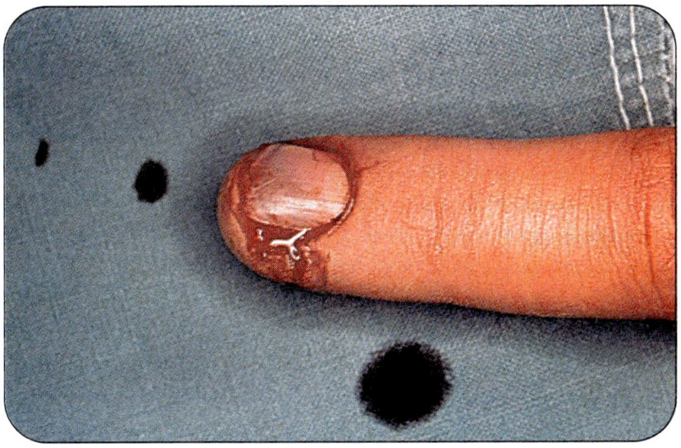

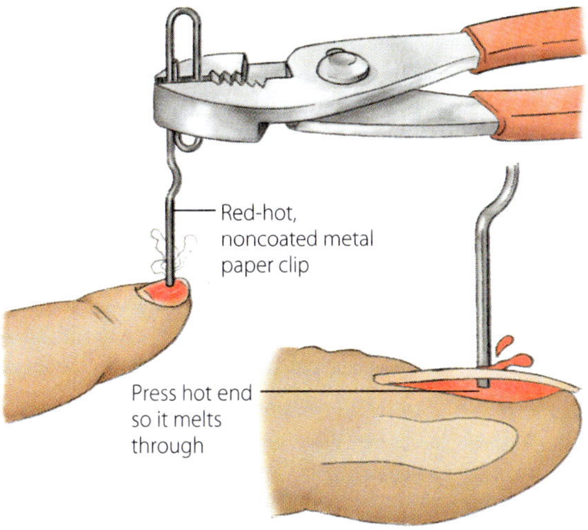

Figure 5 Making a hole in a fingernail

3. Apply a dressing to absorb the draining blood and to protect the injured nail.

Ring Strangulation

Sometimes a finger is so swollen that a ring cannot be removed. Ring strangulation can be a serious problem if it cuts off circulation long enough. Try one or more of the following methods to remove a ring:

- Lubricate the finger with grease, oil, butter, petroleum jelly, or some other slippery substance, and then try to remove the ring.
- Immerse the finger in cold water or apply an ice pack for several minutes to reduce the swelling.
- Massage the finger from the tip to the hand to move the swelling; lubricate the finger again and try removing the ring.
- Call 9-1-1 or your local emergency number. They can use a ring-cutter to remove the ring when all else fails.

Learning Activities

Fractures

Directions: Circle Yes if you agree with the statement, and circle No if you disagree.

Yes No **1.** For a suspected arm or leg fracture, check blood flow and nerves.

Yes No **2.** Apply cold on a suspected fracture.

Yes No **3.** A splint can help stabilize (keep in place) a fracture.

Scenario: While changing a light bulb in a high ceiling lighting fixture, an electrician falls off a 10-foot ladder. The victim complains about a pain in his left leg. You check the left leg and find some deformity, tenderness, and swelling. What should you do?

Dislocations and Sprains

Yes No **1.** The letters RICE represent the treatment for sprains and dislocations.

Yes No **2.** When using ice, place it directly on the skin.

Yes No **3.** Applying heat too soon to the injury is a common mistake.

Yes No **4.** An elastic bandage, if used correctly, can help control swelling in a joint.

Scenario: Your husband comes home limping and in pain. He says he twisted his ankle at work. One of his co-workers told him that it was best to "walk it out." What should you do?

Muscle Injuries

Yes No **1.** Give salt tablets to a person suffering muscle cramps.

Yes No **2.** Apply heat initially to a muscle injury.

Yes No **3.** An elastic bandage, if used correctly, can help limit swelling.

Scenario: During a company softball game, a batter loses her grip while swinging at a pitch. The bat flies through the air and hits a nearby player hard on the thigh. Although the skin is not broken, there is tenderness and some swelling. What should you do?

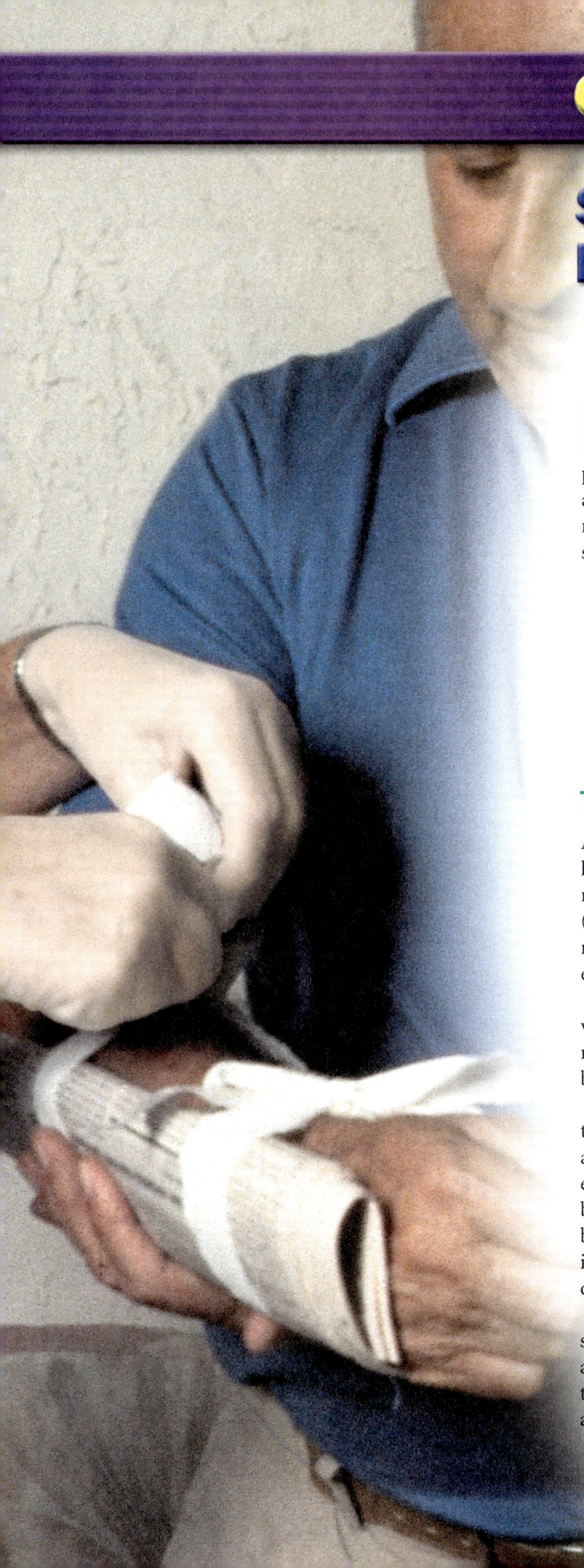

Chapter 11

Splinting Extremities

Most extremity fractures are minor. Because medical help is usually nearby, the injury can be stabilized by splinting the extremity in the position in which it was found. To stabilize means to use any method to hold a body part still and prevent movement. Before a victim is moved, all fractures should be stabilized to:

- reduce pain
- prevent damage to muscle, nerves, and blood vessels
- prevent a closed fracture from becoming an open fracture
- reduce bleeding and swelling

Types of Splints

A splint is any device used to stabilize a fracture or a dislocation. Such a device can be improvised from a folded newspaper, for example, or it can be a commercial splints (eg, SAM Splint™). Lack of a commercial splint should never prevent you from properly stabilizing an injured extremity ▶Skill Scans.

Splinting sometimes requires improvisation. Improvised splints can be made from folded newspapers, magzines, heavy cardboard, wood, pillow, folded blanket, baseball bat, or an umbrella.

A rigid splint is an inflexible device attached to an extremity to maintain stability. It may be a padded board, a piece of heavy cardboard, or a SAM Splint™ to fit the extremity. Whatever its construction, a rigid splint must be long enough so that it can be secured well above and below the fracture site. A soft splint, such as an air splint, is useful mainly for stabilizing fractures of the lower leg or the forearm.

A self, or anatomic, splint is almost always available. A self splint is one in which the injured body part is tied to an uninjured part. For example, an injured finger can be tied to an adjacent finger, the legs can be tied together, an injured arm can be tied to the chest.

Splinting Guidelines

All fractures and dislocations should be stabilized before the victim is moved. When in doubt, apply a splint.

Caution:

DO NOT straighten dislocations or fractures of the spine, elbow, wrist, hip, or knee because of the proximity of major nerves and arteries. Instead, if the CSM (circulation-sensation-movement) is all right, splint joint injuries in the position found.

What to Do

1. Cover all open wounds, if any, with a dry, sterile dressing before applying a splint.
2. Check CSM in the extremity. If the pulses are absent, and medical help is hours away, try to straighten a mid-shaft fracture or dislocations of the shoulder or knee cap to restore blood flow.
3. As a general rule, a splint should extend to stabilize the joints above and below the area of the broken bone. For example, stabilize the wrist and elbow for a fractured radius or ulna (bone in the lower arm); stabilize both shoulder and elbow for a fractured humerus (upper arm bone); stabilize both knee and ankle for a fractured tibia or fibula (lower leg bones). An upper extremity fracture, in addition to being splinted, should be placed in an arm sling and a swathe (binder).
4. If two first aiders are present, one should support the injury site and minimize movement of the extremity until splinting is completed.
5. When possible, place splint materials on both sides of the injured part, especially when two bones are involved such as the lower arm's radius and ulna or the lower leg's tibia and fibula. This "sandwich splint" prevents the injured extremity from rotating and keeps the two bones from touching. With rigid splints, use extra padding in natural body hollows and around any deformities.
6. Apply splints firmly but not so tightly that blood flow into an extremity is affected. Check CSM before and after the splint is applied. If the pulse disappears, loosen the splint enough so you can feel the pulse. Leave the fingers or toes exposed so CSM can be checked easily.
7. Use RICE on the injured part. When practical, elevating the injured extremity after stabilization promotes gravity-induced drainage from the limb and reduces swelling. *Do not, however, apply ice packs if a pulse is absent.*

Most fractures do not require rapid transportation. An exception is an arm or a leg without a pulse, which means there is insufficient blood flow to that extremity. In that case, *immediate* medical attention is necessary.

Skill Scan Splinting—Upper Extremities

Arm Sling: Shoulder and Clavicle Injuries

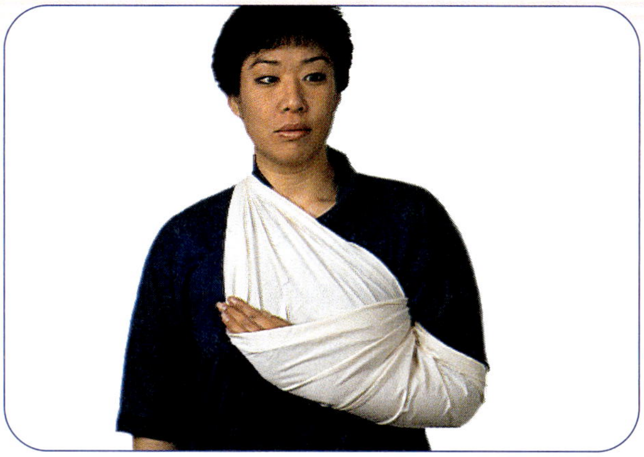

Upper Arm (Humerus)

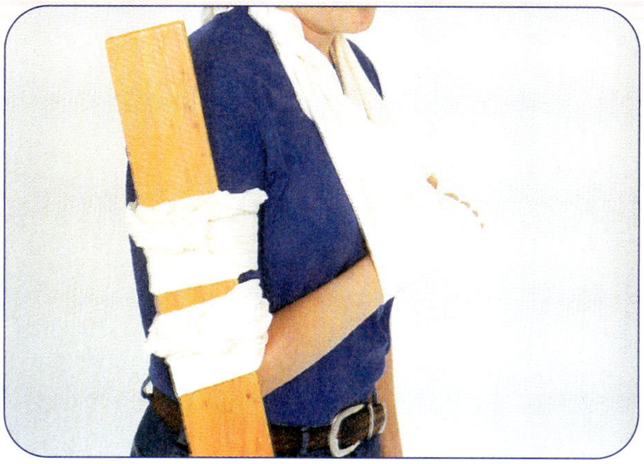

Arm Sling and Swathe for Upper Extremity Injuries

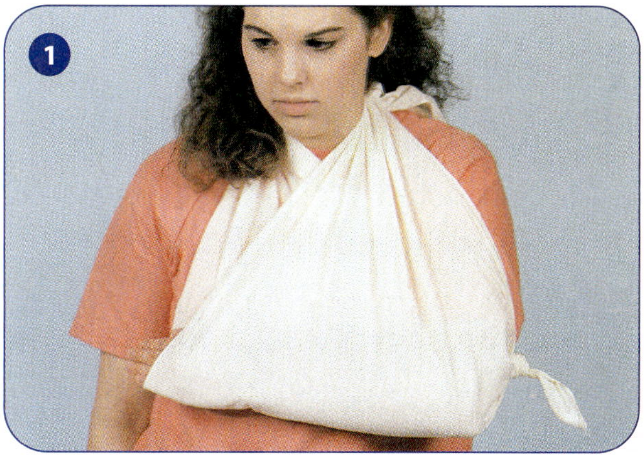

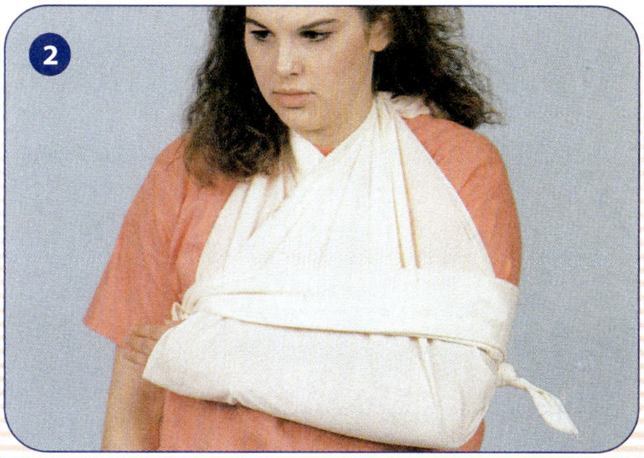

Forearm (Radius/Ulna)

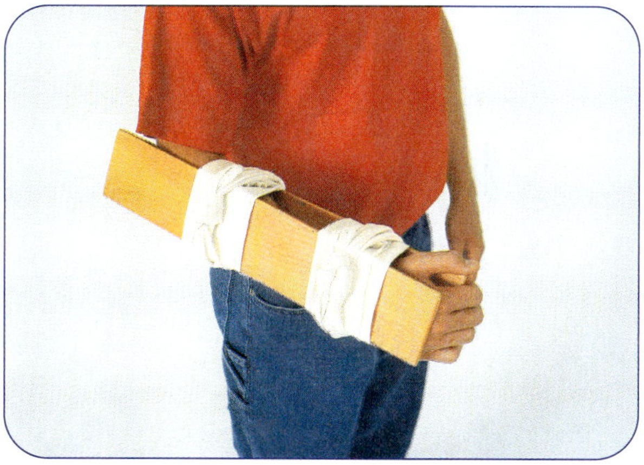

Fingers and Hand (Position of Function)

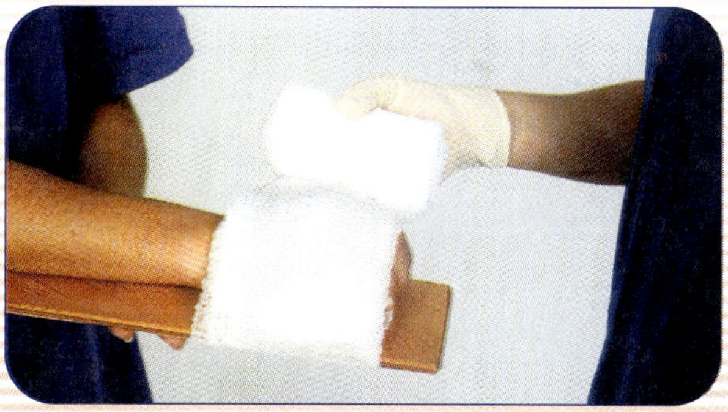

Skill Scan Splinting—Elbow and Knee

Elbow in Bent Position

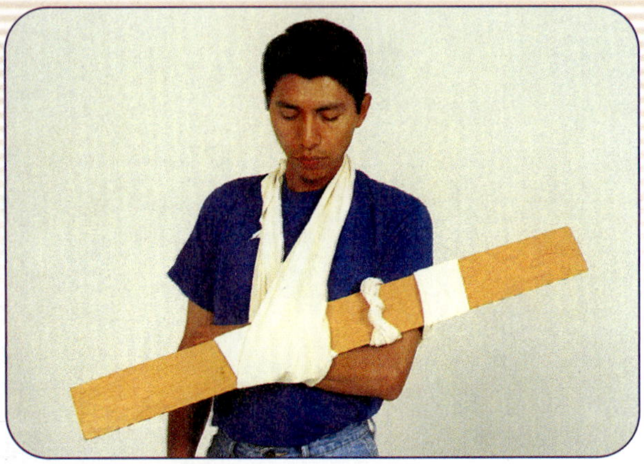

Knee in Bent Position

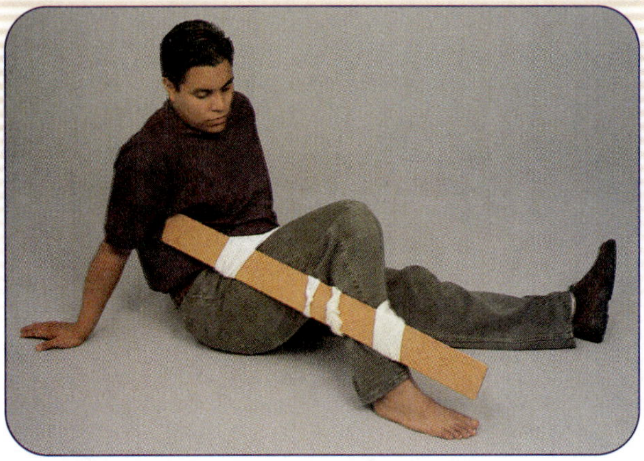

Elbow in Straight Position

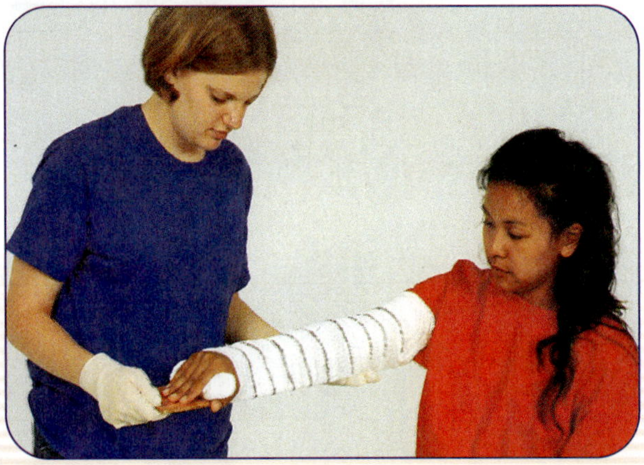

Knee in Straight Position

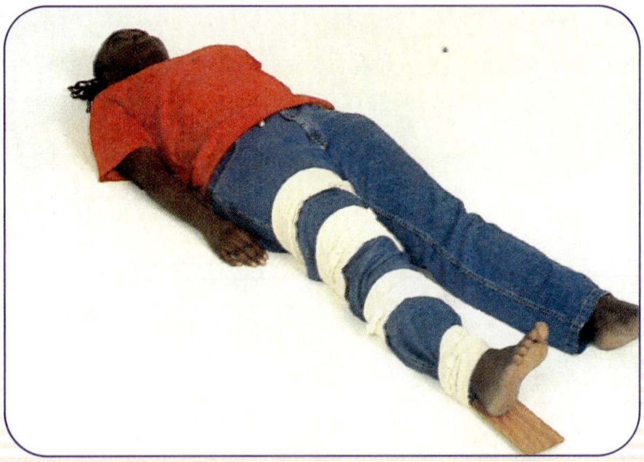

Skill Scan Splinting—Lower Extremities

Lower Leg (Tibia/Fibula)—Rigid Splint

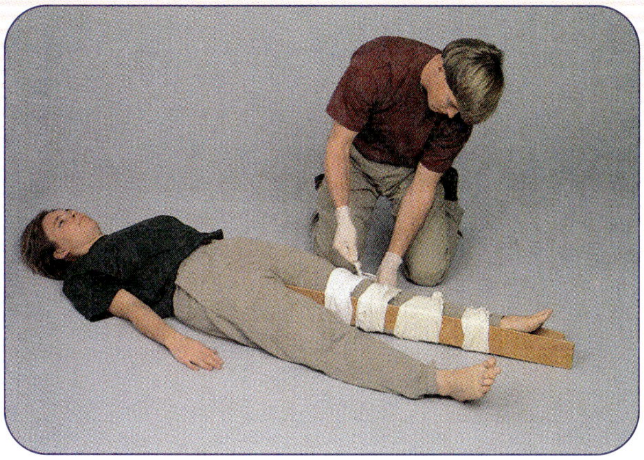

Thigh (Femur)—Rigid Splint

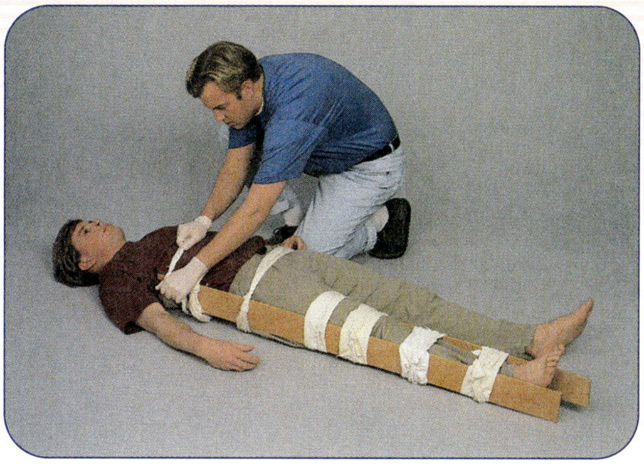

Soft Splint: Ankle/Foot

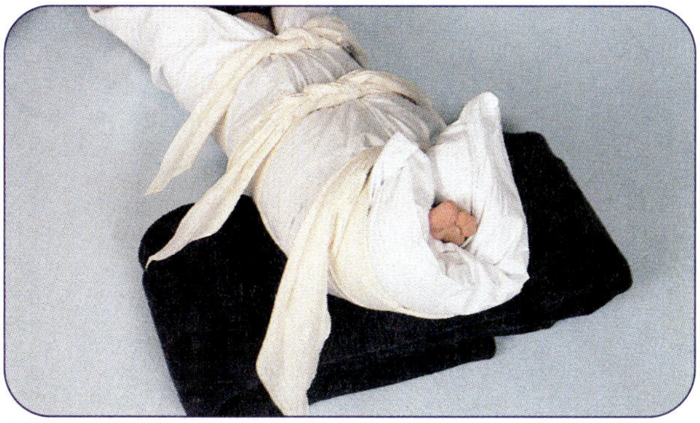

Self-Splint: Leg

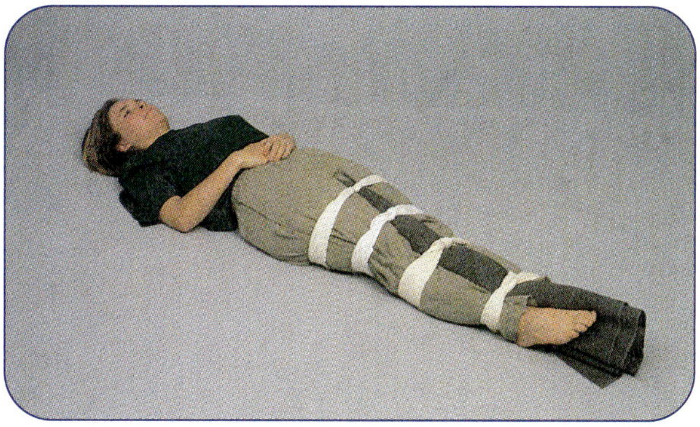

Self-Splint: Fingers/Toes

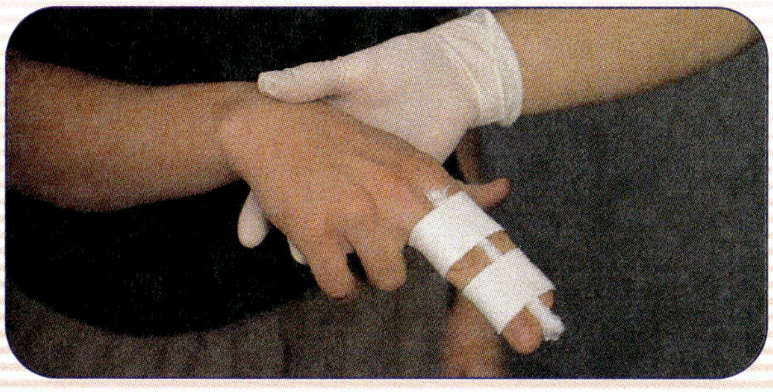

Learning Activities

Splinting the Extremities

Directions: Circle Yes if you agree with the statement, and circle No if you disagree.

Yes No **1.** A splint is a device that can be used to help stabilize a fractured bone.

Yes No **2.** A padded board is a type of self-splint.

Yes No **3.** When splinting, you should check CSM before and after applying the splint.

Yes No **4.** You should attempt to straighten all extremity fractures.

Yes No **5.** Splints should only be placed on one side of injured area to maintain adequate circulation.

Yes No **6.** Splints should be applied snugly enough to reduce circulation.

Yes No **7.** Extremity fractures rarely need more advanced medical attention

Yes No **8.** Splints should extend beyond the joints above and below the injured area.

Scenario: A home builder has fallen from a ladder and possibly broken his wrist. What should you do?

____

____

____

Chapter 12

Sudden Illnesses

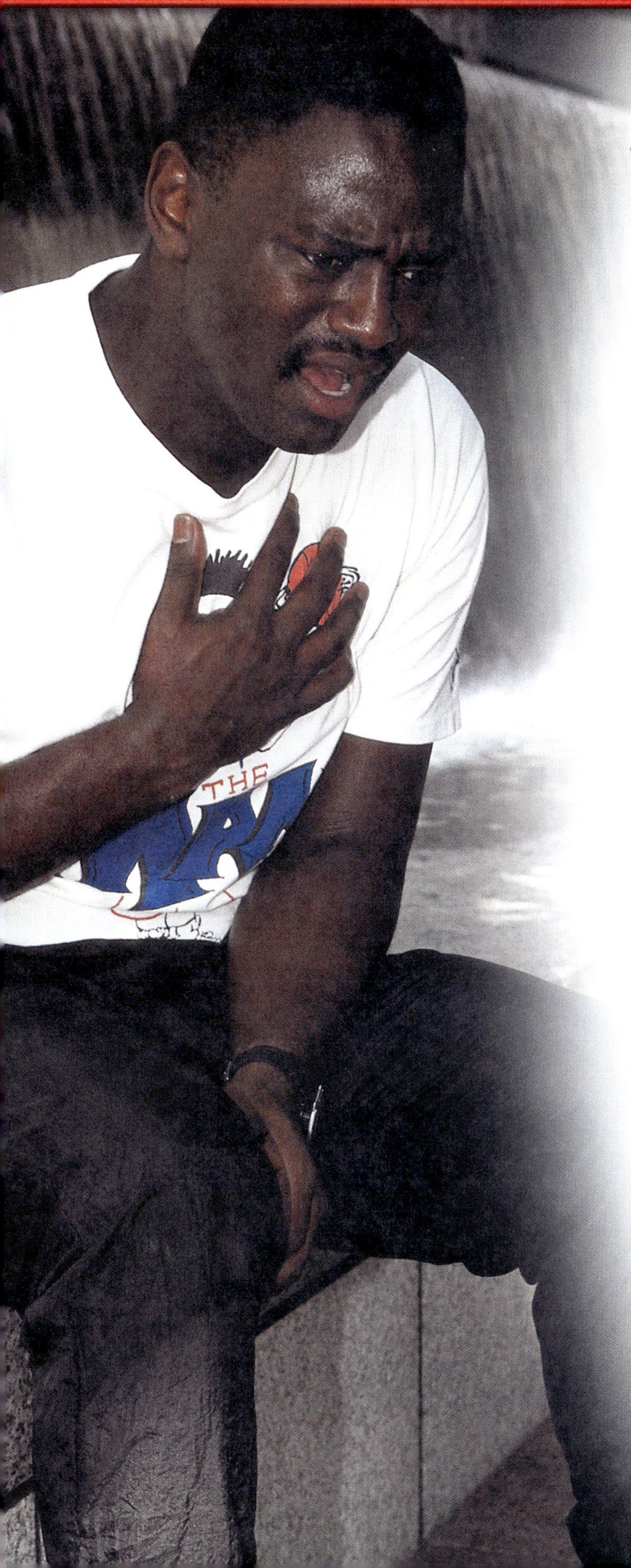

Heart Attack

A heart attack happens when the blood supply to part of the heart muscle is severely reduced or stopped. Usually that happens when one of the coronary arteries (the arteries that supply blood to the heart muscle) is blocked by an obstruction or a spasm.

What to Look For

Heart attacks are difficult to determine. Because medical care at the onset of a heart attack is vital to survival and the quality of recovery, if you suspect a heart attack for any reason, seek medical attention *at once.*

Possible signs and symptoms of a heart attack include:

- uncomfortable pressure, fullness, squeezing, or pain in the center of the chest that lasts more than a few minutes or that goes away and comes back
- pain spreading to the shoulders, neck, or arms
- chest discomfort with lightheadedness, fainting, sweating, nausea, or shortness of breath

Not all these warning signs occur in every heart attack. It is difficult to determine if someone is having a heart attack. Many victims will deny that they are experiencing something as serious as a heart attack. Delay can seriously increase the risk of major damage. Insist on taking prompt action.

What to Do

1. Call EMS or get to the nearest hospital emergency department with 24-hour emergency cardiac care.
2. Monitor victim's condition.
3. Help the victim to the least painful position, usually sitting with legs up and bent at the knees ▶Figure 1. Loosen clothing around the neck and midriff. Be calm and reassuring.
4. Determine if the victim is known to have coronary heart disease and is using nitroglycerin. Nitroglycerin tablets or spray under the tongue or

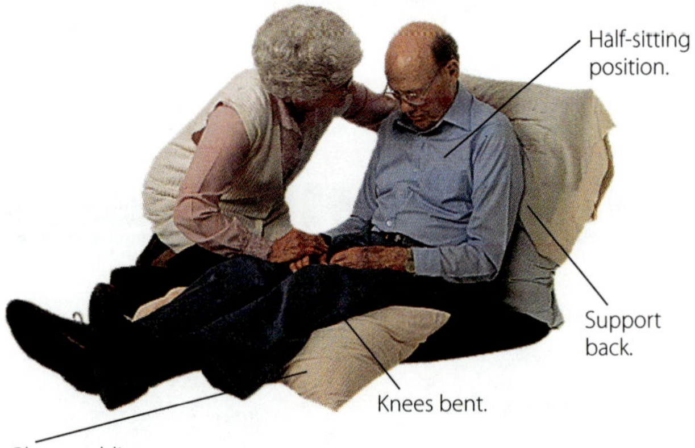

Figure 1 Help the victim into a relaxed position to ease strain on heart.

nitroglycerin ointment on the skin may relieve chest pain. Nitroglycerin dilates the coronary arteries, which increases blood flow to the heart muscle, and lowers blood pressure and dilates the veins, which decreases the work of the heart and the heart muscle's need for oxygen.

Caution: Because nitroglycerin lowers blood pressure, the victim should sit or lie down once it is taken.

5. If the victim is unresponsive, check ABCs and start CPR, if needed.

Angina

Chest pain called angina pectoris can result from coronary heart disease just as a heart attack does. Angina happens when the heart muscle does not get as much blood as it needs (which means a lack of oxygen).

Angina is brought on by physical exertion, exposure to cold, emotional stress, or the ingestion of food. It seldom lasts longer than 10 minutes and almost always is relieved by nitroglycerin. (In contrast, chest pain from a heart attack is as likely to happen at rest as during activity; the pain lasts longer than 10 minutes and is not relieved by nitroglycerin.)

Stroke (Brain Attack)

A stroke, also referred to as a brain attack or cerebrovascular accident (CVA), occurs when blood vessels that deliver oxygen-rich blood to the brain rupture or become plugged, so part of the brain does not get the blood flow it needs (▼**Figure 2**). Deprived of oxygen, nerve cells in the affected area of the brain cannot function and die within minutes. Because dead brain cells are not replaced, the devastating effects of a stroke often are permanent.

Transient ischemic attacks (TIAs) are closely associated with strokes. Because TIAs have many of the same signs and symptoms, they often are confused with strokes. The main difference between a TIA and a stroke is that the symptoms of TIA are transient, lasting from several minutes (75% last less than five minutes) to several hours, with a return to normal neurologic function. TIAs are "mini-strokes." A TIA should be considered a serious warning sign of a potential stroke—about one third of all TIA cases will suffer a stroke within 2 to 5 years after their first TIA. Any signs and symptoms of a TIA should be reported to a physician.

What to Look For

- weakness, numbness, or paralysis of the face, an arm, or a leg on one side of the body
- blurred or decreased vision, especially in one eye
- problems speaking or understanding
- dizziness or loss of balance
- sudden, severe, and unexplained headache
- deviation of the pupils of the eyes from PEARL (**P**upils **E**qual **A**nd **R**eactive to **L**ight), which may mean the brain is being affected by lack of oxygen

What to Do

First aid for a stroke victim is limited to supportive care:

1. If victim is unresponsive, check the ABCs.
2. Call EMS.

Figure 2 Severe brain hemorrhage causing a stroke

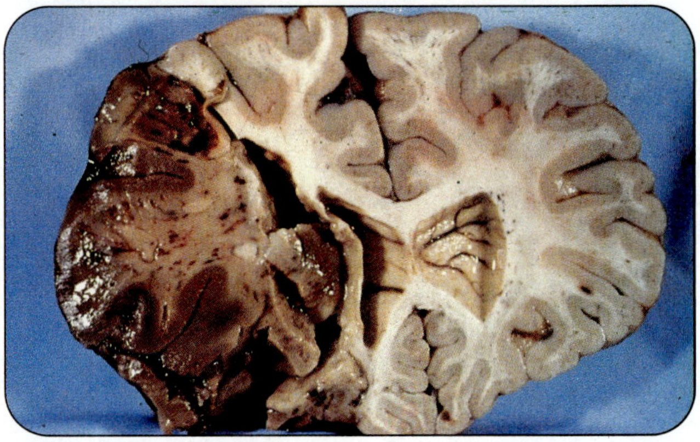

3. If the victim does not have any injury (from a fall), lay the victim down with the head and shoulders slightly elevated, to reduce blood pressure on the brain. Place a victim who is unresponsive but breathing in the recovery position, which is on the side (to keep the airway open and to permit secretions and vomit to drain from the mouth).

Caution:

DO NOT give a stroke victim anything to drink or eat. The throat may be paralyzed, which restricts swallowing.

Asthma

What to Look For

- coughing
- cyanosis (bluish skin color)
- inability to speak in complete sentences without pausing for breath
- nostrils flaring with each breath
- difficulty breathing including wheezing (high-pitched whistling sound during breathing)

What to Do

1. Keep the victim in a comfortable upright position that makes it easier to breathe.
2. Monitor the ABCs.
3. Ask the victim about any asthma medication he or she may be using (▼Figure 3). Most asthma sufferers will have some form of asthma medication, usually administered through physician-prescribed, hand-held inhalers.
4. If the victim does not respond well to his or her inhaled medication or is having an extreme asthma attack (known as status asthmaticus), seek medical attention immediately.

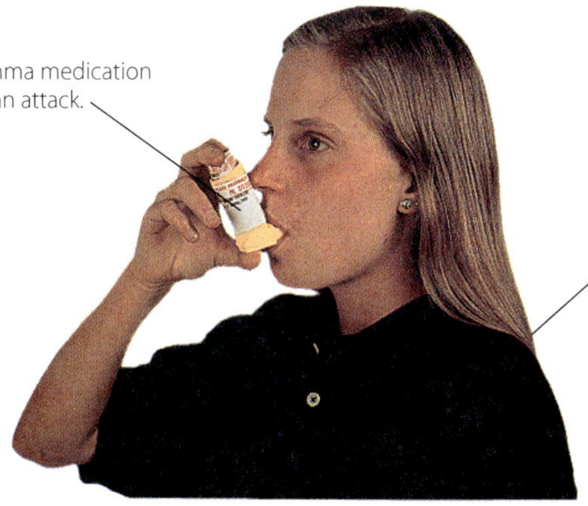

Figure 3 Taking asthma medication

Hyperventilation

Fast, deep breathing is common during emotional stress.

What to Look For

- dizziness or lightheadedness
- numbness
- tingling of the hands and feet
- shortness of breath
- breathing rates faster than 40/min

What to Do

1. Calm and reassure the victim.
2. Encourage the victim to breathe slowly, using the abdominal muscles. Inhale through the nose; hold the full inhalation for several seconds; then exhale slowly. Do NOT have the victim breathe into a paper bag.

Fainting

Most fainting is associated with decreased blood flow to the brain. The decreased blood flow may be caused by low blood sugar (hypoglycemia), slow heart rate (vagal reaction, in which the vagus nerve, which slows the heart rate, is overstimulated by fright, anxiety, drugs, or fatigue), heart-rhythm disturbances, dehydration, heat exhaustion, anemia, or bleeding.

Sitting or standing for a long time without moving, especially in a hot environment, can cause blood to pool in dilated vessels. That results in a loss of effective circulating blood volume, and blood pressure drops. As the blood flow to the brain decreases, the person loses consciousness and collapses.

What to Do

1. Check ABCs.
2. If the victim is unresponsive, but breathing, place the victim in the recovery position.

3. Loosen tight clothing and belts.
4. If the victim has fallen, check for any sign of injury. After recovery, have the victim sit for a while. When he or she is able to swallow, give cool, sweetened liquids to drink, and help the victim slowly regain an upright posture.
5. Fresh air and a cold, wet cloth for the face usually aid recovery.

Most fainting episodes are not serious, and the victim recovers quickly. Seek medical attention, however, if the victim

- has had repeated attacks of unconsciousness.
- does not quickly regain consciousness.
- loses consciousness while sitting or lying down.
- faints for no apparent reason.

Seizures

A seizure is the result of an abnormal stimulation of the brain's cells. A variety of medical conditions increase the instability or irritability of the brain and can lead to seizures, including the following:

- epilepsy
- heatstroke
- poisoning
- electric shock
- hypoglycemia
- high fever in children
- brain injury, tumor, or stroke
- alcohol withdrawal, drug abuse/overdose

Epilepsy is not a mental illness, and it is not a sign of low intelligence. It also is not contagious. Between seizures, a person with epilepsy functions normally.

What to Do

The Epilepsy Foundation lists the following first aid procedures for seizures:

1. Cushion the victim's head (a rolled towel or jacket works well); remove items that could cause injury if the person bumped into them.
2. Loosen any tight clothing, especially around the neck.
3. Roll the victim onto his or her side.
4. As the seizure ends, offer your help. Most seizures in people with epilepsy are not medical emergencies. They end after a minute or two without harm and usually do not require medical attention.
5. Call EMS if any of the following exists:
   - A seizure happens to someone who is not known to have epilepsy (eg, there is no "epilepsy" or "seizure disorder" identification). It could be a sign of serious illness.
   - A seizure lasts more than five minutes.
   - The victim is slow to recover, has a second seizure, or has difficulty breathing afterward.
   - The victim is pregnant or has another medical condition.
   - There are any signs of injury or illnesses.

Diabetic Emergencies

Diabetes is a condition in which insulin, a hormone produced by the pancreas that helps the body use the energy in food, is either lacking or ineffective ▼Figure 4. Insulin is needed to take sugar from the blood and carry it into the cells to be used. If the sugar remains in the blood, the body cells must rely on fat as fuel. Blood sugar (glucose) is a major body fuel, and when it cannot be used, it builds up in the blood, overflows into the urine, and passes out of the body unused so the body loses an important source of fuel. Diabetes develops. Diabetes is not contagious.

Figure 4 Diabetic emergencies

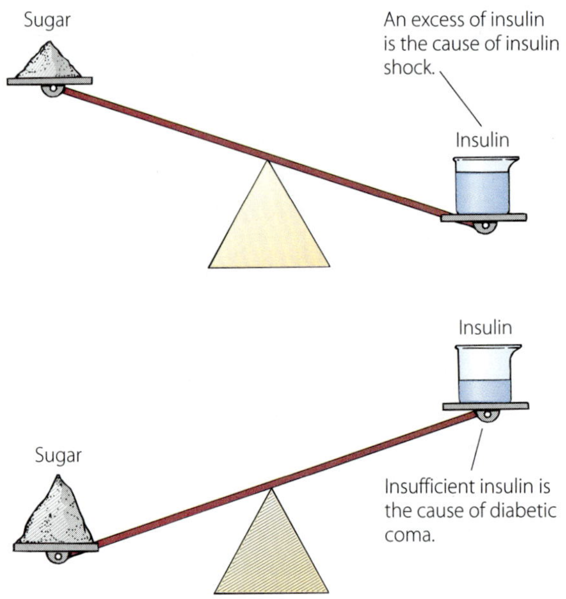

There are two types of diabetes:

- *Type I: juvenile-onset or insulin-dependent* diabetes. Type I diabetics require external (not made by the body) insulin to allow sugar to pass from the blood into cells. When deprived of external insulin, the diabetic becomes quite ill.
- *Type II: adult-onset or non-insulin-dependent* diabetes. Type II diabetics tend to be overweight. They are not dependent on external insulin to allow sugar into cells. However, if their insulin level is low, the lack of sugar in the cells increases sugar production and sugar in the blood to very high levels. That causes glucose to spill into the urine, drawing fluid with it and resulting in dehydration.

The body is continuously balancing sugar and insulin. Too much insulin and not enough sugar leads to low blood sugar, possibly insulin shock. Too much sugar and not enough insulin leads to high blood sugar, possibly diabetic coma.

Low Blood Sugar

Very low blood sugar, called hypoglycemia, is sometimes referred to as an "insulin reaction." This condition can be caused by too much insulin, too little or delayed food, exercise, alcohol, or any combination of these factors.

The American Diabetes Association lists the following signs and symptoms of insulin reaction and hypoglycemia as diabetic emergencies requiring first aid:

- sudden onset
- staggering, poor coordination
- anger, bad temper
- pale color
- confusion, disorientation
- sudden hunger
- excessive sweating
- trembling
- eventual unconsciousness

What to Do

Use the "Rule of 15s" for giving sugar if the victim is a known diabetic, mental status is changed, and is awake to swallow:

1. Give 15 grams of sugar (eg, 2 large teaspoons or lumps of sugar, or one half can of regular soda, or 4 ozs. of orange juice, or two to five glucose tablets, or one tube of glucose gel) ►Figure 5.

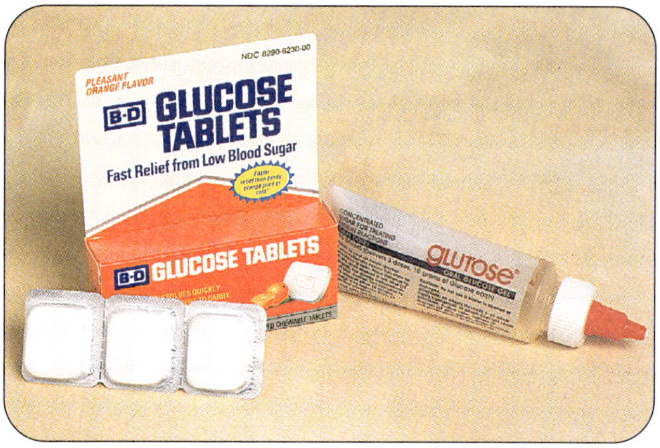

Figure 5 Glucose tablets and gel

2. Wait 15 minutes.
3. If no improvement, give 15 more grams of sugar (carbohydrate).
4. If no improvement, seek immediate medical attention.

High Blood Sugar

Hyperglycemia—also known as diabetic coma—is the opposite of hypoglycemia. Hyperglycemia occurs when the body has too much sugar in the blood. This condition may be caused by insufficient insulin, overeating, inactivity, illness, stress, or a combination of these factors.

The American Diabetes Association lists the following signs and symptoms of diabetic coma and hyperglycemia as diabetic emergencies requiring first aid:

- gradual onset
- drowsiness
- extreme thirst
- very frequent urination
- flushed skin
- vomiting
- fruity breath odor
- heavy breathing
- eventual unconsciousness

What to Do

1. If you are uncertain whether victim has high or low blood-sugar level, give the person food or drink containing sugar.
2. If you do not see improvement in 15 minutes, seek medical care.

DIABETIC EMERGENCIES

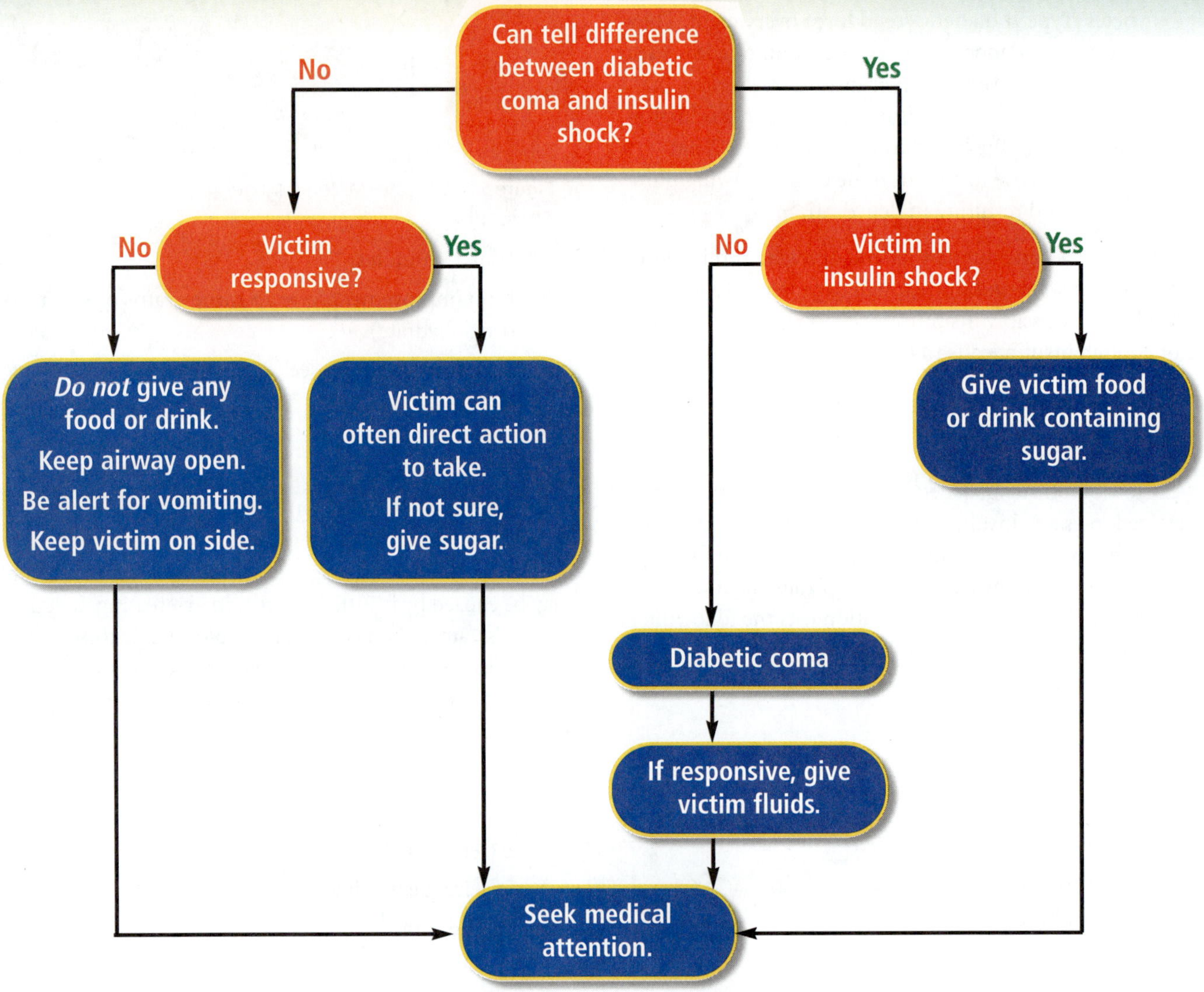

Emergencies During Pregnancy

Most pregnancies are normal and occur without complications. However, sometimes problems do arise and medical attention is required. It is essential that you remain calm, focused, and considerate of the mother during this unforeseen and stressful situation.

What to Look For

Immediately notify a doctor to report the following signs and symptoms in a pregnant woman:

- vaginal bleeding
- cramps in lower abdomen
- swelling of the face or fingers
- severe continuous headache
- dizziness or fainting
- blurring of vision or seeing spots
- uncontrollable vomiting

What to Do

If the victim is experiencing vaginal bleeding or abdominal pain:

1. Keep quiet, warm, and on her left side
2. Have victim or another woman place a sanitary napkin or any sterile or clean pad over the opening of the vagina.
3. Have victim or another woman replace but save any blood-soaked pads and all tissues that are passed. Send this with the woman to medical help for examination by the physician.
4. Arrange for immediate transportation to a medical facility.

If the victim has injuries to her lower abdomen:

1. Keep the woman quiet, warm, and on her left side.
2. Monitor ABCs.
3. Arrange for immediate transportation to a medical facility.

Learning Activities

Sudden Illnesses

Directions: Circle Yes if you agree with the statement, and circle No if you disagree.

Yes No **1.** Heart attack victims experience the least amount of chest pain when lying down.

Yes No **2.** When taking doctor-prescribed nitroglycerin for chest pain, the person should be sitting or lying down.

Yes No **3.** A stroke victim should have his or her head slightly raised.

Yes No **4.** Most asthma victims will usually have a physician-prescribed inhaler.

Yes No **5.** A victim who is breathing fast (hyperventilation) should be encouraged to breathe slowly by holding inhaled air for several seconds, then exhaling slowly.

Yes No **6.** Splash or sprinkle water on a person who has fainted.

Yes No **7.** Have a fainted victim inhale smelling salts or ammonia inhalants.

Yes No **8.** Place a strong stick or similar object between a seizure victim's teeth.

Yes No **9.** A person having seizures always requires medical attention.

Yes No **10.** If in doubt about whether a victim is having an insulin reaction or is in a diabetic coma, give sugar to a responsive victim who can swallow.

Yes No **11.** During a diabetic emergency, if you do not see improvement in 15 minutes, seek medical attention for the victim.

Scenario #1: A 50-year-old co-worker complains about chest pain. He says that it started about an hour ago and has not let up. He is sure that it is just a little indigestion and feels silly about talking about it. He says the pain feels like "something pressing on my chest," and he feels nauseous. What should you do?

Scenario #2: You are working in an office cubicle next to a co-worker who suddenly collapses. You rush to help and find him confused, with numbness and paralysis on one side. Another co-worker says that he earlier complained of a severe headache. What should you do?

Scenario #3: During a first aid training video showing a bloodied victim, a young man suddenly falls from his chair to the floor. He is breathing and has a pulse, but is unresponsive. No other injuries from the fall are detected. What should you do?

Scenario #4: You see some of your co-workers holding down another employee on the floor. They are trying to force a couple of pencils between her teeth. The person is unresponsive and is having severe muscle jerks. What should you do?

Scenario #5: After work, the car-pool driver is driving fast and erratically. When she stops to let her first rider out, she just sits in the car staring ahead. She then slumps over onto the steering wheel. Her skin is cold and sweaty. You are aware the driver is diabetic. What should you do?

Chapter 13

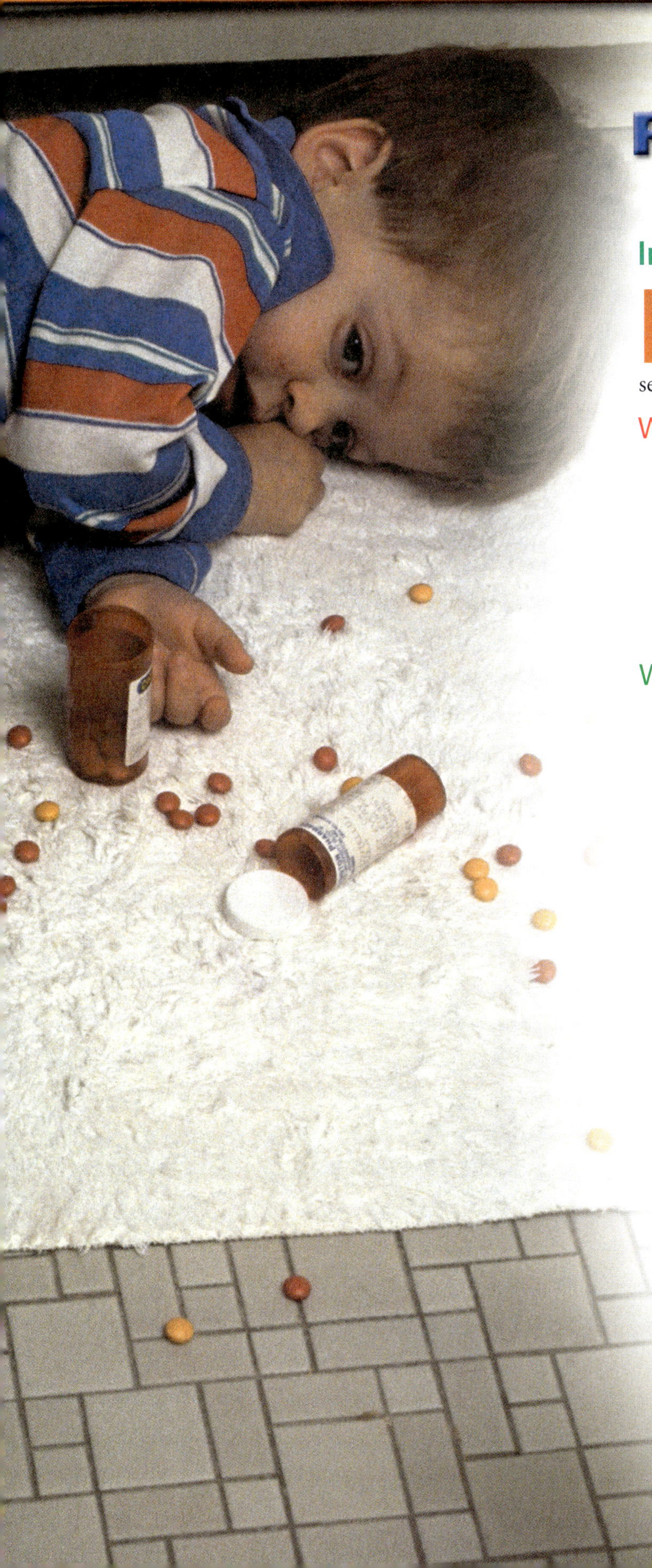

Poisoning

Ingested (Swallowed) Poisons

Fortunately, most poisons ingested have low toxicity or are swallowed in amounts so small that severe poisoning rarely occurs. However, the potential for severe or fatal poisoning is always present.

What to Look For

- abdominal pain and cramping
- nausea or vomiting
- diarrhea
- burns, odor, stains around and in mouth
- drowsiness or unconsciousness
- poison containers nearby

What to Do

1. Determine critical information:
   - Age and size of the victim?
   - What was swallowed? (Read container label; save vomit for analysis.)
   - How much was swallowed (eg, a "taste," half a bottle, a dozen tablets)?
   - When was it swallowed?
2. If a corrosive or caustic (ie, acid or alkali) substance was swallowed, immediately dilute it by having the victim drink at least one or two eight-ounce glasses of water or milk. (*Cold* milk or water tends to absorb heat better than room-temperature or warmer liquids.)
3. *For a responsive victim,* call a poison control center *immediately.* Some poisons do not cause harm until hours later, while others do damage immediately. More than 75% of poisonings can be treated by following the instructions given over the telephone from a poison control center. The center also will advise you if medical attention is needed. Poison control centers routinely follow up calls to check whether additional symptoms or unexpected effects are occurring. The inside front covers of telephone directories contain the number for local poison control centers.

SWALLOWED POISON

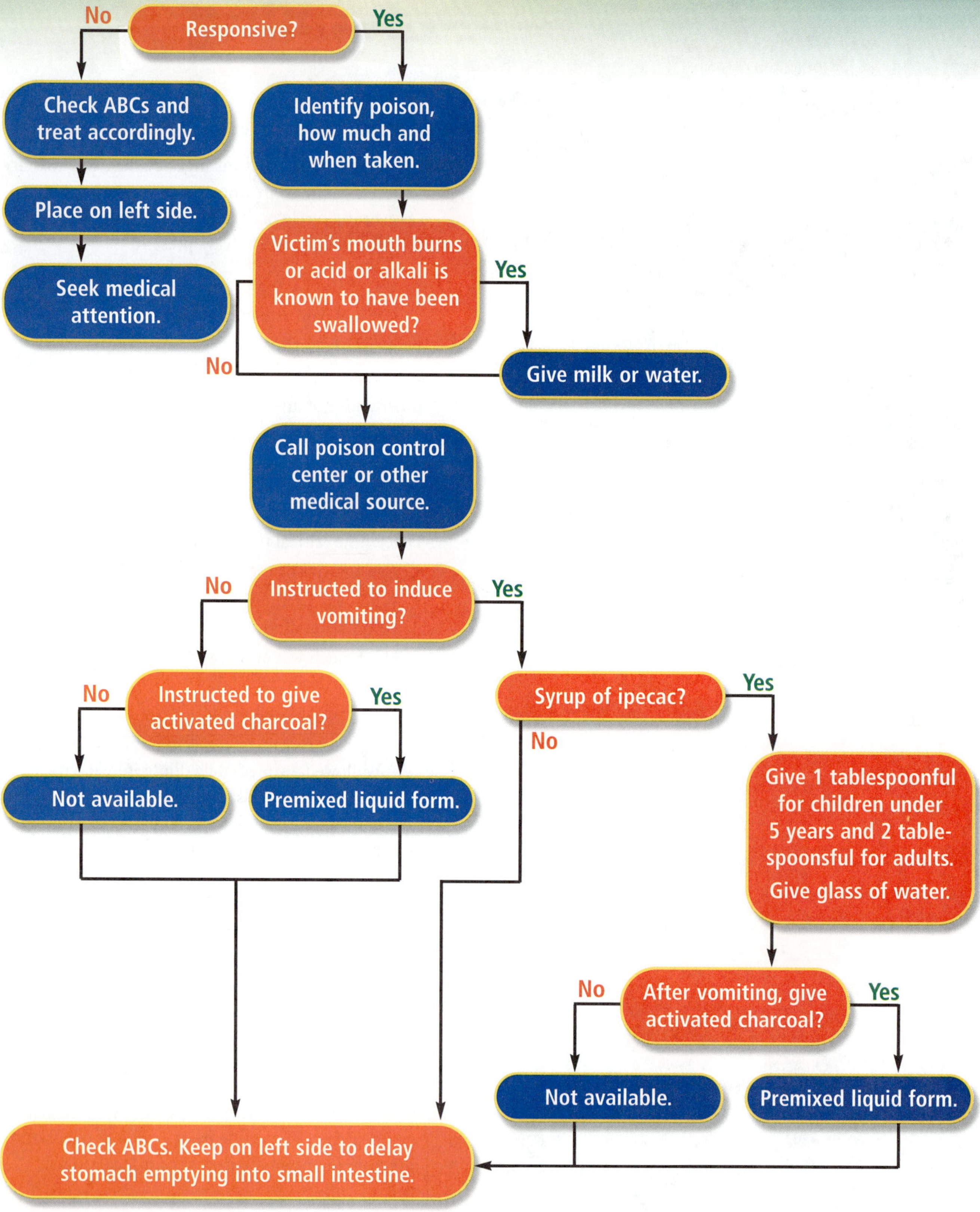

Material Safety Data Sheets (MSDS)

- For each hazardous chemical in the workplace, an employer is required by law to maintain a copy of the MSDS. An MSDS lists the hazardous ingredients of a product, its physical and chemical characteristics (eg, flammability), its effects on human health, the chemicals with which it can adversely react, handling precautions, measures that can be used to control exposure, emergency and first aid procedures, and methods to contain a spill.

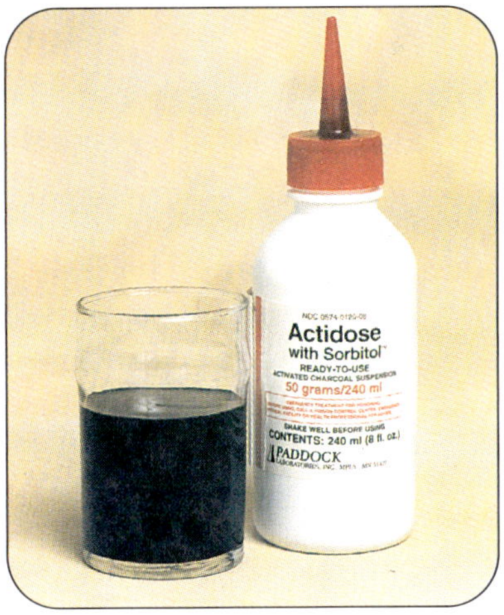

Figure 2 Activated charcoal

4. *For an unresponsive victim,* check ABCs and treat accordingly. Call 9-1-1 or the local emergency number. Monitor ABCs often.
5. Place the victim on his or her *left* side. This positions the end of the stomach where it enters the small intestine (pylorus) straight up. In this position, gravity will delay (by as much as two hours) the poison's advance into the small intestine, where absorption into the victim's circulatory system is faster ▼Figure 1. The side position also helps prevent breathing foreign materials into the lungs if vomiting begins.
6. Induce vomiting *only* if a poison control center or a physician advises it. Inducing must be done within 30 minutes of swallowing.

   If you are instructed by a poison control center or a physician to induce vomiting, use syrup of ipecac. It can be purchased without a prescription and is easily given. Follow the directions carefully. Ipecac will not work unless you also give sufficient water.
7. Give activated charcoal if a poison control center advises ►Figure 2. It is the single most effective agent for most swallowed poisons. Activated charcoal acts like a sponge to bind and keep the poison in the digestive system, thus preventing its absorption into the blood.

   Although activated charcoal may appear similar to burnt-toast scrapings and charcoal briquettes, they *cannot* be used for poisoning.

   Not all chemicals, however, are absorbed well by activated charcoal, including acids and alkalis (eg, bleach, ammonia), potassium, iron, alcohol, methanol, kerosene, cyanide, malathion, and ferrous sulfate.

   Major drawbacks of activated charcoal are its grittiness and its appearance. Trying to improve the taste or consistency by adding chocolate syrup, sherbet, ice cream, milk, or other flavoring agents only decreases the charcoal's binding capacity. Place the charcoal mixture in an opaque container and have the victim sip it through a straw so it will be more palatable. First aiders should give only the pre-mixed form. Some common names for the pre-mixed form are Actidose™, InstaChar™, and LiquiChar™

   Although activated charcoal is an inexpensive, safe, and effective means for decreasing poison absorption, pharmacies do not routinely stock it.
8. Save poison containers, plants, and the victim's vomit to help medical personnel identify the poison.

Figure 1 The left-side position delays the poison from advancing into the small intestine.

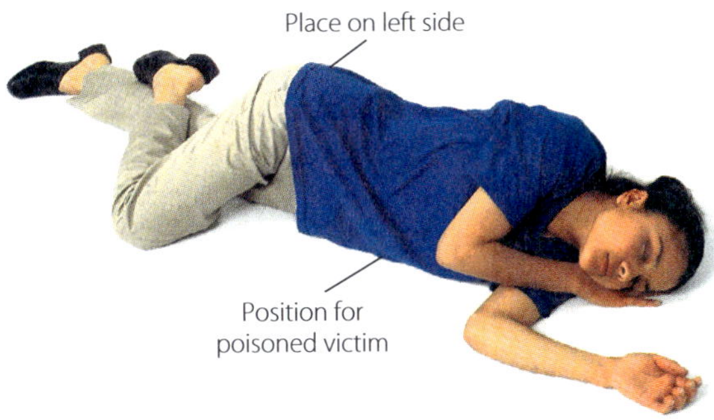

Caution:

DO NOT give water or milk to dilute poisons unless instructed to do so by a poison control center. Fluids may dissolve a dry poison (eg, tablets or capsules) more rapidly and fill up the stomach, forcing stomach contents (ie, the poison) into the small intestine, where poisons are absorbed faster.

Alcohol and Other Drug Emergencies

Alcohol Intoxication

Helping an intoxicated person is often difficult since the individual may be belligerent and combative. Also, personal hygiene is sometimes less than optimal. However, it is important that alcohol abusers be helped and not just labeled as "drunks." Their condition may be quite serious, even life-threatening.

What to Look For

Although the following signs indicate alcohol intoxication, some may also mean illness or injury other than alcohol abuse, such as diabetes or heat injury:

- the odor of alcohol on a person's breath or clothing
- unsteady, staggering walking
- slurred speech and the inability to carry on a conversation
- nausea and vomiting
- flushed face

Caution:

DO NOT let an intoxicated person sleep on his or her back.

DO NOT leave an intoxicated person alone.

DO NOT try to handle a hostile drunk by yourself. Find a safe place, then call the police for help.

What to Do

First aid for an intoxicated person includes these steps:

1. Look for any injuries. Alcohol can mask pain.
2. Check ABCs and treat accordingly.
3. If the intoxicated person is lying down, place him or her in the recovery position. Rolling the victim onto the left side not only reduces the likelihood of vomiting and aspiration of vomit , but also delays absorption of alcohol into the bloodstream.
4. Call the poison control center for advice or the local emergency number for help.
5. Provide emotional support, but if the victim becomes violent, leave the scene and find a safe place until police arrive.
6. If the intoxicated victim has been exposed to the cold, suspect hypothermia and move the person to a warm environment whenever possible. Remove wet clothing and cover the individual with warm blankets. Handle a hypothermic victim gently, because rough handling could induce a heart attack.

Drugs Other Than Alcohol

What to Do

1. Check ABCs
2. Call the poison control center for advice or EMS for help.
3. Check for injuries.
4. Keep the person on the *left* side to reduce the likelihood of vomiting and aspiration of vomit and to delay the absorption of drugs into the bloodstream.
5. Provide reassurance and emotional support.
6. If the person becomes violent, find a safe place until the police arrive. Let law enforcement officers handle dangerous situations.

Carbon Monoxide Poisoning

Carbon monoxide (CO) victims are often unaware of its presence. The gas is invisible, tasteless, odorless, and nonirritating. It is produced by the incomplete burning of organic material such as gasoline, wood, paper, charcoal, coal, and natural gas.

What to Look For

It is difficult to tell if a person is a CO victim. Sometimes, a complaint of having the "flu" is really a symptom of CO poisoning. Although many symptoms of CO poisoning resemble those of the flu, there are differences. For example, CO poisoning does not cause low-grade fever or generalized aching or involve the lymph nodes as the flu does.

The following conditions indicate possible CO poisoning:

- The symptoms come and go.
- The symptoms worsen or improve in certain places or at certain times of the day.
- People around the victim have similar symptoms.
- Pets seem ill.

The signs and symptoms of CO poisoning are as follows:

- headache
- ringing in the ears (tinnitus)
- chest pain (angina)
- muscle weakness
- nausea and vomiting
- dizziness and visual changes (blurred or double vision)

- unconsciousness
- respiratory and cardiac arrest

What to Do

1. Get the victim out of the toxic environment and into fresh air *immediately.*
2. Call EMS personnel, who will be able to give the victim 100% oxygen, improving oxygenation.
3. Monitor ABCs.
4. Place an unresponsive victim in the recovery position.
5. Seek medical attention. All suspected CO victims should obtain a blood test to determine the level of CO.

Plant-Induced Dermatitis: Poison Ivy, Poison Oak, and Poison Sumac

Most people cannot identify these irritating plants ▼**Figure 3A–B**. A helpful method of identifying these plants is the "black-spot test." When the sap is exposed to the air, it turns brown in a matter of minutes and by the next day is black.

Figure 3A Poison ivy, found in all 48 contiguous U.S. states

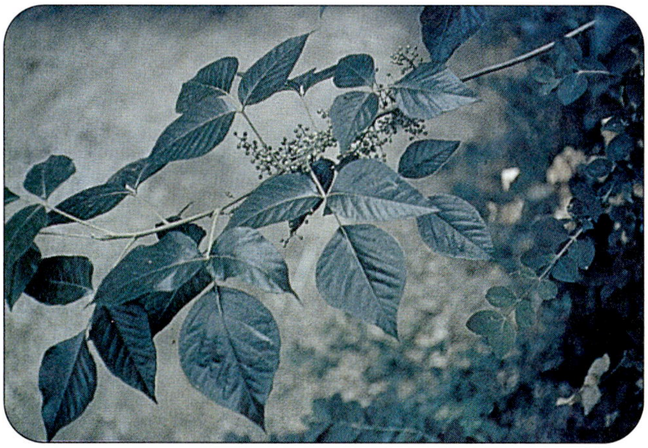

Figure 3B Poison ivy dermatitis

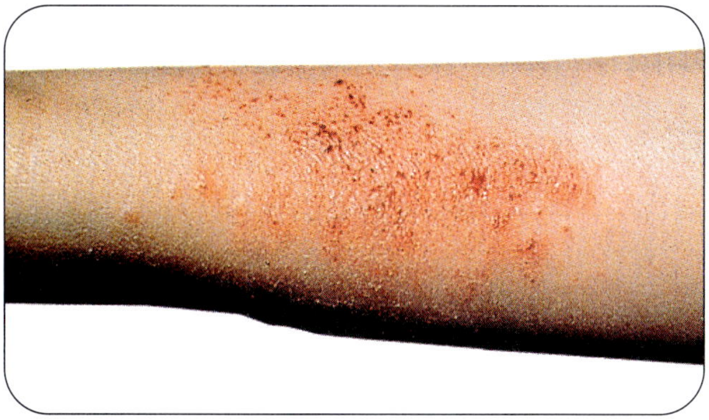

What to Do

1. Those who know they have been in contact with a poisonous plant should decontaminate the skin as soon as possible (within five minutes for sensitive people, up to one hour for moderately sensitive individuals). Use soap and cold water to clean the skin of the oily resin or apply rubbing (isopropyl) alcohol liberally (not in swab-type dabs). If too little isopropyl alcohol is used, the oil will actually spread to another site and enlarge the injury. Other solvents (eg, paint thinner) can be used, but they are hard on the skin and may be flammable. Rinse with water to remove the solubilized material. Water removes the urushiol (plant resin) from the skin, oxidizes and inactivates it, and does not penetrate the skin as do solvents. Unfortunately, most victims do not know about their contact until several hours or days later, when the itching and rash begin.
2. If the reaction is mild, the person can soak in a lukewarm bath sprinkled with one to two cups of colloidal oatmeal, such as Aveeno™ Colloidal oatmeal, which makes a tub slick, so take appropriate precautions, or apply any of the following:
   - calamine lotion (calamine ointment if the skin becomes dry and cracked) or zinc oxide
   - baking soda paste: one teaspoon of water mixed with three teaspoons of baking soda
3. If the reaction is mild to moderate, care for the skin as you would for a mild reaction and use a physician-prescribed corticosteroid ointment.
4. For a severe reaction, follow the same care guidelines for the skin and use a physician-prescribed oral corticosteroid (eg, prednisone). Apply a topical corticosteroid ointment or cream, cover it with a transparent plastic wrap, and lightly bind the area with an elastic or self-adhering bandage.

Caution:

DO NOT use nonprescription hydrocortisone creams, ointments, and sprays in strengths of less than 1%. They offer little benefit.

DO NOT use over-the-counter anti-itch lotions like Caladryl™ because they may cause further skin irritation. Oral antihistamines such as Benadryl™ often are used in conjunction with prescription creams to help decrease itching.

DO NOT let the victim rub or scratch the rash or itching skin.

Learning Activities

Poisoning

Directions: Circle Yes if you agree with the statement, and circle No if you disagree.

Yes No **1.** If a corrosive or caustic substance was swallowed, immediately dilute it by having the victim drink water or milk.

Yes No **2.** For a poisoned victim, call a poison control center immediately.

Yes No **3.** Induce vomiting with ipecac syrup only if advised by a poison control center or a doctor.

Yes No **4.** Place a swallowed poison victim on his or her left side to delay the poison from going into the small intestine.

Yes No **5.** Do NOT let an intoxicated person sleep on his or her back.

Yes No **6.** If an intoxicated or drugged person becomes violent, leave the scene and let law enforcement officers handle the situation.

Yes No **7.** Seek medical attention for all carbon monoxide victims.

Yes No **8.** Calamine lotion can help relieve itching caused by poison ivy, oak, or sumac.

Yes No **9.** Some cases of poison ivy, oak, or sumac require medical attention.

Scenario #1: You find your two-year-old son, Scott, vomiting. You notice the top of a nearby medicine container is off. The label on the container indicates that the medicine belongs to your mother who is visiting. You realize that Scott must have swallowed some of the highly potent medicine. What should you do?

____

____

Scenario #2: At a party given by your boss, one of the guests becomes quite drunk. He vomits and is now unresponsive. What should you do?

____

____

Scenario #3: A 25-year-old co-worker seems to be "freaking out." Another co-worker says she saw the victim take some "pills." After she finally calms down, she tells you that she took some drugs. What should you do?

____

____

Scenario #4: A driver is waiting in his truck until the building workers can load it. He's left the motor running to keep the heater on and has closed all the windows and doors because of the subfreezing outside temperatures. When the building workers come to tell him they're ready, he is slumped over the wheel. They move him to fresh air just as you arrive. What should you do?

____

____

Scenario #5: While weeding around a vacant lot, you pull up a batch of weeds with shiny leaves in clusters of three. You finish the job about an hour later. The next morning your arms are itching, and you notice a rash beginning to appear. What should you do?

____

____

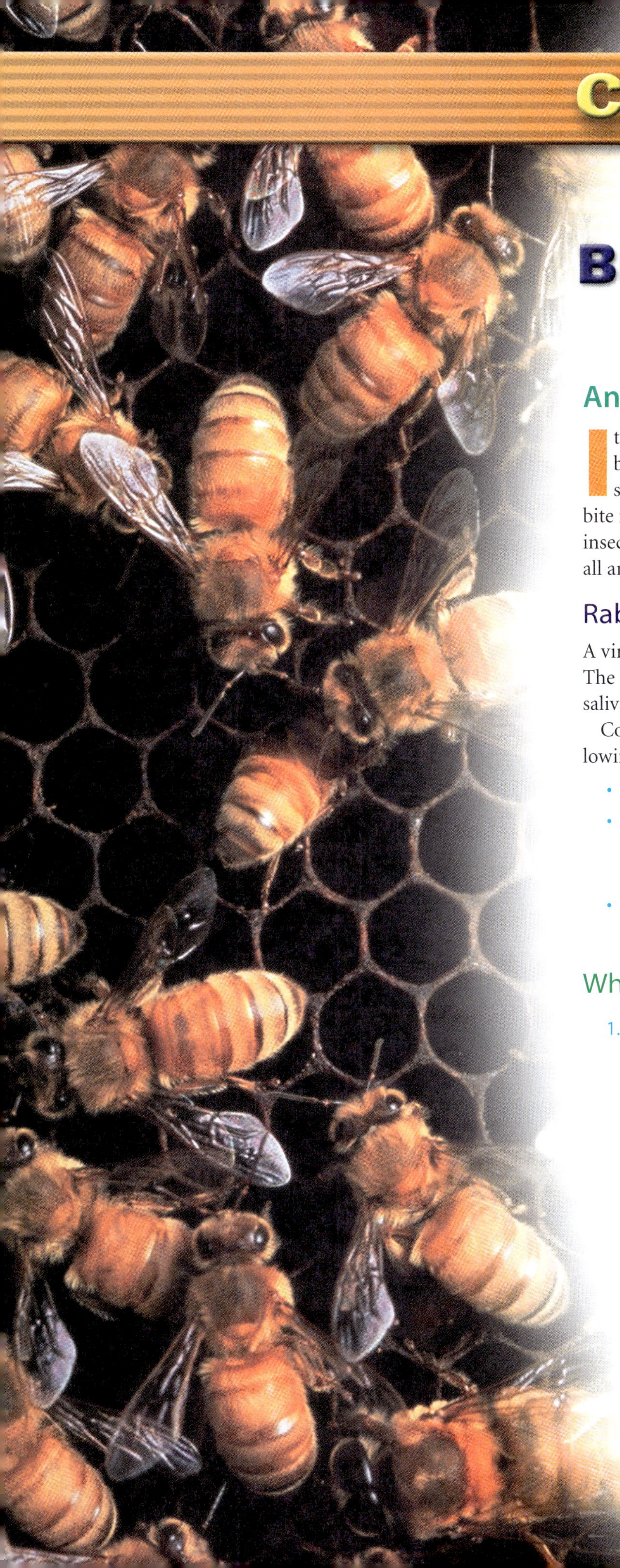

Chapter 14

Bites and Stings

Animal Bites

It is estimated that one of every two Americans will be bitten at some time by an animal or by another person. As it is commonly interpreted, the term animal bite in this section refers to a bite by a mammal, not by an insect or reptile. Dogs are responsible for about 80% of all animal-bite injuries ▶Figure 1.

Rabies

A virus found in warm-blooded animals causes rabies. The disease spreads from one animal to another in the saliva, usually through a bite or by licking.

Consider an animal as possibly rabid if any of the following applies:

- The animal attacked without provocation.
- The animal acted strangely, that is, out of character (eg, a usually friendly dog is aggressive, or a wild fox seems docile and "friendly").
- The animal was a high-risk species (skunk, raccoon, or bat).

What to Do

1. If the victim was bitten in the United States (except for the area along the border with Mexico) by a healthy domestic dog or cat, the animal will likely be confined and observed for 10 days for any illness. If necessary, a veterinarian will kill the animal (domesticated or wild), decapitate it, and send the head to a laboratory for analysis. If the animal is dead when you find it, transport the entire body; do not attempt decapitation (precautions must be taken to prevent exposure to potentially infected tissues and saliva).

   Report animal bites to the police or animal control officers; they should be the ones to capture the animal for observation. If the dog or cat escapes and is not suspected to be rabid, consult local public health officials.

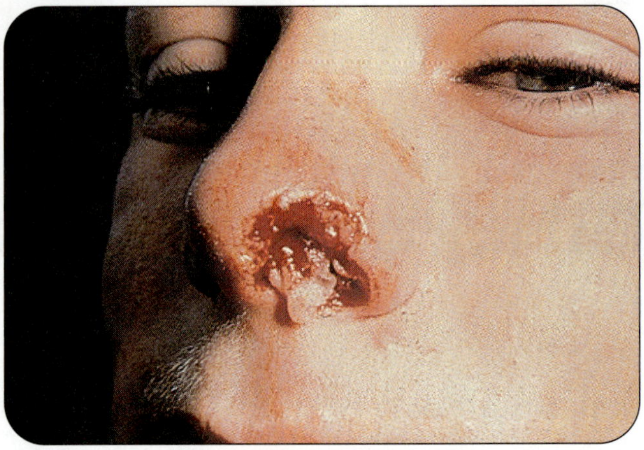

Figure 1 Dog bite

If the victim was bitten in the United States by a skunk, raccoon, bat, fox, or other mammal, it should be considered a rabies exposure and treatment should be started immediately. The only exception is when the bite occurred in a part of the continental United States known to be free of rabies. If the wild animal is captured, it should be killed and its head shipped to a qualified laboratory immediately.

2. Clean the wound with a soap solution and rinse it with water under pressure.
3. Stop the bleeding and give wound care.
4. Seek medical attention for further wound cleaning and a possible tetanus shot. The physician will determine if sutures are needed to close the wound. If needed, a vaccination series against rabies will be started.

Human Bites

The human mouth contains a wide range of bacteria, so the chance of infection is greater from a human bite than from bites of other warm-blooded animals.

What to Do

1. If the wound is not bleeding heavily, wash it with soap and water (under the pressure from a faucet) for 5 to 10 minutes. Avoid scrubbing, which can bruise tissues.
2. Rinse the wound thoroughly with running water under pressure.
3. Control bleeding with direct pressure.
4. Cover the wound with a sterile dressing. Do not close the wound with tape or butterfly bandages, which traps bacteria in the wound and increases the chance of infection.
5. Seek medical attention for possible further wound cleaning, a tetanus shot, and sutures to close the wound (if needed).

Snakebites

Only four snake species in the United States are venomous: rattlesnakes (which account for about 65% of all venomous snakebites and nearly all the snakebite deaths in the United States), copperheads, water moccasins (also known as cottonmouths), and coral snakes ▼Figure 2. The first three are pit vipers. The coral snake is small and colorful, with a black snout and a series of bright red, yellow, and black bands around its body (every other band is yellow).

Pit Viper Bites

What to Look For

- severe burning pain at the bite site
- two small puncture wounds about $^{1}/_{2}$ inch apart (some cases may have only one fang mark) ►Figure 3
- swelling (happens within five minutes and can involve an entire extremity)
- discoloration and blood-filled blisters possibly developing in 6 to 10 hours ►Figure 4

Figure 2 Rattlesnake

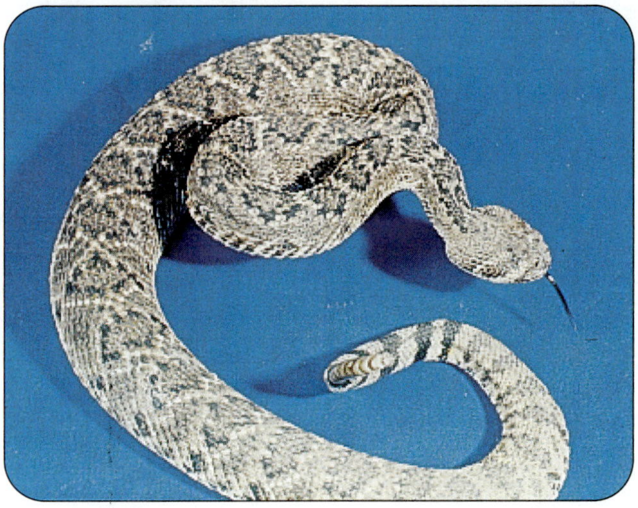

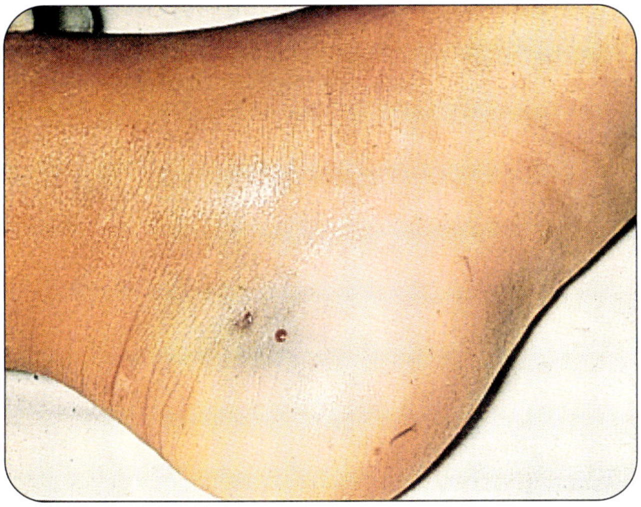

Figure 3 Rattlesnake bite (Note two fang marks)

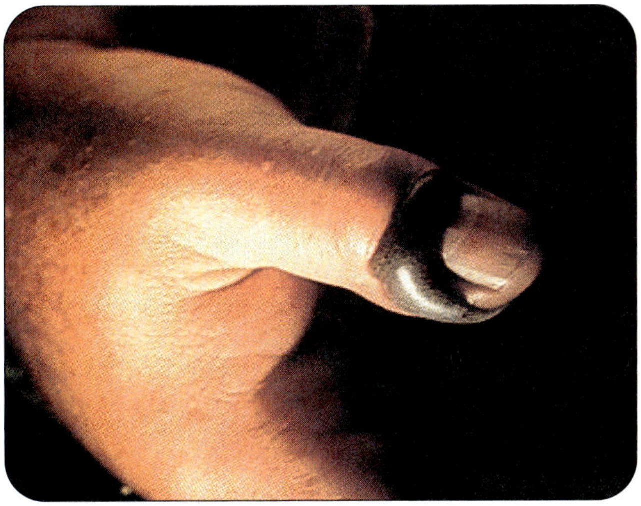

Figure 4 Copperhead bite two hours after bite

- in severe cases, nausea, vomiting, sweating, and weakness

In about 25% of poisonous snakebites, there is no venom injection, only fang and tooth wounds (known as a "dry" bite).

What to Do

Identifying the type of pit viper is of minimal importance, because the same antivenin is used in all cases in North America.

The Wilderness Medical Society lists the following guidelines for dealing with bites by pit vipers:

1. Get the victim and bystanders away from the snake. Snakes have been known to bite more than once. Pit vipers can strike as far away as one half of their body length. Be careful around a decapitated snake head—head reactions can persist for 20 minutes or more.
2. Keep the victim quiet. If possible, carry the victim or have the victim walk very slowly to help.
3. Gently wash the bitten area with soap and water.
4. If you are more than 1 hour from a medical facility with antivenin or if the snake was large and the victim's skin is swelling rapidly, immediately apply suction with the Sawyer Extractor™ ▼Figure 5. It does not require cutting the skin.
5. Seek medical attention immediately. This is the most important thing to do for the victim.

Coral Snake Bites

The coral snake is America's most venomous snake, but it rarely bites people. The coral snake has short fangs and tends to hang on and "chew" its venom into the victim rather than to strike and release, like a pit viper.

What to Do

1. Keep the victim calm.
2. Gently clean the bite site with soap and water.

Figure 5 Extractor™ use does not require cutting the skin.

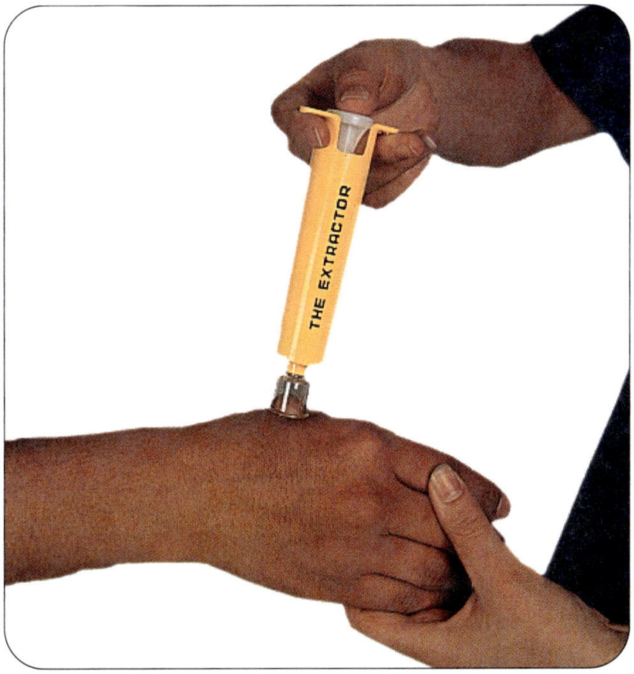

3. Apply mild pressure by wrapping an elastic bandage (eg, Ace™ bandage) over the bite site and the entire arm or leg. You should apply pressure only if the bite is from a coral snake, not any of the pit vipers. Do not cut the victim's skin or use a Sawyer Extractor™.
4. Seek medical attention for antivenin.

Nonpoisonous Snakebites

A nonpoisonous snake leaves a horseshoe shape of toothmarks on the victim's skin. If you are not positive about a snake, assume it was venomous. Some so-called nonpoisonous North American snakes such as hognose and garter snakes have venom that can cause painful local reactions but no systemic (whole-body) symptoms.

What to Do

1. Gently clean the bite site with soap and water.
2. Care for the bite as you would a minor wound.
3. Seek medical advice.

Insect Stings

Severe allergic reactions to insect stings are reported by about 0.5% of the population in the United States. Fortunately, localized pain, itching, and swelling—the most common consequences of an insect bite—can be treated with first aid.

What to Look For

A rule of thumb is that the sooner symptoms develop after a sting, the more serious the reaction will be.

What to Do

Most people who have been stung can be treated on site, and everyone should know what to do if a life-threatening allergic reaction (anaphylaxis) occurs. In particular, those who have had a severe reaction to an insect sting should be instructed on what they can do to protect themselves. They also should be advised to wear a medical-alert identification tag stating they are insect allergic.

1. Check the sting site to see if a stinger and venom sac are embedded in the skin. Bees are the only stinging insects that leave their stingers and venom sacs behind (►Figure 6). If the stinger is still embedded, remove it or it will continue to inject poison for two or three minutes. Scrape the stinger and venom sac away with a hard object such as a long fingernail, credit card, scissor edge, or knife blade. If applied in the first three minutes, a Sawyer Extractor™ can remove a portion of the venom.

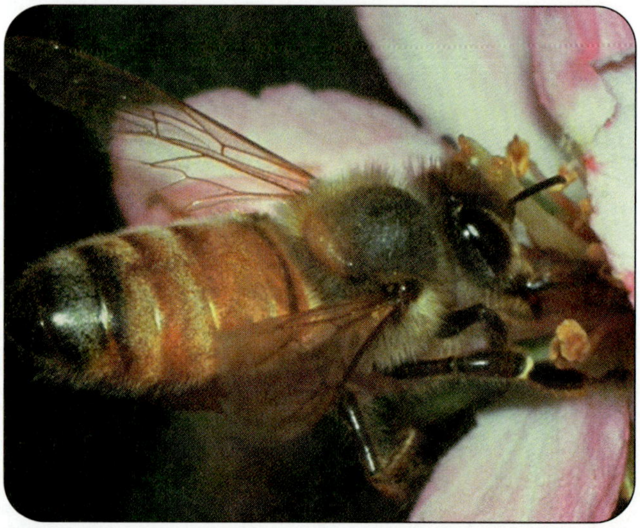

Figure 6 Honeybee

2. Wash the sting site with soap and water to prevent infection.
3. Apply an ice pack over the sting site to slow absorption of the venom and relieve pain. Because bee venom is acidic, a paste made of baking soda and water can help. Sodium bicarbonate is an alkalinizing agent that draws out fluid and reduces itching and swelling.

   Wasp venom, on the other hand, is alkaline, so apply vinegar or lemon juice.
4. To further relieve pain and itching, some type of pain medication usually is adequate. A topical steroid cream, such as hydrocortisone, can help combat local swelling and itching. An antihistamine may prevent some local symptoms and later reactions if given early, but it works too slowly to counteract a life-threatening allergic reaction.
5. Observe the victim for at least 30 minutes for signs of an allergic reaction. Epinephrine is an effective treatment for a person with a severe allergic reaction. A person with a known allergy to insect stings should have a physician-prescribed emergency kit that includes prefilled syringes of epinephrine. Because epinephrine is short-acting, watch the victim closely for signs of returning anaphylaxis. Inject another dose of epinephrine as often as every 15 minutes if needed, available, and consistent with the directions for use in the kit.

Spider Bites

Most spiders are venomous, which is how they paralyze and kill their prey. But spiders lack an effective delivery system (long fangs and strong jaws) to bite a human. Death occurs rarely and only from bites by brown recluse and black widow spiders.

A spider bite is difficult to diagnose, especially when the spider was not seen or recovered, because the bites typically cause little immediate pain.

Black Widow Spiders

Black widow spiders have round abdomens that vary in color from gray to brown to black, depending on the species ▼Figure 7. In the female black widow, the abdomen is shiny black with a red or yellow spot (often in the shape of an hourglass) or white spots or bands. Black widow spiders are found throughout the world.

What to Look For

It is difficult to determine if a person has been bitten by a black widow spider or, for that matter, by any spider.

- The victim may feel a sharp pinprick when the spider bites, but some victims are not even aware of the bite. Within 15 minutes, a dull, numbing pain develops in the bite area.

Figure 7 Black widow spider. Note red hourglass configuration on abdomen.

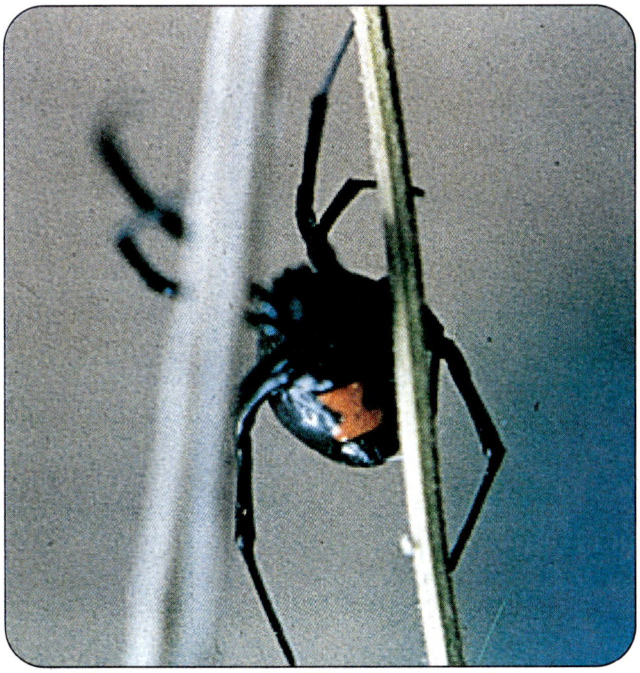

- Two small fang marks might be seen as tiny red spots.
- Within 15 minutes to four hours, muscle stiffness and cramps occur, usually affecting the abdomen when the bite is on a lower part of the body and the shoulders, back, or chest when the bite is on an upper part. Victims often describe the pain as the most severe they have ever experienced.
- Headache, chills, fever, heavy sweating, dizziness, nausea, and vomiting appear next. Severe pain around the bite site peaks in two to three hours and can last 12 to 48 hours.

Brown Recluse Spiders

Brown recluse spiders are also known in North America as fiddle-back or violin spiders ►Figure 8A. They have a violin-shaped figure on their backs (several other spider species have a similar configuration on their backs). Color varies from fawn to dark brown, with darker legs.

Brown recluse spiders are found primarily in the southern and midwestern states, with other, less toxic, related spiders throughout the rest of the country. They are absent from the Pacific Northwest where the aggressive house spider, also known as the hobo spider, is found and causes injuries similar to those of the brown recluse

What to Look For

- A local reaction usually occurs within two to eight hours with mild to severe pain at the bite site and redness, swelling, and local itching.
- In 48 to 72 hours, a blister develops at the bite site, becomes red, and bursts. During the early stages, the affected area often takes on a bull's-eye appearance, with a central white area surrounded by a reddened area, ringed by a whitish or blue border ►Figure 8B. A small, red crater remains, over which a scab forms. When that scab falls away in a few days, a larger crater remains. That also scabs over and falls off, leaving a yet larger crater. The craters are known as volcano lesions. This process of slow tissue destruction can continue for weeks or even months. The ulcer sometimes requires skin grafting.
- Fever, weakness, vomiting, joint pain, and a rash may occur.
- Stomach cramps, nausea, and vomiting may occur.

Tarantulas

Tarantulas bite only when vigorously provoked or roughly handled. The bite varies from almost painless to a deep throbbing pain lasting up to 1 hour. The tarantula, when upset, will roughly scratch the lower surface of its abdomen with its legs and flick hairs onto the invader's skin. The hairs cause itching and hives that can last several weeks. Treatment is cortisone cream and antihistamines.

What to Do (for All Spider Bites)

1. If possible, catch the spider to confirm its identity. Even if the body has been crushed, save it for identification (although most spider-bite victims never see the spider). The species helps determine the treatment, so the dead spider (if it can be found) should be taken with the victim to the hospital.
2. Clean the bite area with soap and water or rubbing alcohol.
3. Place an ice pack over the bite to relieve pain and delay the effects of the venom.
4. Monitor ABC.
5. Seek medical attention immediately. An antivenin exists for black widow spider bites. It is usually reserved for children (under 6 years), the elderly (over 60 and with high blood pressure), pregnant women, and victims with severe reactions. The antivenin will give relief within 1 to 3 hours. Antivenin for brown recluse and other spider bites is not currently available.

Figure 8A Brown recluse spider. Note violin or fiddle configuration on back.

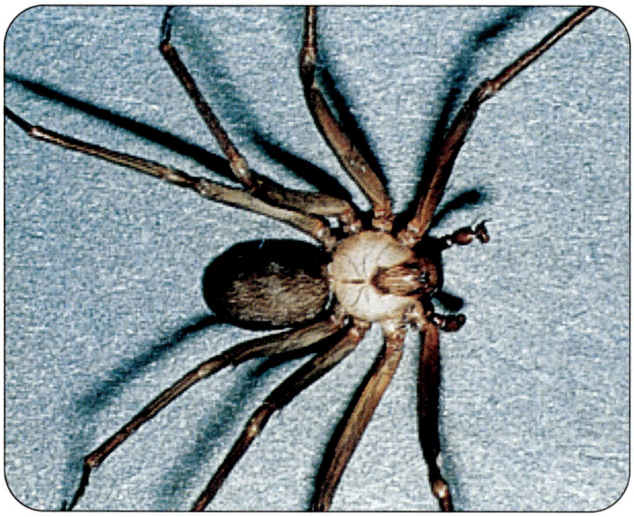

Figure 8B Brown recluse spider bite. Note bull's-eye approach.

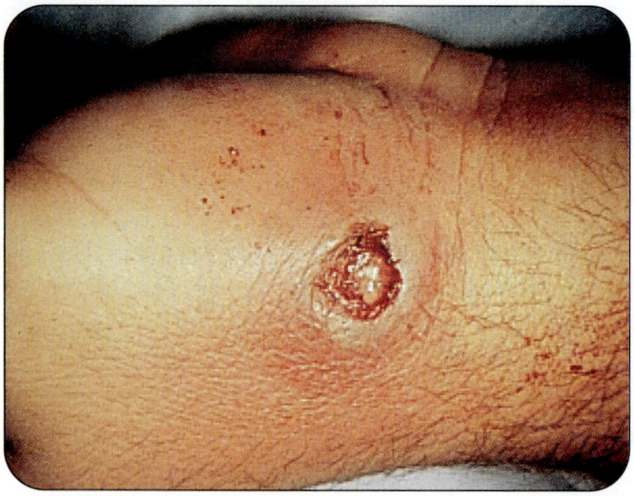

Scorpion Stings

Scorpions look like miniature lobsters, with lobster-like pincers and a long upcurved "tail" with a poisonous stinger ▼Figure 9. Several species of scorpions inhabit the southwestern United States, but only the bark scorpion poses a threat to humans.

What to Look For

The most frequent symptom of a scorpion sting, especially in an adult victim, is local, immediate pain and burning around the sting site. Later, numbness or tingling occurs.

Figure 9 Scorpion

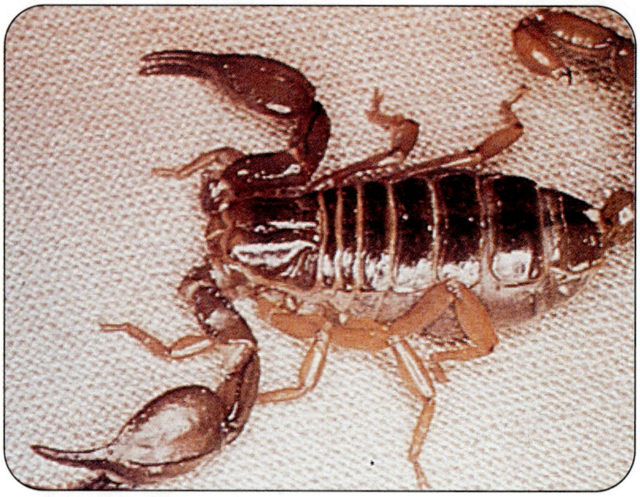

What to Do

1. Monitor ABCs.
2. Gently clean the sting site with soap and water or rubbing alcohol.
3. Apply an ice pack over the sting site.
4. Seek medical attention. Small children are prime candidates for receiving antivenin. An antivenin is available only in Arizona.

Embedded Ticks

Removing Ticks

Remove ticks as soon as possible. If a tick is carrying a disease, the longer it stays embedded, the greater the chance of the disease being transmitted.

Because its bite is painless, a tick can remain embedded for days without the victim's realizing it ▼Figure 10. Most tick bites are harmless, although ticks can carry serious diseases.

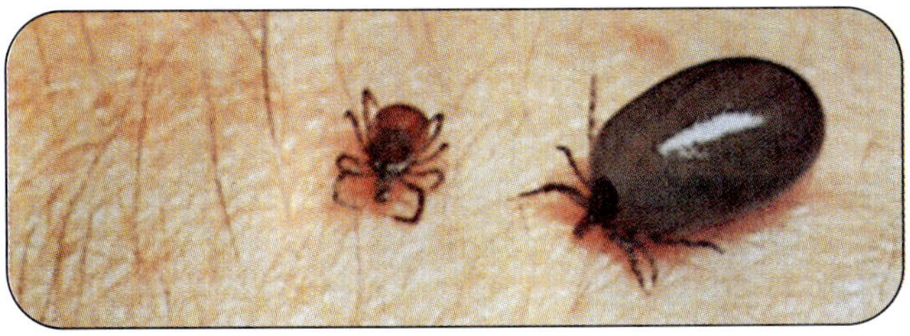

Figure 10 Deer ticks: not engorged and blood engorged

1. To pull a tick off ▼Figure 11,
   - Use tweezers or one of the specialized tick-removal tools. Grasp the tick as close to the skin as possible and lift the tick with enough force to "tent" the skin surface. Hold in this position until the tick lets go. This may take several seconds.
2. Wash the bite site with soap and water. Apply rubbing alcohol to further disinfect the area.
3. Apply an ice pack to reduce pain.
4. Apply calamine lotion to relieve any itching. Keep the area clean.
5. Continue to watch the bite site for one month for a rash. If a rash appears, see a physician. Watch for other signs such as fever, muscle aches, sensitivity to bright light, and paralysis that begins with leg weakness.

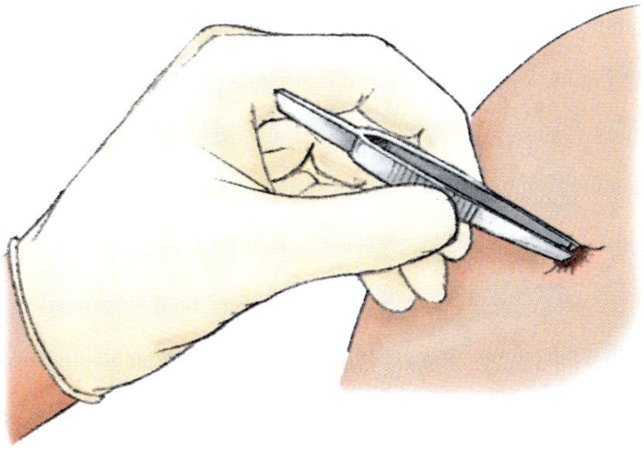

Figure 11 Removing a tick with tweezers

Learning Activities

Bites and Stings

Directions: Circle Yes if you agree with the statement, and circle No if you disagree.

Yes No **1.** Report animal bites to the police or animal control officers.

Yes No **2.** Apply cold or ice over a snakebite.

Yes No **3.** Use the "cut-and-suck" method for a snakebite.

Yes No **4.** In remote settings, suction snake venom out with a Sawyer Extractor™.

Yes No **5.** Apply a cold or ice pack over an insect sting or a suspected spider bite.

Yes No **6.** A baking soda paste can help reduce the itching and swelling from an insect sting.

Yes No **7.** A victim's doctor-prescribed epinephrine may have to be given if the victim has a life-threatening reaction to an insect sting.

Yes No **8.** Spider bite antivenin is available for only black widow spider bites, and not all victims need it.

Yes No **9.** A capsule with antihistamine or cortisone ointment or tablet can be useful for mosquito bites.

Yes No **10.** Applying a blown-out, glowing match head or heated needle will cause an embedded tick to back out of a victim's skin.

Yes No **11.** Cover an embedded tick with heavy oil or grease to make the tick back out because of lack of oxygen.

Scenario #1: A mail carrier is heard crying for help while being attacked by a neighbor's large dog. The dog's owner calls off the dog and takes it inside his house. You run up the street and help the victim over to a nearby yard. You find several severe bite marks on the mail carrier's legs and arms. What should you do?

____

____

Scenario #2: You rush to a vacant lot to help a young woman who is calling for help. She says that some type of snake bit her on the leg. You see two puncture wounds (fang marks) on her leg. What should you do?

____

____

Scenario #3: A garden shop employee complains about her face swelling and a feeling of tightness across her chest. She is having some breathing difficulty. She says a bee stung her. She has a medical alert tag around her neck indicating an allergy to insects. She tells you that she has medication for such an emergency. There is an ice machine nearby. What should you do?

____

____

Scenario #4: While resting during lunch in the patio behind your office building, you feel a sharp pinprick on your arm. About 15 minutes later, a dull, numbing pain develops in your back. You look at your arm and see two tiny red spots. About an hour later, abdominal cramping starts and steadily gets worse. What should you do?

____

____

Scenario #5: On a Monday morning, one of your co-workers returns from a weekend camping trip. When he rubs the back of his head, he feels a bump and asks you to look at it. You see a tick embedded in his scalp. What should you do?

____

____

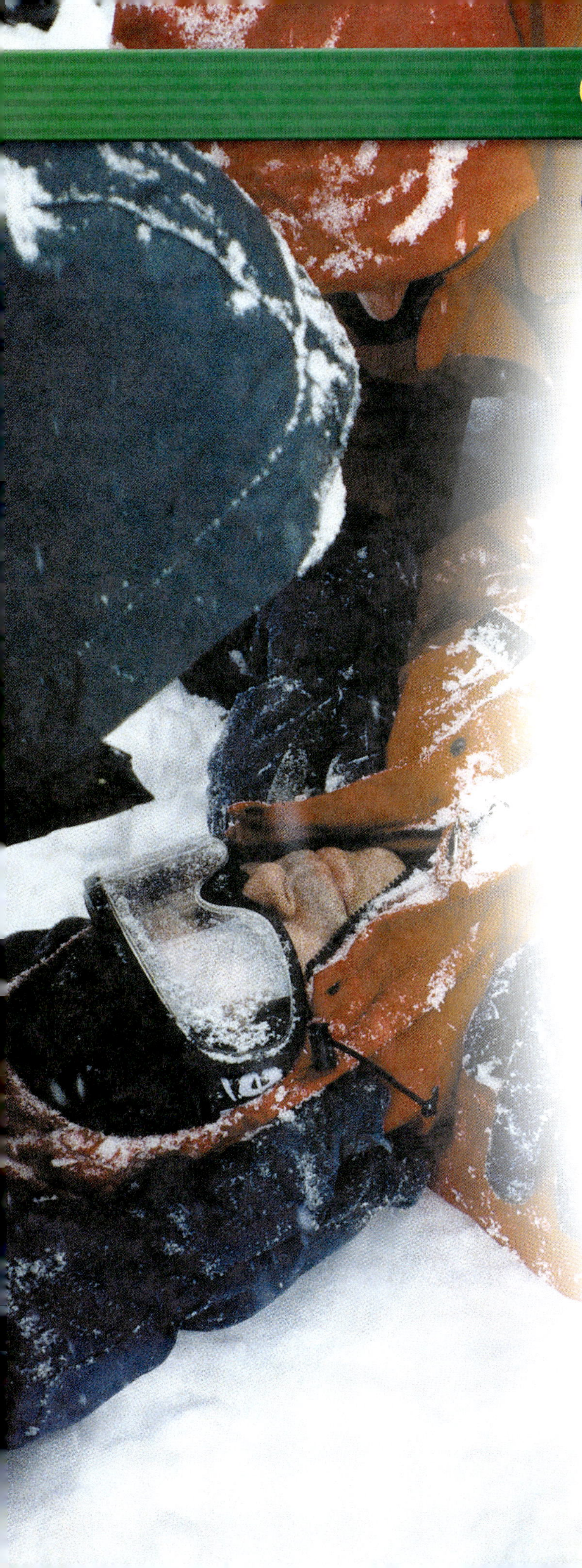

Chapter 15

Cold-Related Emergencies

Freezing Injuries

Most injuries from cold are confined to exposed areas of the body, such as the face, or to extremities such as the fingers, and toes ▶Figure 1. Freezing cold injuries can occur whenever the air temperature is below freezing (32°F). Freezing limited to the skin surface is frostnip. Freezing that extends deeper through the skin and into the flesh is frostbite.

Frostnip is caused by water freezing on the skin surface. The skin becomes reddened and possibly swollen. Although frostnip is painful, there usually is no further damage after rewarming. Repeated frostnip in the same spot can dry the skin, causing it to crack and to become sensitive. It is difficult to tell the difference between frostnip and frostbite. Frostnip should be taken seriously because it may be the first sign of impending frostbite.

To treat frostnip:

1. Gently warm the affected area by placing it against a warm body part (eg, put bare hands under the armpits or on the stomach or blow warm air on the area).
2. Do not rub the area. After rewarming, the affected area may be red and tingling.

Frostbite occurs when temperatures drop below freezing. Frostbite affects mainly the feet, hands, ears, and nose. These areas do not contain large heat-producing muscles and are some distance from the body's heat-generating sources. The most severe consequences of frostbite are gangrene and amputation.

What to Look For

The exact severity and extent of frostbite are difficult to judge until hours after thawing, although before thawing it can be classified as *superficial* or *deep*. Even physicians have to wait until thawing has occurred before they can judge the extent of the injury.

FROSTBITE

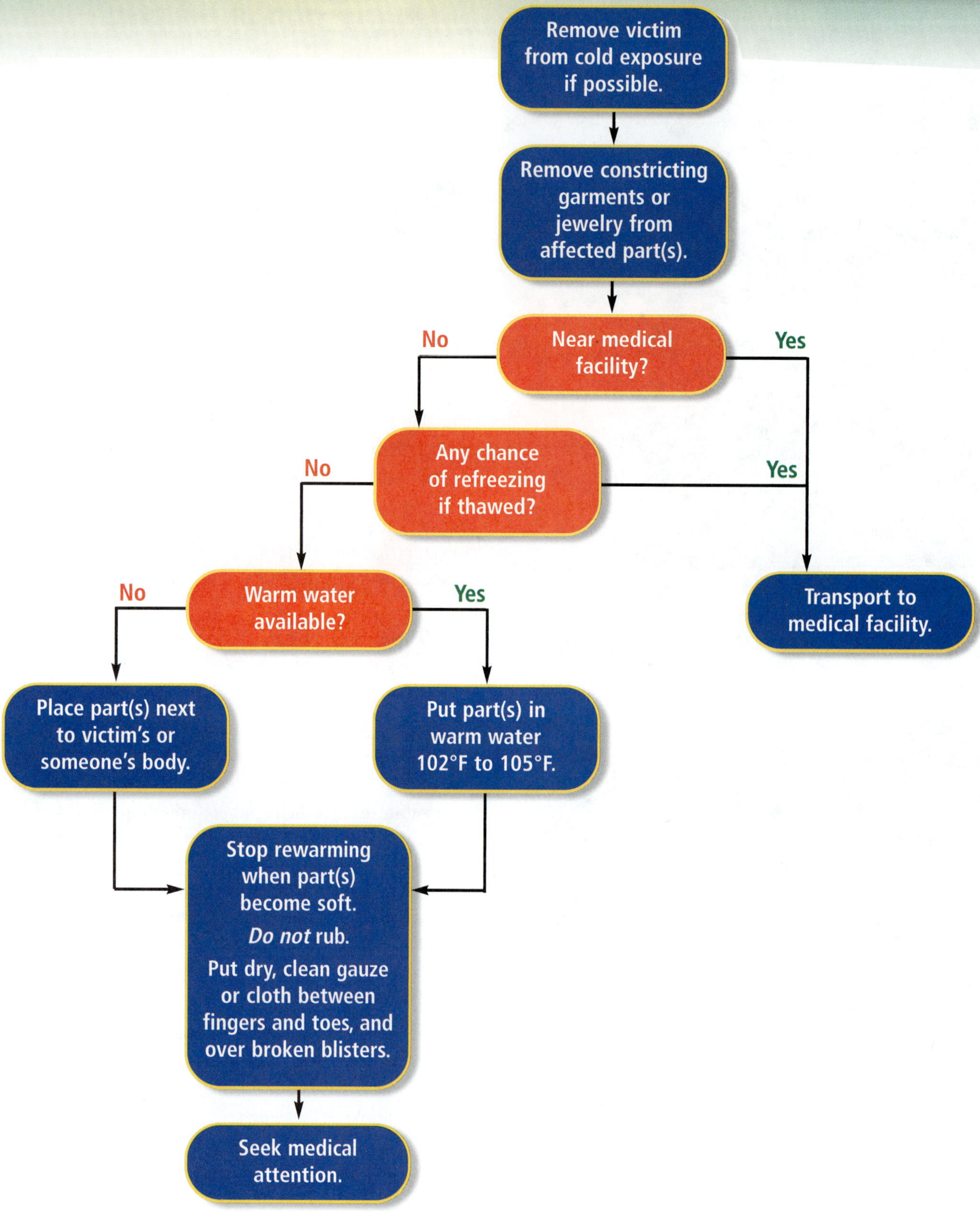

Remove victim from cold exposure if possible.
Remove constricting garments or jewelry from affected part(s).
Near medical facility?
No
Yes
Any chance of refreezing if thawed?
No
Yes
Transport to medical facility.
Warm water available?
No
Yes
Place part(s) next to victim's or someone's body.
Put part(s) in warm water 102°F to 105°F.
Stop rewarming when part(s) become soft.
Do not rub.
Put dry, clean gauze or cloth between fingers and toes, and over broken blisters.
Seek medical attention.

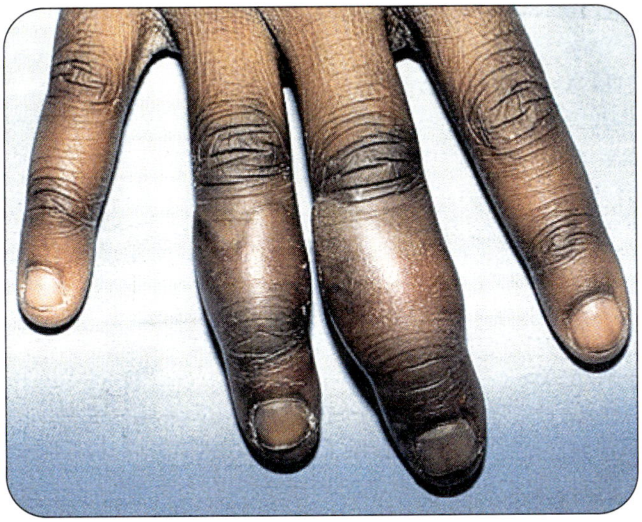

Figure 1 Frostbitten fingers, 6 hours after rewarming in 106° water

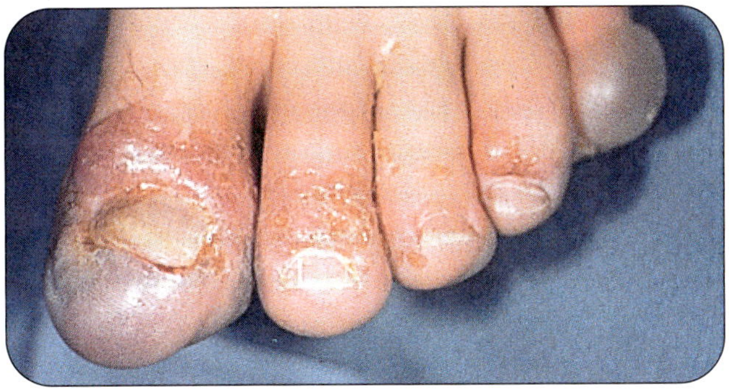

Figure 2 Second-degree frostbite

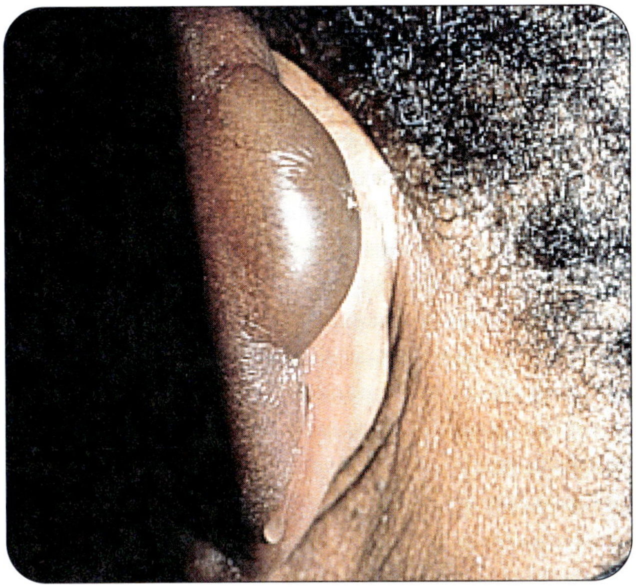

Figure 3 Frostbitten ear 8 hours old

The signs and symptoms of superficial frostbite are as follows:

- Skin color is white, waxy, or grayish-yellow.
- The affected part feels very cold and numb. There may be tingling, stinging, or aching sensations.
- The skin surface feels stiff or crusty and the underlying tissue feels soft when depressed gently and firmly.

Deep frostbite is indicated by the following signs and symptoms:

- The affected part feels cold, hard, and solid and cannot be depressed.
- The affected part is cold, with pale, waxy skin.
- A painfully cold part suddenly stops hurting.
- Blisters may appear after rewarming ▶Figures 2 and 3.

After a part has thawed, frostbite can be categorized by degrees, similar to the burn classifications.

What to Do

Frostbite injuries require the following first aid treatment.

1. Get the victim out of the cold and into a warm place.
2. Remove any clothing or constricting items that could impair blood circulation (eg, rings).
3. Seek immediate medical attention.
4. Place dry, sterile gauze between toes and the fingers to absorb moisture and to keep them from sticking together.
5. Slightly elevate the affected part to reduce pain and swelling.

If the victim is in a remote or wilderness situation (more than 1 hour from a medical facility), and you have warm water, use the following wet, rapid rewarming method.

1. Place the frostbitten part in warm (102°F to 105°F) water. If you do not have a thermometer, pour some of the water over the inside of your arm or put your elbow into it to test that it is warm, not hot. Maintain water temperature by adding warm water as needed. Rewarming usually takes 20 to 40 minutes or until the tissues are soft. For ear or facial injuries, apply warm moist cloths, changing them frequently.
2. After thawing,
   - Treat victim as a "stretcher" case—the feet will be impossible to use after they are rewarmed.

- Protect the affected area from contact with clothing and bedding.
- Place dry, sterile gauze between the toes and the fingers to absorb moisture and to keep them from sticking together.
- Slightly elevate the affected part to reduce pain and swelling.
- Apply aloe vera gel to promote skin healing.
- Give the victim aspirin (adults only) or ibuprofen to limit pain and inflammation.

Hypothermia

Body temperature falls when the body cannot produce heat as fast as it is being lost. Hypothermia is a life-threatening condition when the body's core temperature falls below 95°F.

Hypothermia can happen indoors, in the southern states, and even on a summer day. It does not require subfreezing temperatures.

What to Look For

- *Change in mental status.* This is one of the first symptoms of developing hypothermia. Examples are disorientation, apathy, and changes in personality, such as unusual aggressiveness.
- *Shivering.* Shivering is the first and most important body defense against a falling body temperature. *Shivering* starts when the body temperature drops 1°F *and can produce more heat than many rewarming methods.* As the core temperature continues to fall, however, shivering stops at about 90°F. Shivering also stops as body temperature rises. If shivering stops as responsiveness decreases, assume that the core temperature is falling. If, on the other hand, shivering stops as the victim is becoming more coordinated and feeling better, assume that the core temperature is rising.
- *Cool abdomen.* Place the back of your hand between the clothing and the victim's abdomen to assess the victim's temperature. When the victim's abdominal skin under clothing is cooler than your hand, consider the victim hypothermic until proved otherwise.
- *Low core body temperature.* The best indicator of hypothermia is a thermometer reading of the core body temperature. Normal thermometers do not register below 94°F and so do not indicate whether the hypothermia is mild or severe. While thermometers exist that register below 90°F, measuring rectal temperatures is seldom done, mainly because low-reading rectal thermometers usually are not readily available, and taking a rectal temperature can be difficult, inconvenient, and embarrassing to victim and rescuer. If done outdoors, such a procedure can expose the already cold victim.

Types of Hypothermia

In severe hypothermia, the victim becomes so cold that shivering stops. That means the victim's body cannot rewarm itself internally and will require external heat for recovery.

Victims of mild hypothermia have a core body temperature above 90°F. Symptoms are shivering, slurred speech, memory lapses, and fumbling hands. Victims frequently stumble and stagger, but they are usually responsive and can talk. Mild hypothermia victims will have the "-umbles": grumbles, mumbles, fumbles, and stumbles.

What to Do

1. For all hypothermic victims, stop further heat loss:
   - Get the victim out of the cold.
   - Add insulation such as blankets, towels, pillows, or newspapers beneath and around the victim. Cover the victim's head (50% to 80% of the body's heat loss is through the head).
   - Replace wet clothing with dry clothing.
   - Handle the victim gently. Rough handling can cause cardiac arrest.
   - Keep the victim in a horizontal (flat) position.
2. Call EMS. Remember that hypothermia is more common in urban settings than in the wilderness.

Adding heat to a victim is extremely difficult. The longer the victim is exposed to the cold, the longer it will take to raise the core temperature to normal. Trying to rewarm a hypothermic victim may cause cardiac arrest.

Although surface rewarming suppresses shivering, it may be the only option when the victim is far from medical care. In that case, the victim must be warmed by any available external heat source.

HYPOTHERMIA

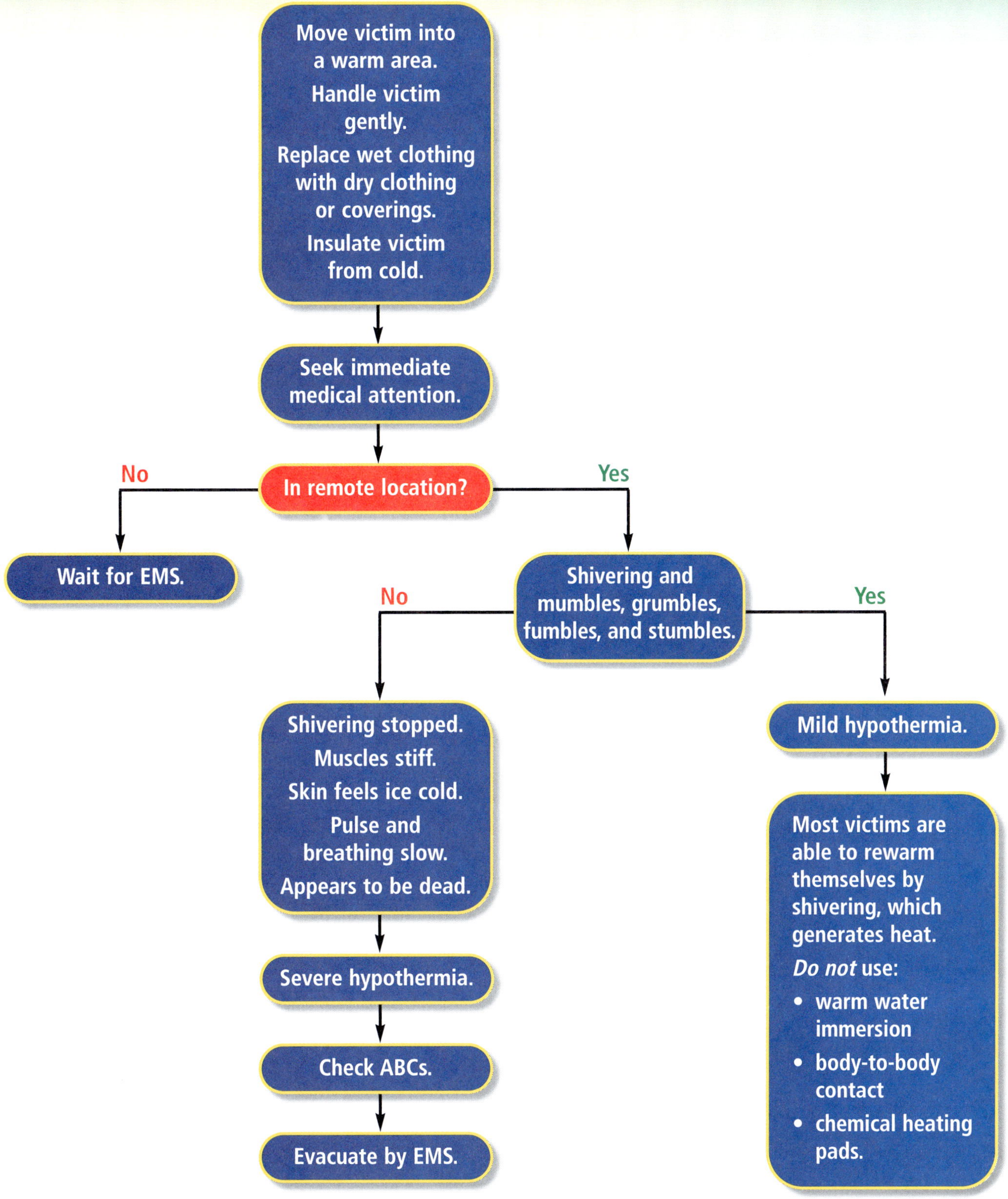

Learning Activities

Frostbite

Directions: Circle Yes if you agree with the statement, and circle No if you disagree.

Yes No **1.** Rub or massage to rewarm a frostbitten part.

Yes No **2.** Frostbite damage becomes more severe if the affected area thaws and then refreezes.

Yes No **3.** It's best to rewarm a frostbitten part by using warm water.

Yes No **4.** Placing frostbitten hands in another person's armpits is the best rewarming method.

Yes No **5.** When near a hospital, it's best to let medical personnel thaw the frostbitten part.

Scenario: In subfreezing temperatures during a snowstorm, you find a stalled truck on a little-used road. Inside the truck is an elderly man, who tells you that his truck is out of gasoline and that when he tried to refill the truck's gas tank he dropped the gas can and some of the gasoline spilled on his hands. He has been stranded for over 3 hours. The man complains of numb fingers and cold feet. He did not know about a cabin about a quarter mile away. What should you do?

____

____

____

____

Hypothermia

Yes No **1.** Add insulation (blankets) around and under the victim.

Yes No **2.** Replace wet clothing with dry clothing.

Yes No **3.** Shivering is sufficient to rewarm a mild hypothermic victim.

Yes No **4.** For mild hypothermia, applying chemical heat packs or using a rescuer's body heat are preferred methods of rewarming a victim.

Yes No **5.** Severe hypothermic victims should be transported to a hospital for rewarming.

Yes No **6.** Check the pulse of a severely hypothermic victim for at least 30 to 45 seconds.

Scenario: It is a cold winter day so you decide to check on your 80-year-old grandfather, who lives alone. As you enter his home, you notice that it is not much warmer inside the house than it is outside. You find your grandfather wrapped in a blanket lying on top of his bed. You speak to him, but you get only mumbling. He is severely shivering. What should you do?

____

____

____

____

Chapter 16

Heat-Related Emergencies

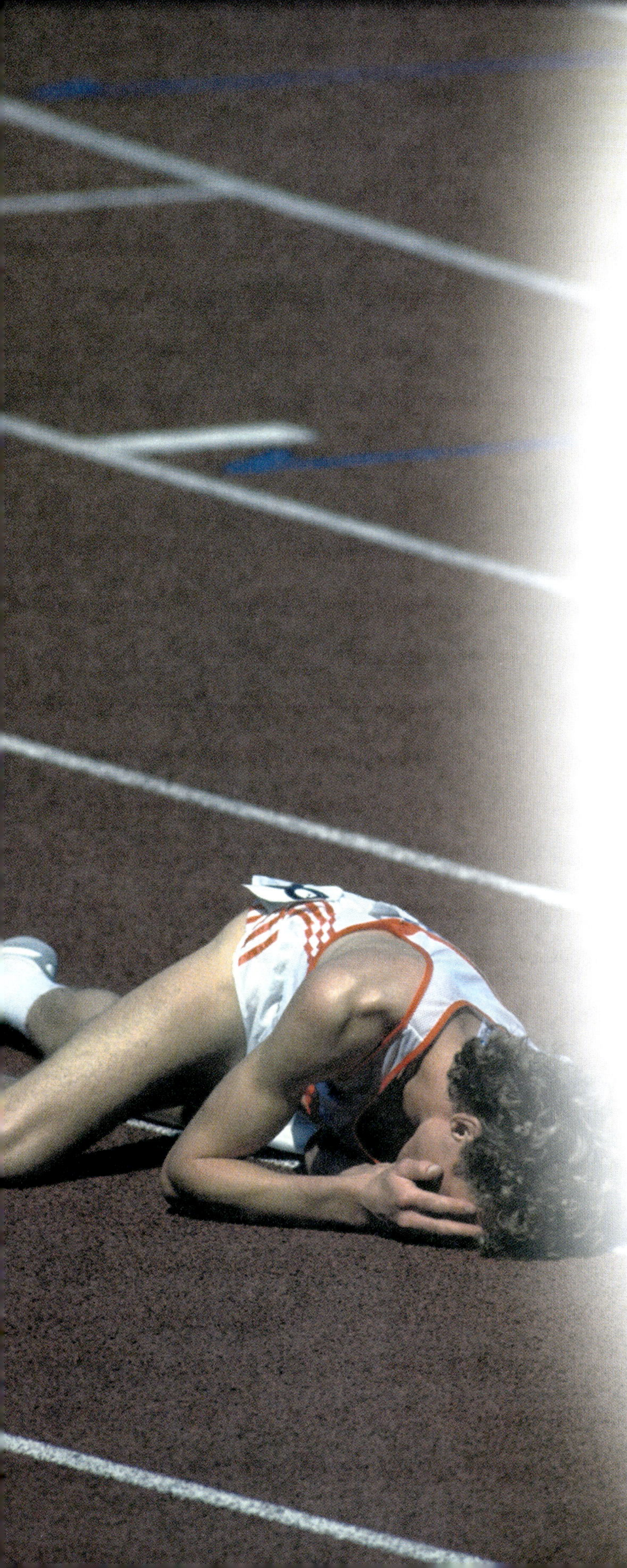

Heat Illnesses

Heat illnesses include a range of disorders. Some of them are common, but only heatstroke is life-threatening. Untreated heatstroke victims always die.

Heat Cramps

Heat cramps are painful muscular spasms that happen suddenly, usually immediately after exertion. They usually involve the muscles in the back of the leg (calf and hamstring muscles) or the abdominal muscles. Some experts claim they are caused by salt depletion. Victims may be drinking fluids that do not have adequate salt content. However, other experts disagree, claiming the typical American diet is heavy with salt.

Heat Exhaustion

Heat exhaustion is characterized by heavy perspiration with normal or slightly above normal body temperatures. It is caused by water or salt depletion or both. Some experts believe that a better term would be severe dehydration. Heat exhaustion affects workers and athletes who do not drink enough fluids while working or exercising in hot environments. Symptoms include severe thirst, fatigue, headache, nausea, vomiting, and sometimes diarrhea. The affected person often mistakenly believes he or she has the flu. Uncontrolled heat exhaustion can evolve into heatstroke.

Heatstroke

Two types of heatstroke exist: classic and exertional. Classic heatstroke, also known as the "slow cooker," may take days to develop. It is often seen during summer heat waves and typically affects the poor, elderly, chronically ill, alcoholic, or obese. Because the elderly, who often have medical problems, are frequently afflicted, this type of

HEAT-RELATED EMERGENCIES

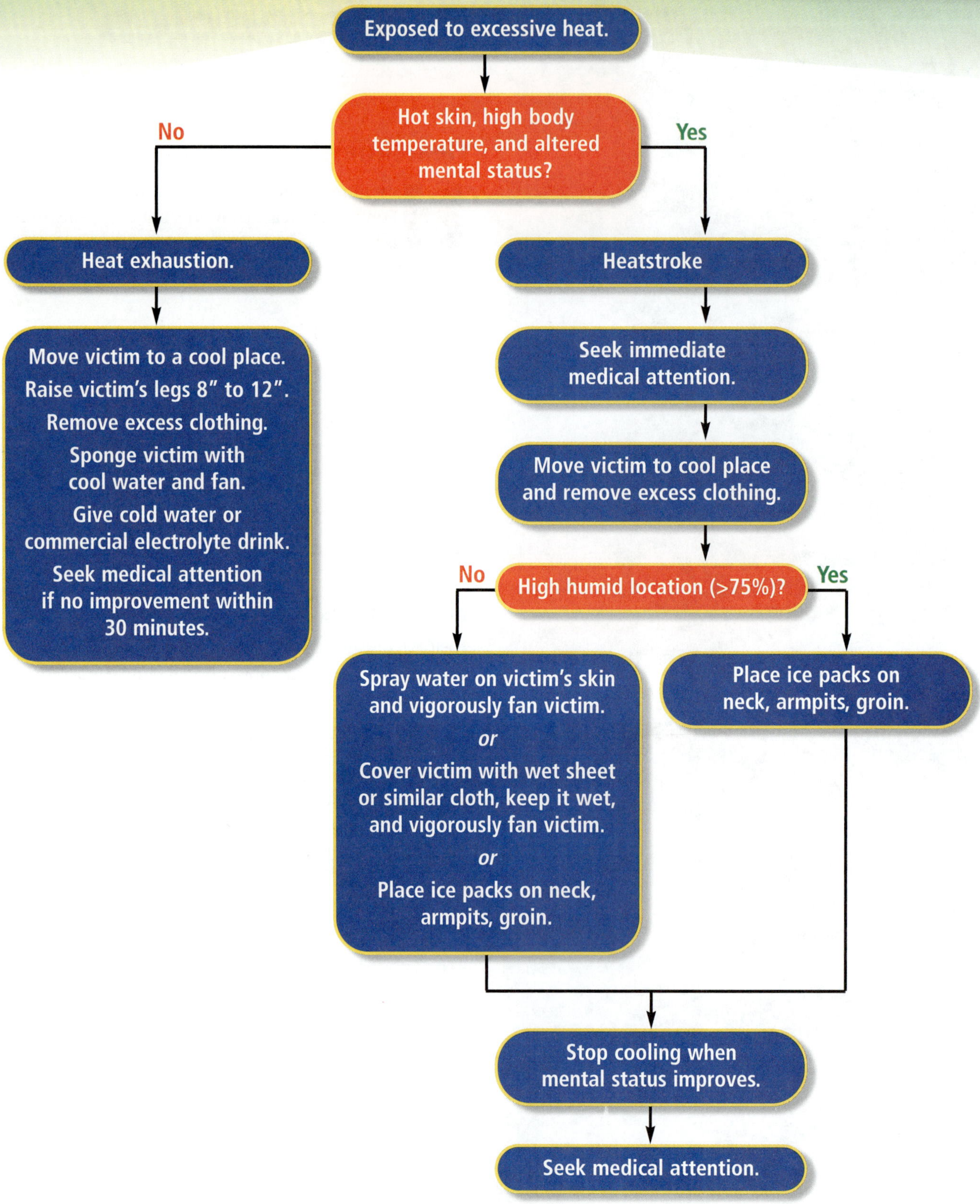

heatstroke has a 50% death rate, even with medical care. It results from a combination of a hot environment and dehydration. Exertional heatstroke is also more common in the summer. It is frequently seen in athletes, laborers, and military personnel, all of whom often sweat profusely. This type of heatstroke is known as the "fast cooker." It affects healthy, active individuals who are strenuously working or playing in a warm environment. Because its rapid onset does not allow enough time for severe dehydration to occur, 50% of exertional heatstroke victims usually are sweating. (Classic heatstroke victims are not sweating.)

There are several ways to tell the difference between heat exhaustion and heatstroke. First, if the victim's body feels extremely hot when touched, suspect heatstroke. Another major mark of heatstroke is altered mental status (behavior), ranging from slight confusion and disorientation to coma. Between those extreme conditions, victims usually become irrational, agitated, or even aggressive and may have seizures. In severe cases, the victim can go into a coma in less than an hour. The longer a coma lasts, the less the chance for survival.

A third way to distinguish heatstroke from heat exhaustion is by rectal temperature. That is not very practical, however, because a responsive heatstroke victim may not cooperate. Taking a rectal temperature can be embarrassing to both victim and rescuer. Moreover, rectal thermometers are seldom available.

What to Do

Heat Cramps

To relieve heat cramps (it may take several hours), follow these steps:

1. Rest in a cool place.
2. Drink lightly salted cool water (dissolve ¼ teaspoon salt in a quart of water) or a commercial sports drink.
3. Stretch the cramped calf muscle, or try an acupressure method: pinch the upper lip just below the nose.

Heat Exhaustion

1. Move the victim immediately out of the heat to a cool place.
2. Give cool liquids, adding electrolytes (lightly salted water or a commercial sports drink) if plain water does not improve the victim's condition in 20 minutes. Do not give salt tablets; they can irritate the stomach and cause nausea and vomiting.
3. Raise the victim's legs 8 to 12 inches (keep the legs straight).
4. Remove excess clothing.
5. Sponge with cool water and fan the victim.
6. If you don't see any improvement within 30 minutes, seek medical attention.

Heatstroke

Heatstroke is a medical emergency and must be treated rapidly! Every minute delayed increases the likelihood of serious complications or death.

1. Seek immediate medical attention, even if the victim seems to be recovering.
2. Move the victim immediately out of the heat to a cool place.
3. Remove all clothing down to the victim's underwear.
4. Keep the victim's head and shoulders slightly elevated.
5. The only way to prevent damage is to cool the victim quickly and by any means possible. Cooling methods include the following:
   - *Spraying* the victim with water and then *fanning*. The water droplets act as artificial sweat and will cool through evaporation. This method is not effective in high-humidity (more than 75%) conditions.
   - Place ice bags against the large veins in the groin, arm-pits, and sides of the neck to cool the body regardless of the humidity.

Learning Activities

Heat-Related Emergencies

Directions: Circle Yes if you agree with the statement, and circle No if you disagree.

Yes No **1.** For heat cramps, stretch a cramped leg muscle.

Yes No **2.** Salt tablets can be given to victims of any heat illness.

Yes No **3.** Move heat illness victims out of the heat to a cool place.

Yes No **4.** Heat exhaustion victims need immediate medical attention—it's a life-threatening condition.

Yes No **5.** Heatstroke victims need immediate cooling by any means possible.

Yes No **6.** Apply rubbing alcohol on a heatstroke victim's skin for cooling.

Yes No **7.** If in high humidity conditions, wet down or spray and fan the heatstroke victim.

Yes No **8.** In low humidity conditions, only cold or ice packs applied to the neck, armpits, and groin will work well to cool a heatstroke victim.

Scenario #1: A teenager's summer job is mowing lawns for various companies in an industrial park. He is sweating heavily on a very hot, humid day. He complains about being very thirsty, nauseous, and having a headache. What should you do?

____

____

____

Scenario #2: On your vacation, you spend a day at a large amusement park. It is an extremely hot and humid day. During the afternoon, you decide to rest and watch one of the special shows. Soon after you sit down, an elderly man in front of you suddenly falls forward out of his seat. When you reach him, his wife reports that they have been walking around the park practically all day without stopping. His skin feels very hot and dry, and he is unresponsive. What should you do?

____

____

____

Scenario #3: In January, a high-ranking company official from Buffalo has flown to Florida to inspect a new assembly plant. He is accustomed to the cold conditions of the north but not to the heat and humidity of the southeast. He spent the morning inspecting the new plant. Satisfied with what he's seen, he accepts an invitation to golf in the afternoon. While putting at the sixteenth hole, he becomes dizzy and faints, but soon becomes responsive. What should you do?

____

____

____

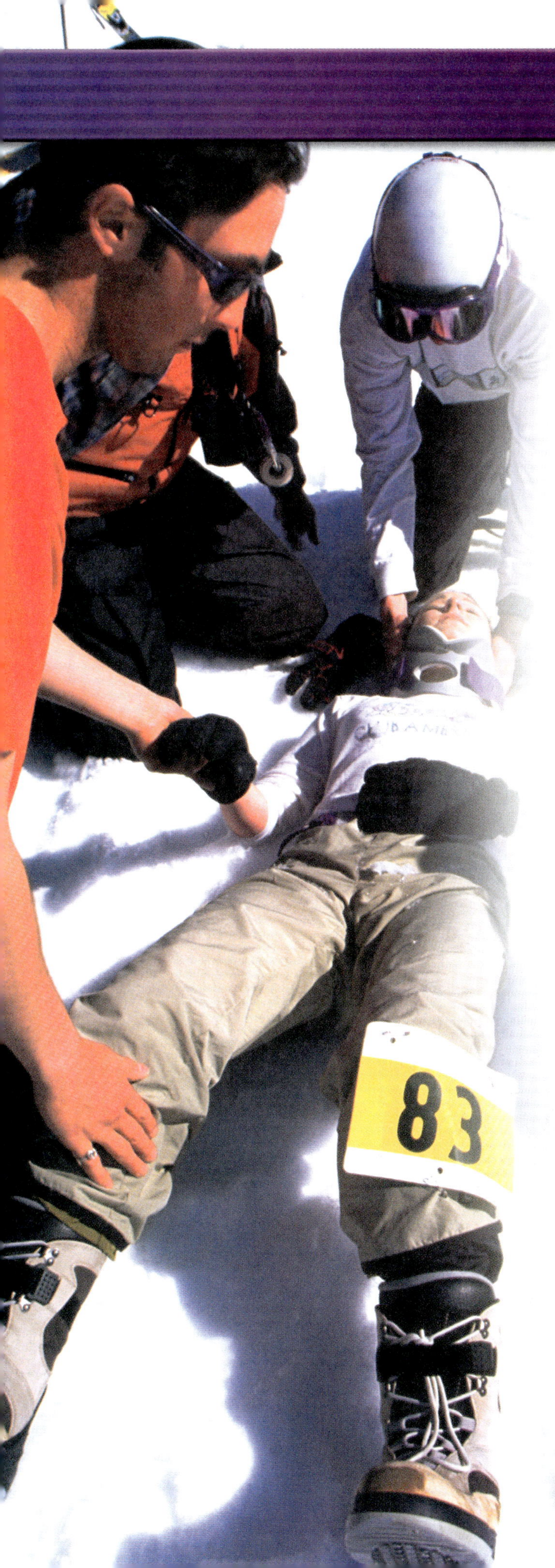

Chapter 17

Rescuing and Moving Victims

Victim Rescue

Water Rescue

Reach-throw-row-go identifies the sequence for attempting a water rescue. The first and simplest rescue technique is to *reach* for the victim. Reaching requires a lightweight pole, ladder, long stick, or any object that can be extended to the victim. Once you have your "reacher," secure your footing and have a bystander grab your belt or pants for stability. Secure yourself before reaching for the victim.

You can *throw* anything that floats—empty picnic jug, empty fuel or paint can, life jacket, floating cushion, piece of wood, inflated spare wheel—whatever is available. If there is a rope handy, tie it to the object to be thrown so you can pull the victim in, or, if you miss, you can retrieve the object and throw it again. The average untrained rescuer has a throwing range of about 50 feet.

If the victim is out of throwing range and there is a rowboat, canoe, motor boat, or boogie board nearby, you can try to *row* to the victim. Maneuvering these craft requires skills learned through practice. Wear a personal flotation device (PFD) for your own safety. To avoid capsizing, never pull the victim in over the side of a boat; pull over the stern (rear end).

If the reach–throw–row techniques are impossible and you are a capable swimmer trained in water lifesaving procedures, you can *go* to the drowning victim by swimming. Entering even calm water makes a swimming rescue difficult and hazardous. All too often a would-be rescuer becomes a victim as well.

Caution:

DO NOT swim to and grasp a drowning person unless you are trained to make the rescue.

Ice Rescue

If a person has fallen through the ice near the shore, extend a pole or throw a line with a floatable object attached to it. When the person has hold of the object, pull him or her toward the shore or the edge of the ice.

If the person has fallen through the ice away from the shore and you cannot reach him or her with a pole or a throwing line, lie flat and push a ladder, plank, or similar object ahead of you. You can tie a rope to a spare tire and the other end to an anchor point, lie flat, and push the wheel ahead of you. Pull the person ashore or to the edge of the ice.

Caution:

DO NOT go near broken ice without support.

Electrical Emergency Rescue

Electrical injuries can be devastating. Just a mild shock can cause serious internal injuries. A current of 1,000 volts or more is considered high voltage, but even the 110 volts of household current can be deadly.

When a person gets an electric shock, electricity enters the body at the point of contact and travels along the path of least resistance (nerves and blood vessels). The current travels rapidly, generating heat and causing destruction.

Most indoor electrocutions are caused by faulty electrical equipment or careless use of electrical appliances. Before you touch the victim, turn off the electricity at the circuit breaker, fuse box, or outside switch box or unplug the appliance (if the plug is undamaged).

If the electrocution involves high-voltage *power lines*, the power must be turned off before anyone approaches a victim. If you approach a victim and feel a tingling sensation in your legs and lower body, stop. You are on energized ground, and an electrical current is entering one foot, passing through your lower body, and leaving through the other foot. If that happens, raise one foot off the ground, turn around, and hop to a safe place. Wait for trained personnel with the proper equipment to cut the wires or disconnect them.

If a power line has fallen over a car, tell the driver and passengers to stay in the car. A victim should try to jump out of the car *only* if an explosion or fire threatens, and then without making contact with the car or the wire.

Caution:

DO NOT touch an appliance or the victim until the current is off.

DO NOT try to move downed wires.

DO NOT use *any* object, even dry wood (broomstick, tools, chair, stool) to separate the victim from the electrical source.

Hazardous Materials Incidents

At almost any highway crash scene, there is the potential danger of hazardous chemicals. Clues that indicate the presence of hazardous materials include:

- signs on vehicles (eg, "explosive," "flammable," "corrosive")
- spilled liquids or solids
- strong, unusual odors
- clouds of vapor

Stay well away and upwind from the area. Only those who are specially trained in handling hazardous materials and who have the proper equipment should be in the area.

Motor Vehicle Crashes

In most states, you are legally obligated to stop and give help when you are involved in a motor vehicle crash. If you come on a crash shortly after it happens, the law does not require you to stop, although it might be argued that you have a moral responsibility to render any aid you can.

1. Stop and park your vehicle well off the highway or road and out of active traffic lanes. Park at least 5 car lengths from the crash. If the police have taken charge, do not stop unless you are asked to do so. If the police or other emergency vehicles have not arrived, call or send someone to call 9-1-1 or the local emergency number as soon as possible. Ways to call include:
   - Find a pay phone or roadside emergency phone.
   - Use a cellular phone or CB radio.
   - Ask to use a phone at a nearby house or business.
2. Turn on your vehicle's emergency hazard flashers. Raise the hood of your vehicle to draw more attention to the scene.
3. Make sure everyone on the scene is safe.

- Ask the driver(s) to turn off the ignition or turn it off yourself.
- Ask bystanders to stand well off the roadway.
- Place flares or reflectors 250 to 500 feet behind the crash scene to warn oncoming drivers of the crash. Do not ignite flares around leaking gasoline or diesel fuel.

4. If the driver or passenger is unresponsive or might have spinal injuries, use your hands to stabilize their heads and necks.
5. Check and keep monitoring the ABCs. Treat any life-threatening injuries.
6. Whenever possible, wait for EMS personnel to extricate the victims from vehicles, because they have training and the proper equipment. In most cases, keep the victims stabilized inside the vehicle.
7. Allow the EMS ambulance to take victims to the hospital.

Caution:

DO NOT rush to get victims out of a car that has been in a crash. Contrary to opinion, most vehicle crashes do not involve fire, and most vehicles stay in an upright position.

DO NOT move or allow victims to move unless there is an immediate danger like fire or oncoming traffic. Treat victims as though every bone in their bodies is broken.

DO NOT transport victims in your car or any other bystander's vehicle.

Fires

If you encounter a fire, you should:

1. Get all the people out fast.
2. Call the emergency telephone number (usually 9-1-1).

Then—and *only* then—if the fire is small and if your own escape route is clear, should you fight the fire yourself with a fire extinguisher. You may be able to put out the fire or at least hold damage to a minimum.

To use a fire extinguisher, aim directly at whatever is burning and sweep across it. Extinguishers expel their contents quickly, in 8 to 25 seconds for most home models containing dry chemicals.

Caution:

DO NOT get trapped while fighting a fire. Always stay close to an open door so you can exit if the fire gets too big.

Confined Spaces

A confined space is an area not intended for human occupancy that also has the potential for containing or accumulating a dangerous atmosphere. There are three types of confined spaces: below-ground, ground-level, and above-ground. Below-ground confined spaces include manholes, below-ground utility vaults, storage tanks, old mines, cisterns, and wells. Ground-level confined spaces include industrial tanks and farm storage silos. Above-ground confined spaces include water towers and storage tanks.

An accident in a confined space demands immediate action. If someone who enters a confined space signals for help or becomes unconscious, follow these steps to help:

1. Call for immediate help.
2. Do *not* rush in to help.
3. Activate EMS.
4. Do *not* enter the confined space unless you have the proper training and equipment, such as self contained air supply, safety harness, and lifeline.
5. Once the victim is removed, provide care.

Triage: What to Do with Multiple Victims

You may encounter emergency situations in which there are two or more victims. This often happens in multiple-car accidents or disasters. After making a quick scene survey, decide who must be cared for and transported first. This process of prioritizing or classifying injured victims is called "triage." *Triage* is a word taken from the French word "trier," which means *to sort.* The goal is to do the greatest good for the greatest number of victims.

Finding Life-Threatened Victims

A variety of systems are used to identify care and transportation priorities. To find those needing immediate care for life-threatening conditions, first tell all victims who can get up and walk to move to a specific area. Victims who can get up and walk rarely have life-threatening injuries. These victims ("walking wounded") are classified as "delayed priority" (see below). Do not force a victim to move if he or she complains of pain.

Find the life-threatened victims by performing only the initial survey (ABC) on all remaining victims. Go to motionless victims first. You must move quickly (spend less than 60 seconds with each victim) from one victim to the next until all have been assessed. Classify victims according to the following care and transportation priorities:

1. *Immediate care.* Victim has life-threatening injuries but can be saved.
   - airway or breathing difficulties (not breathing or breathing rate slower than 8 per minute or faster than 24 per minute)
   - weak or no pulse
   - uncontrolled or severe bleeding
   - unresponsive or unconscious
2. *Urgent care.* Victims not fitting into the immediate or delayed categories. Care and transportation can be delayed up to one hour.
3. *Delayed care.* Victims with minor injuries. Care and transportation can be delayed up to 3 hours.
4. *Dead.* Victims are obviously dead, mortally wounded, or unlikely to survive because of the extent of their injuries, age, and medical condition.

Do not become involved in treating the victims at this point, but ask knowledgeable bystanders to care for immediate life-threatening problems (ie, rescue breathing, bleeding control).

Reassess victims regularly for changes in their condition. Only after victims with immediate life-threatening conditions receive care should those with less serious conditions be given care.

Later, you will usually be relieved when more highly trained emergency personnel arrive on the scene. You may then be asked to provide first aid, to help move victims, or to help with ambulance or helicopter transportation.

Moving Victims

A victim should not be moved until he or she is ready for transportation to a hospital, if required. All necessary first aid should be provided first. A victim should be moved only if there is an immediate danger (▶Skill Scan):

- There is a fire or danger of fire.
- Explosives or other hazardous materials are involved.
- It is impossible to protect the scene from hazards.
- It is impossible to gain access to other victims in the situation (eg, a vehicle) who need lifesaving care.

A cardiac arrest victim is usually moved unless he or she is already on the ground or floor, because CPR must be performed on a firm surface.

Caution:

DO NOT move a victim unless you absolutely have to, such as when the victim is in immediate danger or must be moved to shelter while waiting for the EMS to arrive.

DO NOT make the injury worse by moving the victim.

DO NOT move a victim who could have a spine injury.

DO NOT move a victim without stabilizing the injured part.

DO NOT move a victim unless you know where you are going.

DO NOT leave an unresponsive victim alone unless you are taking a short time to call EMS.

DO NOT move a victim when you can send someone for help. Wait with the victim and send someone else for help.

DO NOT try to move a victim by yourself if other people are available to help.

Emergency Moves

The major danger in moving a victim quickly is the possibility of aggravating a spine injury. In an emergency, every effort should be made to pull the victim in the direction of the long axis of the body to provide as much protection to the spinal cord as possible. If victims are on the floor or ground, you can drag them away from the scene by using various techniques.

Nonemergency Moves

All injured parts should be stabilized before and during moving. If rapid transportation is not needed, it is helpful to practice on another person about the same size as the injured victim.

Skill Scan Drags

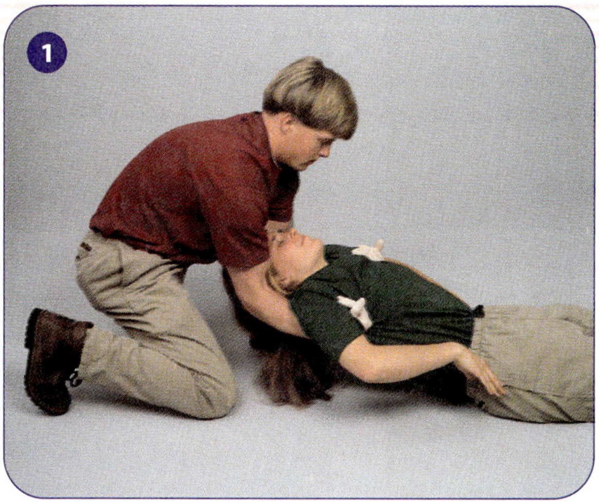

1. *Shoulder drag.* For short distances over a rough surface, stabilize victim's head with your forearms.

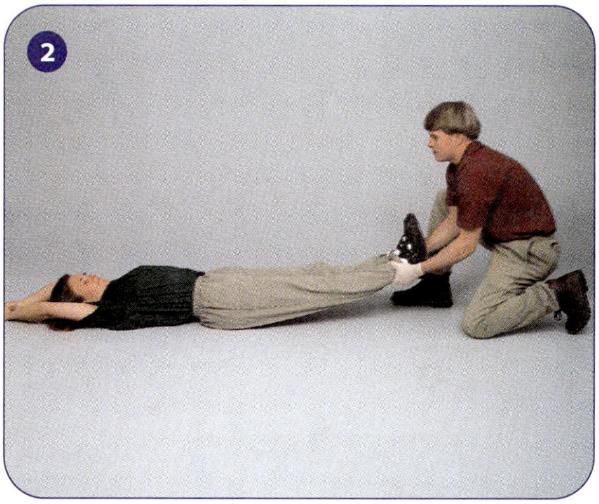

2. *Ankle drag.* The fastest method for a short distance on a smooth surface.

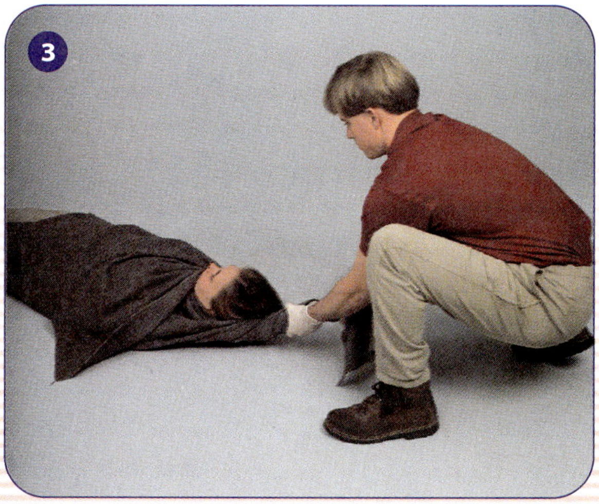

3. *Blanket pull.* Roll the victim onto a blanket and pull from behind the victim's head.

Skill Scan One-Person Moves

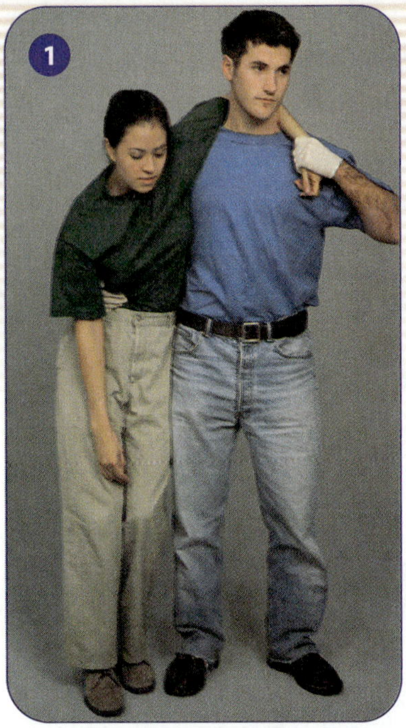

1. *Human crutch (one person helps victim to walk).* If one leg is injured, help the victim to walk on the good leg while you support the injured side.

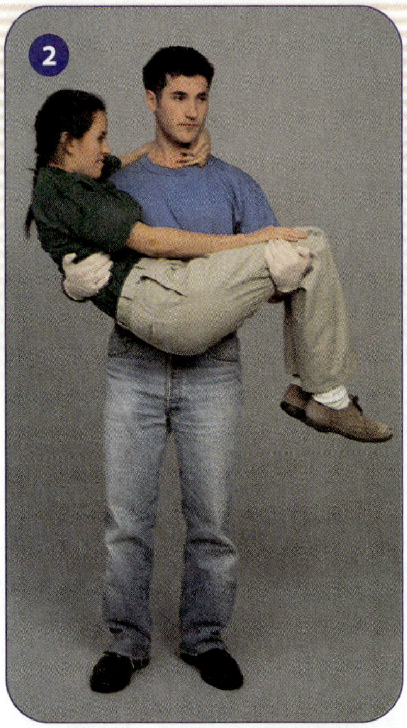

2. *Cradle carry.* Use for children and lightweight adults who cannot walk.

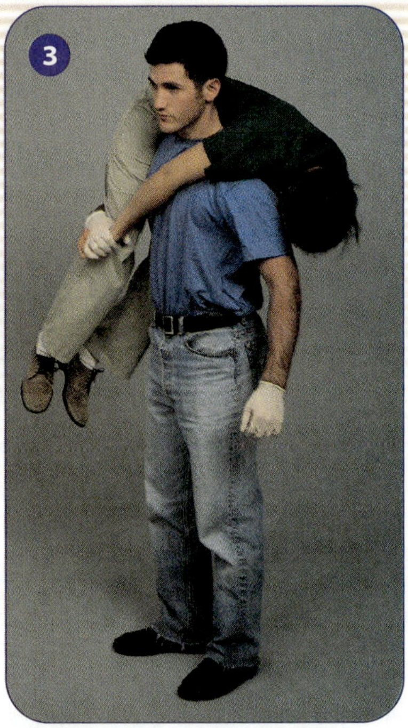

3. *Firefighter's carry.* If the victim's injuries permit, you can travel longer distances if you carry the victim over your shoulder.

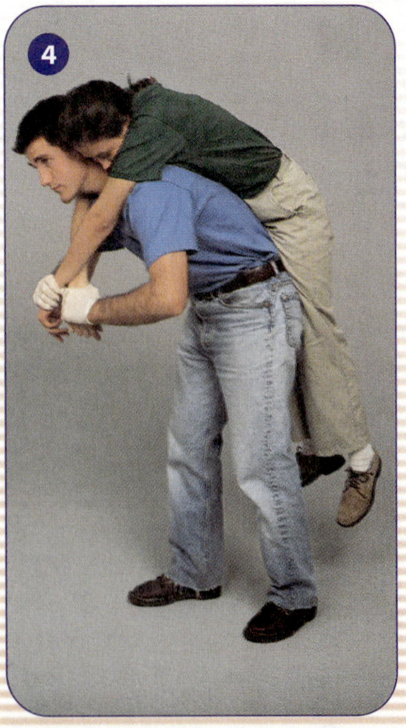

4. *Pack-strap carry.* When injuries make the fireman's carry unsafe, this method is better for longer distances.

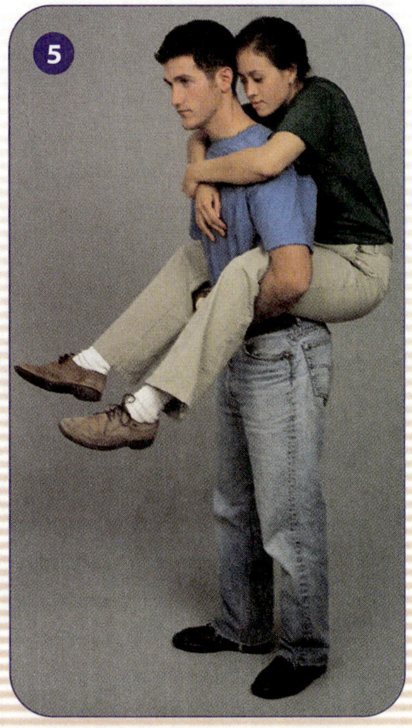

5. *Piggyback carry.* Use this method when the victim cannot walk but can use the arms to hang onto the rescuer.

Skill Scan Two/Three-Person Moves

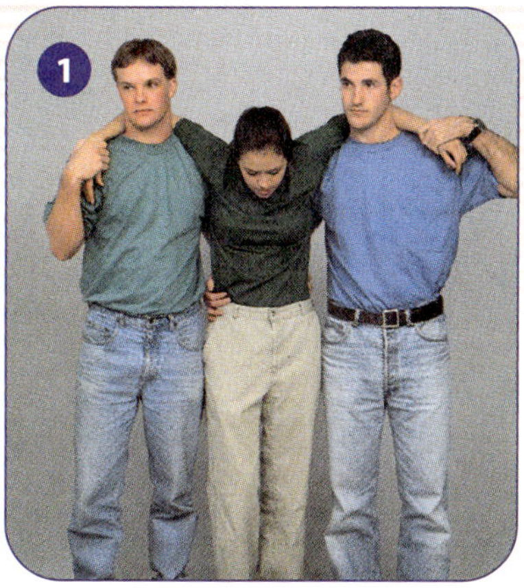

1. *Two-person assist.* Similar to human crutch.

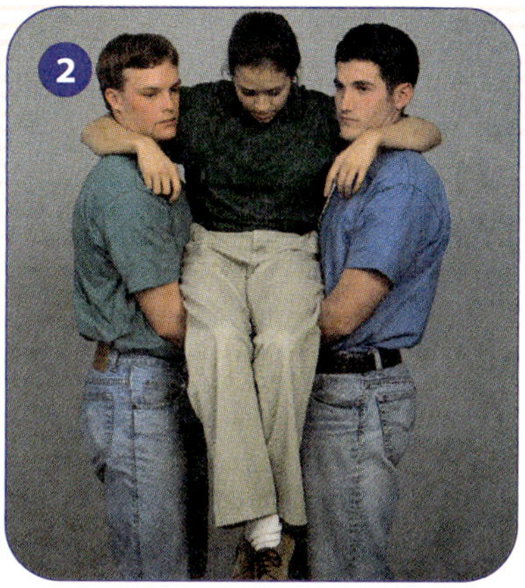

2. *Two-handed seat carry.*

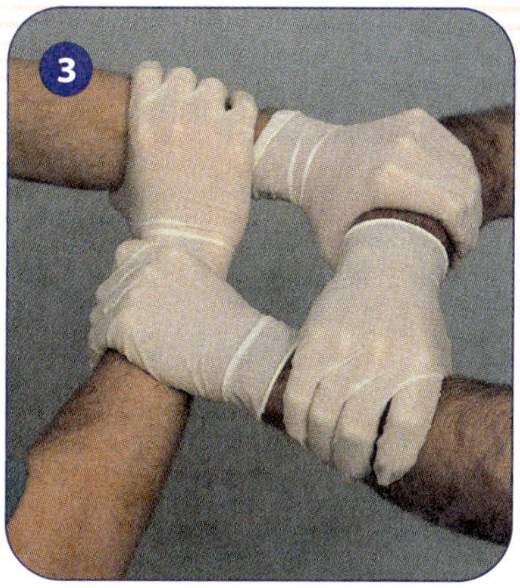

3. *Four-handed seat carry.* The easiest two-person carry when no equipment is available, and the victim cannot walk but can use the arms to hang onto the two rescuers.

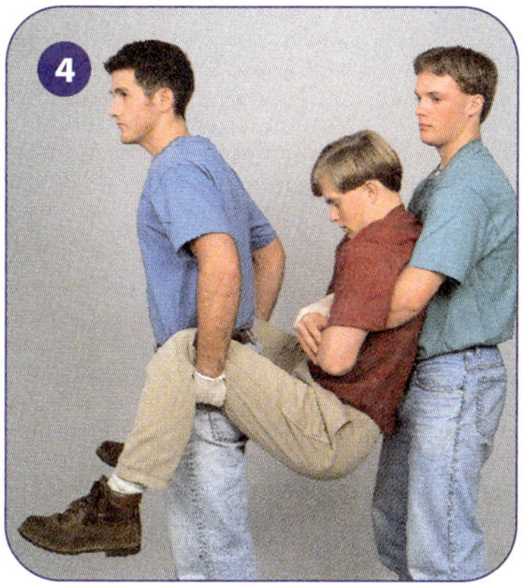

4. *Extremity carry.*

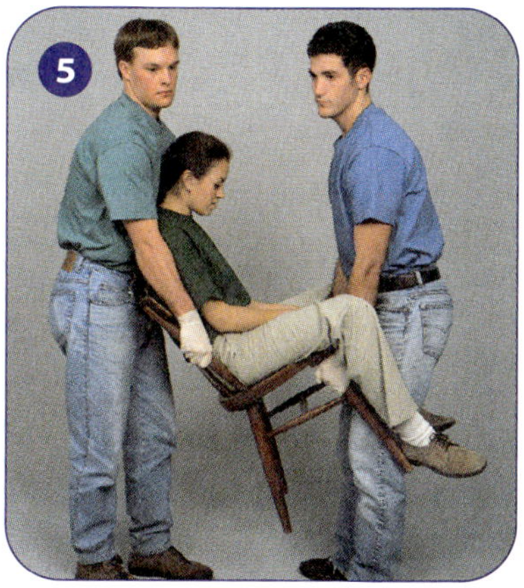

5. *Chair carry.* Useful for a narrow passage or up or down stairs. Use a sturdy chair that can take the victim's weight.

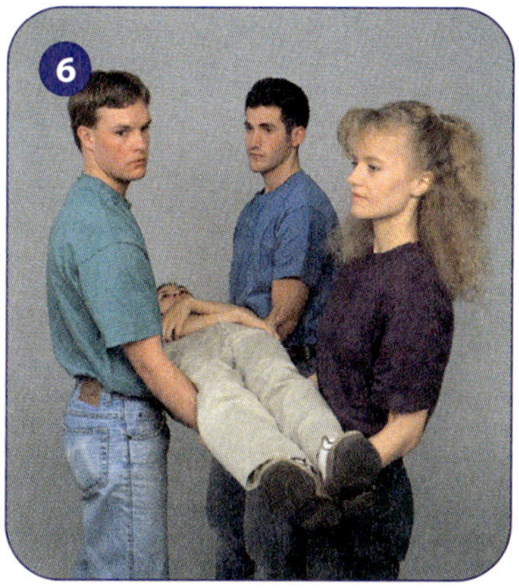

6. *Hammock carry.* Three to six people stand on alternate sides of the injured person and link hands beneath the victim.

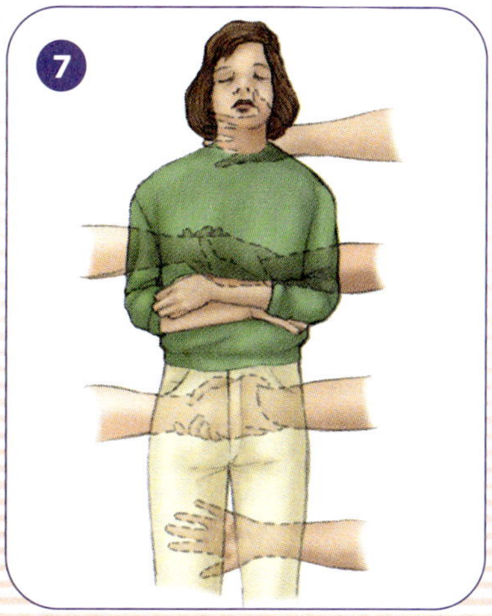

Learning Activities

Rescuing and Moving Victims

Directions: Circle Yes if you agree with the statement, and circle No if you disagree.

Yes No **1.** You should attempt to move downed power lines away from a victim, using a broom or other wooden object.

Yes No **2.** Strong, unusual odors or clouds of vapor are possible indications of the presence of hazardous materials.

Yes No **3.** To keep from getting trapped while attempting to extinguish a fire, you should always keep a door behind you for rapid exit.

Yes No **4.** When triaging victims, airway and breathing difficulties are classified as urgent care priorities.

Yes No **5.** A major concern in moving a victim quickly is the possibility of aggravating a spine injury.

Yes No **6.** "Row – throw – reach – and go" represents the safe order for executing a water rescue.

Yes No **7.** In most states, you are not legally obligated to stop and give help when you are involved in a motor vehicle crash.

Scenario: A co-worker has been hurt in an explosion in a lab. He has been thrown across the room and is lying motionless on the floor. You determine it is safe to help, but are afraid there could be another explosion. What should you do?

____

____

____

Appendix A First Aid Supplies

Workplace First Aid Kit*

Equipment	Minimum Quantity
1. Adhesive strip bandages (1" × 3")	20
2. Triangular bandages (muslin, 36" – 40" × 36" – 40" × 52" – 56")	4
3. Sterile eye pads (2 1/8" × 2 5/8")	2
4. Sterile gauze pads (4" × 4")	6
5. Sterile nonstick pads (3" × 4")	6
6. Sterile trauma pads (5" × 9")	2
7. Sterile trauma pads (8" × 10")	1
8. Sterile conforming roller gauze (2" width)	3 rolls
9. Sterile conforming roller gauze (4 1/2" width)	3 rolls
10. Waterproof tape (1" × 5 yards)	1 roll
11. Porous adhesive tape (2" × 5 yards)	1 roll
12. Elastic roller bandages (4" and 6")	1 each
13. Antiseptic skin wipes, individually wrapped	10
14. Medical-grade exam gloves (medium, large, extra large), conforming to FDA requirements	2 pairs per size
15. Mouth-to-barrier device, either a face mask with a one-way valve or a disposable face shield	1
16. Disposable instant-activating cold packs	2
17. Resealable plastic bags (quart size)	2
18. Padded malleable splint (SAM splint™, 4" × 36")	1
19. Emergency blanket, Mylar	1
20. Paramedic shears (with one serrated edge)	1
21. Splinter tweezers (about 3" long)	1
22. Biohazard waste bag (3 1/2 gallon capacity)	2
23. First aid and CPR manual and list of local emergency telephone numbers	1

* This list does not include over-the-counter ointments, topicals, or internal medicines; consult the workplace's medical director for these.

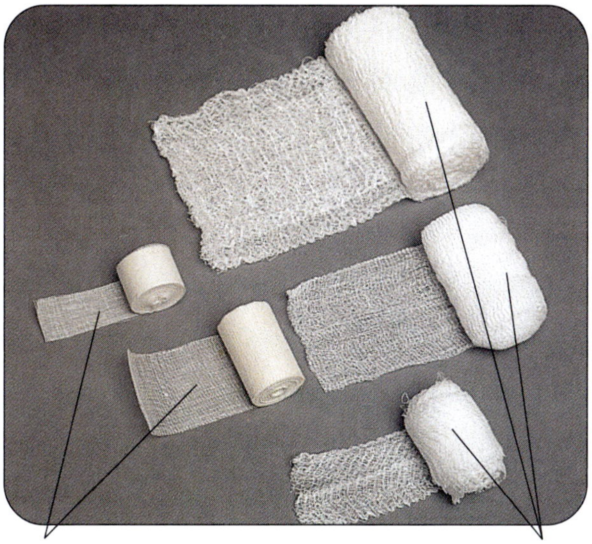

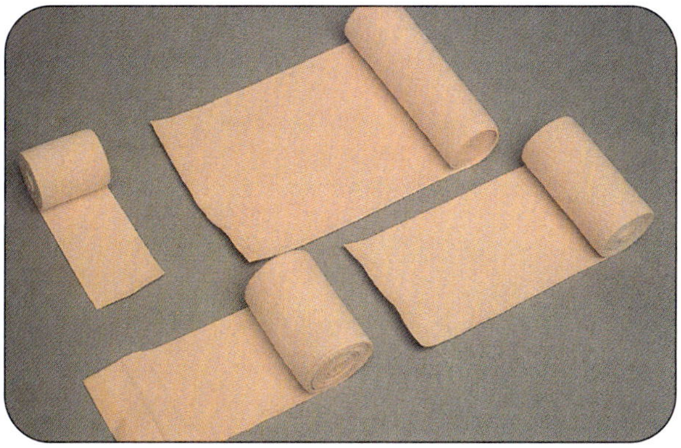

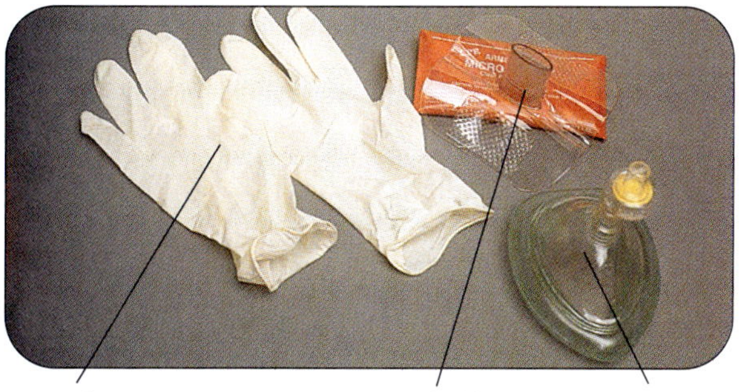

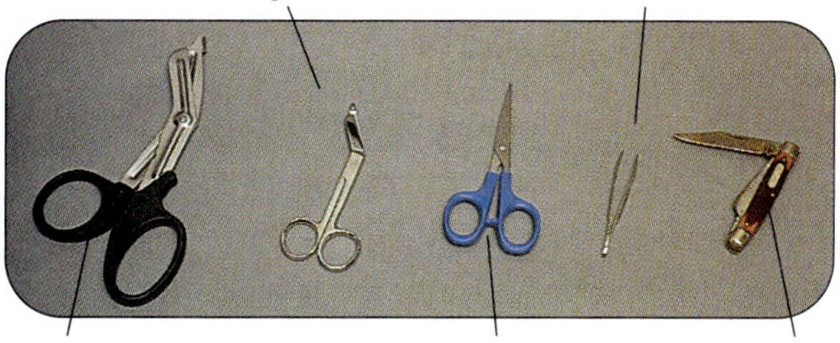

Photo and Illustration Credits

Chapter 1
Opener © Mark E. Gibson; **Figure 1** courtesy of Ellis and Associates

Chapter 2
Opener © Brian Pieters, Masterfile

Chapter 3
Opener © 1998 Bob Winsett/Index Stock Imagery/PictureQuest; **Figures 1, 4** courtesy of American Academy of Orthopaedic Surgeons (AAOS)

Chapter 4
Opener © 1988 Peter Menzel/Stock, Boston/PictureQuest

Chapter 5
Opener © Christopher Morris/Black Star Publishing/PictureQuest; **Figures 1B, 5** courtesy of AAOS; **Figure 2** © Howard Backer

Chapter 6
Opener © Frank Pedrick/Index Stock Imagery/PictureQuest

Chapter 7
Opener © Owen Franken/Stock, Boston/PictureQuest; **Figure 2** courtesy of AAOS

Chapter 8
Opener © 1992 Tim Lynch/Stock, Boston/PictureQuest

Chapter 9
Opener © Custom Medical Stock Photo

Chapter 10
Opener © 1999 Jim Pickerell/Stock Connection/PictureQuest

Chapter 11
Opener © Custom Medical Stock Photo

Chapter 12
Opener © Wedgworth, Custom Medical Stock Photo; **Figure 5** courtesy of AAOS

Chapter 13
Opener © 1991 Stephen Agricola/Stock, Boston/PictureQuest; **Figure 2** courtesy of AAOS

Chapter 14
Opener © David Dennis, Animals Animals

Chapter 15
Opener © Howard Backer

Chapter 16
Opener © Bob Daemmrich/Stock, Boston/PictureQuest

Chapter 17
Opener © Mark E. Gibson

Appendix B
Figure 1 courtesy of AAOS

Quick Emergency Index

National Safety Council®

INSTRUCTOR'S RESOURCE MANUAL FOR

First Aid

Fourth Edition

JONES AND BARTLETT PUBLISHERS
Sudbury, Massachusetts
BOSTON TORONTO LONDON SINGAPORE

World Headquarters
Jones and Bartlett Publishers
40 Tall Pine Drive
Sudbury, MA 01776
978-443-5000
nsc@jbpub.com
Internet: http://www.jbpub.com/nsc/

Jones and Bartlett Publishers Canada
2406 Nikanna Road
Mississauga, ON L5C 2W6
CANADA

Jones and Bartlett Publishers International
Barb House, Barb Mews
London W6 7PA
UK

The first aid procedures in this book are based on the most current recommendations of responsible medical sources. The National Safety Council and the publisher, however, make no guarantee as to, and assume no responsibility for, the correctness, sufficiency or completeness of such information or recommendations. Other or additional safety measures may be required under particular circumstances.

Printed in the United States of America

05 04 03 02 01 10 9 8 7 6 5 4 3 2 1

INSTRUCTOR'S RESOURCE MANUAL FOR FIRST AID

TABLE OF CONTENTS

What Is the National Safety Council?

The National Safety Council dedicates itself to saving lives and preventing injuries. Its mission statement includes the mitigating of human and economic losses from injuries. Emergency response training is one way of mitigating injuries.

Every National Safety Council first aid/CPR instructor should know:

- The National Safety Council was founded in 1913. Its main offices are in the Chicago area.
- The Council is a not-for-profit, nongovernmental public service organization. The Council has no authority to legislate or regulate.
- An Act of Congress in 1953 formally established the Council as a federally chartered organization. The Charter mandates that the National Safety Council be nonpolitical and not contribute to or otherwise support or assist any political party or candidate for office.
- The Council is dedicated to the safety and health of all people.
- Chapters established throughout the United States and Canada provide their members with services and offer education and information to meet a variety of safety and health needs.
- The Council is the leader in the nation's voluntary safety movement.
- The Council reaches millions of people each year. Industrial programs involve more than 18,000 companies and their 40 million employees.
- Annually, the Council's national convention, known as the National Safety Congress and Exposition, attracts more than 20,000 people, with more than 500 sessions and 1,000 exhibitors.
- The Council publishes magazines, newsletters, and a variety of technical manuals. The latest publication, *Every Second Counts,* provides information for the first aid/CPR instructor. It is the only such publication of its kind and purpose.
- The Council is recognized as the nation's most extensive and reliable source of injury information.
- The Council has more than 10,000 first aid and CPR instructors and 4,000 training centers worldwide.

SECTION 1: INTRODUCTION

This instructor's manual is designed to help National Safety Council instructors teach first aid for adults. The manual provides all the information and materials needed to conduct the first aid training.

Section 2 of this manual provides on overview of teaching strategies, including teaching to objectives, and teaching methods.

Section 3 of this manual provides the course outlines for the First Aid (Adult) and First Aid and CPR, Standard courses. These outlines include the topics being presented, whether video segments are available, and the recommended times. The outlines also identify the various skills that are to be practiced in the course.

Section 4 of this manual provides lesson plans that contain the following components:

- Objectives—Each lesson begins by providing objectives indicating what participants should learn.
- Approximate Length—The approximate length for each lesson is provided to assist instructors in pacing the class.
- Equipment for Skill Practice—Equipment needed for various skill practice sessions, such as bleeding control or splinting is listed here.
- Scenarios—Scenarios are provided to help with each lesson.
- Teaching Points—These points provide the minimal information that must be covered to ensure participants can meet the educational objectives for the lesson. These points are covered in many video segments, but if the video is not used or does not cover a particular topic, the instructor must cover these points.
- Skill Practice Sessions—Skill practice sessions are identified in each appropriate lesson. These activities are designed to help reinforce the information being presented.
- Assessing Progress—Answers to the learning activities at the end of each chapter of the participant's manual are provided.

Section 5 of this manual provides standardized participant course exams and instructor answer keys to be used when teaching this program.

For additional information on how to conduct National Safety Council courses and other administrative information, refer to the *Instructor's Administrative Guide for First Aid Institute Programs.*

SECTION 2: TEACHING STRATEGIES

TEACHING TO OBJECTIVES

It is important for you, as an instructor, to know what to present in a particular course. You will also need to be able to address specific needs of the audience you are addressing. Although it may be difficult to meet everyone's needs, the information presented should meet the needs of the majority of the class. You will not be able to be all things to all people at all times. The number of participants, time restrictions, available equipment, and facility limitations can pose challenges for you.

Some people get confused when *objectives* are mentioned. The term has been put through the mill—abused by some, misused by others, and unused by others. Objectives (or outcomes) must be carefully spelled out for the benefit of the learner and the instructor.

Objectives are the road maps that help the learners know what their destination should be, and they provide the instructor with guidelines and direction for designing learning activities that will move the learners in that direction. Learning objectives describe the learning that is expected to occur during the course.

If you, the instructor, specify the course objectives, and the learners attain those objectives, effective learning will occur. When people contribute their experiences to a situation, they may carry learning above and beyond that specified in the objectives.

A behavioral objective means that some observable change is to take place as a result of the training provided. Such an objective identifies not what the instructor will be doing but rather what the learner will have learned or will be able to do upon finishing the course.

For most courses, the learner will need only two basic objectives:

1. Be able to recognize a specific problem (e.g., heart attack or fracture) through various signs and symptoms.
2. Be able to describe and/or apply proper procedures to care for the problem.

How much material should be covered in a specified time period, and the manner in which it should be presented, differs from person to person. This is especially true with adults, who bring to each learning situation different personal and professional goals, requirements, attitudes, and needs. Consequently, a particular course outline or objectives that work well for one group of participants may not work well with another group.

As the instructor, you must constantly be aware of your pace and then be prepared to speed up or slow down as needed. You must be flexible, ready to modify your program to meet the needs of the group. Your outline should be the servant, not the master.

TEACHING METHODS

As objectives provide the road map for the learning destination, teaching methods provide the vehicle to reach the destination. The number of participants, their backgrounds, time restrictions, available equipment, and facility will also affect the teaching method that is used.

Various teaching methods can be used in first aid and CPR programs:

- Lecture
  There are certain situations, such as when initially discussing a new skill, in which lectures are necessary. Although lecturing is a traditional teaching method, it limits instructor–participant interaction and does not always create the most effective learning environment.
- Discussion
  Material can be presented by involving participants in discussions. This allows for good group interaction and allows participants to learn from each other.
- Group Activities
  Participants can work in small groups to solve a problem or determine a course of action for a given scenario. This method also creates good interaction.
- Demonstration
  Using step-by-step techniques, instructor demonstrations help participants understand proper care techniques. Videos should be used to show proper care techniques. This also allows for a standardized demonstration from class to class.
- Skill Practice Sessions
  Participants usually learn more from actual hands-on practice. Providing participants with time to practice skills will greatly enhance their understanding and ability to perform when needed.
- Case Studies
  In case studies, participants are presented with a situation that they need to solve. Participants are then asked to analyze it. In their analysis, they identify what went well and what could have been done differently. They also identify and discuss the principles being presented.
- Role Playing
  In role playing, participants role play various situations and attempt to deal with the situation they are faced with. This method provides for great interaction; however, it will not be effective if participants are shy and not willing to actively participate.

As an instructor, you need to identify the best methods to use for the group you are presenting to. No one method is superior to another. You and your participants will benefit from various teaching methods. Try some of the following suggestions:

- Explain what will be covered and in what time frame you anticipate it being covered.

- Keep the course interesting, and keep it moving. Participants remember information that is presented in an interesting, challenging, and even entertaining way. Making the best use of audiovisual aids will help keep the course interesting and standardize the presentation.
- Remember that adult learners bring a wealth of experience to the classroom. Draw on this experience and keep participants actively involved.
- Make participants responsible for their own learning. Give them enough information, but don't tell them where to dot the "I's" and cross the "T's".

SECTION 3: FIRST AID COURSE OUTLINES

First Aid (Adult) — **3½ Hours**

Topic	*Skills*	*Video*	*Approximate Length*
Introduction/pre-course check			10 min
Background information			5 min
Action at an emergency		✔	10 min
Finding out what's wrong	✔	✔	20 min
Bleeding and shock	✔	✔	15 min
Wounds		✔	5 min
Dressings and bandages	✔		10 min
Burns		✔	10 min
Head and spinal injuries			15 min
Chest, abdominal, and pelvic injuries			10 min
Bone, joint, and muscle injuries		✔	10 min
Splinting the extremities	✔	✔	15 min
Sudden illnesses		✔	15 min
Poisoning		✔	10 min
Bites and stings		✔	10 min
Cold-related emergencies		✔	5 min
Heat-related emergencies		✔	5 min
Rescuing and moving victims	✔	✔	10 min
Post-course check and course review			5 min
Final written exam			15 min

First Aid and CPR, Standard **5 Hours**

Topic	*Skills*	*Video*	*Approximate Length*
Introduction/pre-course check			10 min
Background information			5 min
Action at an emergency		✔	10 min
Finding out what's wrong	✔	✔	20 min
Basic Life Support • Adult Rescue Breathing, Choking, and CPR	✔	✔	75 min
Bleeding and shock	✔	✔	15 min
Wounds		✔	5 min
Dressings and bandages	✔		10 min
Burns		✔	10 min
Head and spinal injuries			15 min
Chest, abdominal, and pelvic injuries			10 min
Bone, joint, and muscle injuries		✔	10 min
Splinting the extremities	✔	✔	15 min
Sudden illnesses		✔	15 min
Poisoning		✔	10 min
Bites and stings		✔	10 min
Cold-related emergencies		✔	5 min
Heat-related emergencies		✔	5 min
Rescuing and moving victims	✔	✔	10 min
Post-course check and course review			5 min
Final written exam • Adult First Aid • Adult CPR Exam			30 min

SECTION 4: LESSON PLANS

INTRODUCTION/PRE-COURSE CHECK

LESSON: INTRODUCTION/PRE-COURSE CHECK

- Welcome course participants
- Introduce yourself
- Have participants introduce themselves
- Provide a brief overview of the course
  - Length of the course
  - General content to be covered
  - Breaks
  - National Safety Council course completion requirements
- Have participants complete the pre-course check, "Your First Aid IQ," in the front of their manuals. They should select the answers in the "pre-course" column. Do not provide any answers to participants at this time. They will return to this page at the completion of the course and complete the "post-check" column as part of the course review prior to taking the final written exam(s).

Approximate length: 10 minutes
Equipment for Skill Practice: None

LESSON: BACKGROUND INFORMATION

Lesson Objectives

After completing this lesson, participants should be able to:

- Recognize the need for first aid training.
- Define "first aid."
- Identify legal considerations when providing first aid.

Approximate Time: 5 minutes

Equipment for Skill Practice: none

SCENARIOS

Scenario: A child on your baseball team slides into third base and injures his arm during practice. His parents are not present. His arm is swelling and he cannot move his fingers. Other coaches are present.

Scenario: You are summoned to render first aid at your workplace for a co-worker who has had his hand amputated. The work day has just ended and you have an important meeting you want to get to right after work. No one else with your level of first aid training is available to help your co-worker. EMS personnel are enroute to your workplace. You begin providing care, but really want to make the meeting after work.

TEACHING POINTS

Need for First Aid Training

- It is better to know first aid and not need it than to need it and not know it.
- A few minutes' delay in a life-threatening situation can make a difference between life and death.
- Most injuries and illnesses do not require lifesaving efforts.
- Knowing what to do for severe or minor injuries or illnesses makes individuals more confident.
- The four leading causes of death in the United States are heart disease, cancer, stroke, and chronic lung disease.
- Unintentional injuries are the fifth leading cause of death in the United States.

What Is First Aid?

- First aid is the immediate care given to an injured or suddenly ill person.
- First aid does not take the place of proper medical treatment.
- First aid may mean the difference between life and death, rapid recovery and long hospitalization, or temporary disability and permanent injury.

Legal Considerations

- Lay rescuers should not be reluctant to give care for fear of being sued.
- Lay rescuers should be aware of several important legal concepts:
  - Get a victim's consent (permission) before providing care.
  - Identify yourself, the level of first aid training you have, and explain what you would like to do.
  - Permission from the victim may be expressed either with words or gestures.
  - It is "implied" that an unresponsive victim would consent to lifesaving help.
  - If a child has a life-threatening condition, and a guardian is not available, care should be given based on implied consent.
  - Once care is started, do not leave until another competent and trained person takes responsibility for the victim.
  - Avoid negligence by following accepted standards of care.
  - No one is required to render first aid when no legal duty exists.
  - Legal duty to act may occur when employment requires it or when a preexisting responsibility exists.
  - In most cases, lay rescuers are not legally required to give first aid.
  - Good Samaritan laws grant immunity against lawsuits but are not a substitute for competent first aid.

ASSESSING PROGRESS

Have participants complete the "Learning Activities" at the end of the chapter in their manual. Answers to the Learning Activities are listed below.

1. No
2. Yes
3. Yes
4. No
5. Yes

6. No
7. Yes
8. No
9. Yes
10. No
11. B
12. No
13. Yes
14. No
15. Yes

LESSON: ACTION AT AN EMERGENCY

Lesson Objectives

After completing this lesson, participants should be able to:

- Identify the actions that a bystander should take in an emergency.
- Recognize that emotional reactions are common when providing emergency care.
- Describe the steps in performing a scene survey.
- Identify situations in which emergency medical services (EMS) should be called.
- Describe how to call EMS.
- Identify ways to minimize the chance of disease transmission.

Approximate Length: 10 minutes

Equipment for Skill Practice: None

SCENARIO

Scenario: A two-car collision has just occurred in front of you. A victim has been thrown from the car. You have a cell phone handy. The traffic on the road is heavy.

Scenario: A neighbor at a local picnic suddenly complains of dizziness and chest discomfort. She states she has never felt this way before. Other neighbors have gathered to see if they can help.

TEACHING POINTS

Instructor's Note

Video segments cover many of the points in this lesson.

Bystander Intervention

- The bystander is a vital link between EMS and the victim.
- A bystander must quickly and reliability:
  - Recognize an emergency exists.
  - Decide to help.
  - Call EMS personnel, if needed.
  - Assess the victim for problems and what kind of help the victim needs.
  - Provide first aid.

Post-Care Reactions

- Emotional reactions are common during and after providing emergency care.
- Discussing your feelings after an event can help prevent later emotional problems.

Scene Survey

- Survey the scene quickly for:
  - Hazards that could be dangerous to you, the victim(s), or bystanders
  - The cause of the injury or illness
  - The number of victims
- When a serious situation occurs, call EMS right away.
- Knowing when to call for an ambulance is important.
- To receive emergency assistance in most communities, simply phone 9-1-1.
- The dispatcher will often ask for the following information.
  - Caller's name and the phone number calling from
  - Victim's location
  - What happened
  - Number of persons needing help and any special conditions
  - Victim's condition
- Do not hang up the phone unless the dispatcher instructs you to do so.
- The EMS dispatcher may advise how to best care for the victim.

> **Instructor's Not**
> *Review the list of conditions when EMS should be called.*

Disease Precautions

- Lay rescuers should understand the risk of disease transmission.
- Precautions can help protect against bloodborne and airborne diseases.
- Hepatitis and HIV/AIDS are serious bloodborne diseases.
- Tuberculosis is a serious airborne disease.
- Employers are required to offer a free vaccine series for hepatitis B to all employees who may be at risk of exposure.
- Reduce the chance of disease transmission by following universal precautions and body substance isolation (BSI) techniques.
  - BSI assumes that any body fluid is a possible risk for exposure.
  - Universal precautions assume that all blood and certain fluids pose a risk for transmission of HBV and HIV.
  - Wear proper personal protective equipment (PPE).
  - PPE includes medical exam gloves, protective eyewear, mask, and mouth-to-barrier devices.

> **Instructor's Note**
> *Provide examples o barrier devices.*

ASSESSING PROGRESS

Have participants complete the "Learning Activities" at the end of the chapter in their manual. Answers to the Learning Activities are listed below.

1. Yes
2. No
3. Yes
4. Yes
5. Yes
6. Yes
7. a. Recognize the emergency.
   b. Decide to help.
   c. Call EMS personnel, if needed.
   d. Assess the victim.
   e. Provide first aid.
8. a. Hazards that can be dangerous to you or the victim
   b. The cause of the injury or injuries
   c. The number of victims
9. a. Your name and the phone number you are calling from
   b. The victim's location
   c. What happened
   d. Number of persons needing help
   e. Victim's condition
10. a. Use gloves
    b. Protective eyewear
    c. Mouth-to-barrier devices

LESSON: FINDING OUT WHAT'S WRONG

Lesson Objectives

After completing this lesson, participants should be able to:

- Describe and demonstrate how to assess a victim, including conducting an initial assessment and physical exam and SAMPLE history.
- Identify problems that are an immediate threat to life.

Approximate Length: 20 minutes

Equipment for Skill Practice : Blankets, mats

SCENARIOS

Scenario: An office worker has collapsed in the lunchroom. He is lying motionless on the ground.

Scenario: A neighbor has fallen from a height while painting his home. He is in obvious pain.

TEACHING POINTS

Instructor's Not

Video Segments cover many of the points in this lesso

Victim Assessment

- Once the scene survey is complete, assess the victim.
- The next step is the initial victim assessment, in which you identify and correct immediate life-threatening conditions.
- Determine whether the victim's problem is an injury or illness.
- For an injured victim with a significant mechanism of injury (MOI), stabilize the head to keep if from moving.
- Perform a brief physical exam and gather information after completing the initial assessment and providing care for any immediately life-threatening conditions.

Initial Assessment

- Takes less than one minute to complete, unless first aid is required at any point.
- Check for responsiveness:
  - Speak to the victim; tap the victim.
  - If the victim can speak, breathing and heartbeat are present.
  - If the victim does not respond, he or she is unresponsive.
  - If the victim is unresponsive, but breathing, position him or her on his or her side (recovery position).

Immediate Threats to Life

- These include altered level of responsiveness, breathing difficulty/not breathing, chest pain/discomfort (possible heart attack), choking, no signs of circulation, and severe bleeding.
- If a person is unresponsive and bystanders are available, have one of them call EMS.
- If you are alone with an adult victim, and a phone is near, call EMS yourself.

> **Instructor's Note**
> *If alone with a child victim, provide care for up to one minute and then call EMS.*

Airway

- The airway must be open for breathing.
- If a responsive victim cannot talk, cry, or cough forcefully, the airway is probably obstructed and must be checked and cleared.
- In an unresponsive victim lying face up, the most common airway obstruction is the tongue.
- If there is no suspected spinal injury, use the head-tilt, chin-lift technique to open the airway.
- If you suspect spinal injury, use the jaw-thrust without head-tilt technique to open the airway.

Breathing

- Breathing is normally quiet, with a rate between 12 and 20 times per minute for adults.
- Note any obvious breathing difficulties or unusual breathing.
- Check for breathing in an unresponsive victim after opening the airway.
- Look, listen, and feel for about 10 seconds to check for breathing.
- If the victim is not breathing, provide rescue breathing.

> **Instructor's Note**
> *Rescue breathing is discussed in detail in the lesson* Adult Basic Life Support.

Circulation

- After checking and correcting airway and breathing problems check circulation.
- Signs of normal circulation include:
  - Breathing

- Coughing
- Movement
- Normal skin color and temperature

- If there are no signs of circulation, begin CPR.
- Check for severe bleeding by looking over the victim's entire body for blood.
- Control any severe bleeding that may be present.

Instructor's No

CPR is discussed detail in the lesso Adult Basic Life Support.

Physical Exam and SAMPLE History

- The initial assessment is followed by a brief physical exam (head to toe) and gathering information through a SAMPLE history.
- Note any signs and symptoms of injury or illness.
- Use the mnemonic D-O-T-S to perform the physical exam from head to toe:
    - Deformities
    - Open wounds
    - Tenderness
    - Swelling
- For a responsive victim, you should focus the physical exam on the victim's main complaint.
- Gather information using a SAMPLE history:
    - S = Symptoms
    - A = Allergies
    - M = Medications
    - P = Past medical problems
    - L = Last oral intake
    - E = Events leading up to the illness or injury
- Medical information tags may identify allergies, medications, or medical conditions that may be the cause of the victim's problem.

What to do Until EMS Arrives

- Regularly recheck the victim's responsiveness, airway, breathing, circulation, and effectiveness of first aid.
- Briefly report your findings and care to EMS personnel when they arrive.

SKILL PRACTICE SESSION

- Have participants break up into small groups to practice victim assessment.
- Review the Skill Scans on "Initial Assessment" and "Physical Exam."
- Evaluate participant performance and remediate any problems.

ASSESSING PROGRESS

Have participants complete the "Learning Activities" at the end of the chapter in their manual. Answers to the Learning Activities are listed below.

1. Yes
2. No
3. No
4. Yes
5. Yes
6. No
7. Yes
8. No
9. D
10. A
11. B
12. A
13. A
14. D
15. D

LESSON: BASIC LIFE SUPPORT (ADULT)

Lesson Objectives

After completing this lesson, participants should be able to:

- Discuss various methods of rescue breathing.
- Describe and demonstrate how to perform rescue breathing for an adult.
- Identify signs of choking.
- Describe and demonstrate how to care for a choking adult.
- Describe and demonstrate how to perform CPR for an adult.

Approximate Length: 75 minutes

Equipment for Skill Practice: Medical exam gloves, manikins, barrier devices, cleaning supplies

SCENARIOS

Scenario: A 60-year-old female has collapsed in church. She is unresponsive, not breathing, and without signs of circulation.

Scenario: An elderly family member is eating when he begins coughing. His cough gets weaker and he is no longer able to speak or breathe. He is pale and grasping at his throat.

TEACHING POINTS

Instructor's Not

Video segments cover many of the points in this lesso

Rescue Breathing

- Rescue breathing is performed on a victim who is unresponsive, not breathing, but has other signs of circulation.
- Open the airway and check for breathing:
  - Use head-tilt/chin-lift technique if you do not suspect spinal injury.
  - Use jaw-thrust without head-tilt if you suspect spinal injury.
- If not breathing, provide 2 slow breaths.
- Check for signs of circulation. If present, but the victim is still not breathing normally, give one slow breath every 4 to 5 seconds.
- Each breath should be just enough to make the chest rise. Rapid, forceful breathing will result in air in the stomach (gastric distension).
- Methods of rescue breathing include:
  - Mouth-to-mouth breathing
  - Mouth-to-nose breathing

- Mouth-to-barrier device (mask or face shield), used to minimize the chance of disease transmission

If rescue breaths fail to make the chest rise, reposition the head and reattempt breaths. If still unsuccessful, begin CPR.

> **Instructor's Note**
> *For lesson plan on child or infant CPR, see* Instructor's Resource Manual for CPR.

CPR

- CPR is performed when a victim is unresponsive, not breathing, and has no signs of circulation.
- Older adults are most likely to suffer sudden cardiac death (cardiac arrest) and need CPR.
- To perform CPR on an adult:
  - Check responsiveness.
  - If unresponsive, send a bystander to call EMS.
  - Open the airway.
  - Check breathing; give 2 slow breaths if not breathing.
  - Check circulation.
  - If no signs of circulation, give chest compressions between the nipples using two hands.
  - Give 15 chest compressions and 2 breaths.
  - The rate of chest compressions is about 100 per minute.
  - The depth of compressions is 1½ to 2 inches.
  - Continue cycles of CPR for 1 minute and then recheck circulation.
- Provide additional care based on your assessment:
  - If unresponsive, but breathing, place in the recovery position.
  - If unresponsive, not breathing, but has signs of circulation, give rescue breaths.
  - If unresponsive, not breathing, and no signs of circulation, continue CPR.
- If you are unable or unwilling to provide rescue breathing, you can at least perform compression-only CPR until EMS personnel arrive.

Airway Obstruction (Choking)

- Food is the most common foreign body airway obstruction (choking).
- Signs of choking include:
  - Inability to speak, cough, or breathe
  - Grasping at the throat (universal distress sign)

- To care for a responsive choking adult:
  - Determine if the victim can speak.
  - Provide abdominal thrusts (Heimlich maneuver) just above the navel until the object is expelled or the victim becomes unresponsive.
  - Have a bystander call EMS.
- If the victim becomes unresponsive, assess the victim and begin CPR if needed. Each time you open the airway to give a breath, look for an object, and if present, remove it.
- If the victim is large, or in the late stages of pregnancy, use chest thrusts instead of abdominal thrusts.

SKILL PRACTICE SESSION

- Have participants break up into small groups to practice rescue breathing, CPR, and caring for airway obstruction.
- Review the skill sheets on "Adult and Child Rescue Breathing and CPR" and "Responsive Adult and Child Airway Obstruction Victim."
- Evaluate participant performance and remediate any problems.

ASSESSING PROGRESS

Have participants complete the "Learning Activities" at the end of the chapter in their manual. Answers to the Learning Activities are listed below.

1. No
2. No
3. Yes
4. Yes
5. Yes
6. Yes
7. Yes
8. Yes
9. Yes
10. No
11. Yes
12. Yes

13. No
14. Yes
15. Yes
16. Yes
17. Yes

Scenario
Have someone call 9-1-1, open the airway using the jaw-thrust without head-tilt, check breathing, check circulation. If no signs of circulation, begin CPR.

Scenario
Make sure the scene is safe. Have someone call 9-1-1. Assess the ABCs and provide care for what you find. If not breathing, give rescue breathing. If no signs of circulation, begin CPR.

Scenario
Determine if he is choking, give abdominal thrusts until the obstruction is relieved or the victim becomes unresponsive.

LESSON: BLEEDING AND SHOCK

Lesson Objectives

After completing this lesson, participants should be able to:

- Identify three types of external bleeding.
- Describe and demonstrate how to care for external bleeding.
- Identify signs of internal bleeding and describe how to care for internal bleeding.
- Identify signs of shock and describe how to care for shock.
- Recognize the signs of anaphylaxis and how to care for it.

Approximate Length: 15 minutes

Equipment for Skill Practice: Medical exam gloves, gauze pads, roller gauze, tape

SCENARIOS

Scenario: A 25-year-old construction worker has been badly cut on his thigh by a circular power saw. Blood is flowing heavily. The cut is about 5″ long. He appears to be pale, anxious, and restless.

Scenario: A landscaper has disturbed a nest of yellow jackets, which proceed to sting her more than a dozen times. She complains that she feels hot and begins coughing and wheezing. You notice that her face seems to be swelling.

TEACHING POINTS

External Bleeding

> **Instructor's No**
> *Video segments cover many of the points in this lesso*

- External bleeding occurs when blood can be seen coming from a wound.
- There are three types of bleeding:
  - Arterial bleeding, which spurts from a wound and can lead to rapid blood loss.
  - Blood from a vein flows steadily or gushes.
  - Capillary bleeding (most common) in which blood oozes from capillaries.
- Regardless of the type of bleeding, the care is the same:
  - Protect yourself against disease by wearing medical exam gloves.
  - Expose the wound.
  - Cover the wound with clean cloth or gauze pad.
  - Apply direct pressure.
  - Elevate the area.

- Apply a pressure bandage.
- If bleeding is still not controlled, apply pressure at a pressure point.

Internal Bleeding

- Internal bleeding occurs when the skin is not broken and blood is not seen.
- The signs of internal bleeding may take days to appear, and include:
  - Bruising
  - Painful, tender, rigid, bruised abdomen
  - Vomiting or coughing up blood
  - Stool that is black or contains bright red blood
- To care for serious internal bleeding:
  - Monitor ABCs
  - Treat for shock by raising the victim's legs 8 to 12 inches
  - Seek immediate medical attention

Shock

- Shock refers to circulatory system failure, which results when insufficient amounts of oxygenated blood are provided for every body part.
- Shock can result from:
  - Pump (heart) failure
  - Fluid loss (bleeding)
  - Pipe failure (blood vessels)
- Signs of shock include:
  - Altered mental status, anxiety, and restlessness
  - Pale, cold, and clammy skin, lip, and nail beds
  - Nausea and vomiting
  - Rapid breathing and pulse
  - Unresponsive in late stages
- To care for shock:
  - Care for life-threatening conditions.
  - Position the victim on his or her back.
  - Raise the victim's legs 8 to 12 inches.
  - Prevent body heat loss.

- Anaphylaxis is a type of shock—a powerful reaction to substances that enter the body.
- Signs of anaphylaxis include:
  - Sneezing, coughing, and wheezing
  - Shortness of breath
  - Tightness in the throat and/or chest
  - Swelling of the tongue, mouth, and nose
  - Blueness around lips and mouth
  - Dizziness
- To care for anaphylaxis:
  - Check ABCs.
  - Seek immediate medical attention.
  - If the victim has his or her own medication (such as epinephrine), help with its use.

SKILL PRACTICE SESSION

- Have participants break up into small groups to practice controlling external bleeding and caring for shock.
- Review the Skill Scans on "Bleeding Control and Positioning the Shock Victim."
- Evaluate participant performance and remediate any problems.

ASSESSING PROGRESS

Have participants complete the "Learning Activities" at the end of the chapter in their manual. Answers to the Learning Activities are listed below.

Bleeding

1. No
2. No
3. Yes
4. No
5. No

Scenario:

Survey the scene.

Put on gloves and apply direct pressure.

Elevate the wound.

If bleeding is not controlled, apply pressure to the pressure point.

Apply a pressure bandage.

Shock

1. Yes
2. No
3. Yes
4. No
5. No

Scenario:

Have the victim lie down, elevate the victim's legs, prevent heat loss, and seek medical attention.

Anaphylaxis

1. No
2. Yes
3. Yes

Scenario:

Check ABCs, seek immediate medical attention, and assist with any physician-prescribed medication (epinephrine).

LESSON: WOUNDS

Lesson Objectives

After completing this lesson, participants should be able to:

- Identify types of open wounds.
- Describe how to care for a wound to prevent infection.
- Describe how to recognize an infected wound.
- Describe how to care for an amputation.
- Describe how to care for an impaled object.

Approximate Length: 5 minutes

Equipment for Skill Practice: None

SCENARIOS

Scenario: You respond to an injured worker calling for help. The worker has cut his thumb off with a circular power saw.

Scenario: At a construction site, a 38-year-old worker drives a large nail through his left hand with a nail gun.

TEACHING POINTS

Instructor's No

Video segments cover many of the points in this lessc

Types of Open Wounds

- There are several types of open wounds:
  - Laceration
  - Incision
  - Puncture
  - Avulsion
  - Amputation

Caring for a Wound

- To clean a shallow wound:
  - Wash the wound with soap and irrigate with water.
  - If bleeding restarts, apply direct pressure.
  - Apply antibiotic ointment.
  - Cover the area with a sterile dressing.

Wound Infection

- Tetanus can produce a powerful poisonous toxin.
- Signs of infection include swelling, reddening, warmth, throbbing, and pus discharge.
- Seek medical attention for infected wounds.
- Get a tetanus booster shot every 5 to 10 years.

Amputation

- To care for an amputated body part:
  - Control the bleeding with direct pressure.
  - Treat the victim for shock.
  - Recover the amputated part.
  - Wrap the part in gauze, place it in a bag, and keep the bag cool.
  - Transport the part with the victim.

Impaled Objects

- To care for an impaled object:
  - Expose the area.
  - Do not remove or move the impaled object.
  - Control bleeding and stabilize the object with bulky dressings.

Closed Wounds

- To care for a closed wound:
  - Apply ice for up to 20 minutes.
  - Apply an elastic bandage.
  - Check for a possible fracture.
  - Elevate the injured extremity to decrease pain and swelling.

ASSESSING PROGRESS

Have participants complete the “Learning Activities” at the end of the chapter in their manual. Answers to the Learning Activities are listed below.

Wound Care

1. Yes
2. Yes
3. Yes
4. No
5. No

Scenario:

Survey the scene.

Put on gloves and apply direct pressure.

Elevate the wound.

If shallow, clean wound and apply antibiotic ointment and bandage.

Amputations

1. Yes
2. No
3. Yes
4. No
5. Yes

Scenario:

Make sure power is shut off and the scene is safe, and put on medical exam gloves.

Continue to apply direct pressure to control bleeding.

Place the amputated part in a dry sterile dressing, place it in a plastic bag, and place the bag on ice.

Call EMS.

Impaled Objects

1. Yes
2. Yes

Scenario

Stabilize the injury site and control bleeding around the wound.

Seek medical attention.

LESSON: DRESSINGS AND BANDAGES

Lesson Objectives

After completing this lesson, participants should be able to:

- Describe and demonstrate how to use dressings and bandages for various body parts.

Length: 10 minutes

Equipment for Skill Practice: Assorted dressings and bandages.

SCENARIOS

Scenario: A co-worker has lacerated his hand on a piece of machinery. He is holding the hand and blood is flowing. He is looking for something to use to help with the bleeding.

Scenario: A friend has fallen on the steps outside your home and cut her knee. You have a first aid kit available.

TEACHING POINTS

Dressings

- A dressing covers an open wound to control bleeding, prevent infection, absorb any fluid drainage, and protect the wound.
- There are various types of dressings, including:
  - Gauze pads
  - Adhesive strips
  - Trauma dressings
- When applying a dressing, make sure it is large enough to extend over the wound.

Bandages

- A bandage is used to:
  - Hold a dressing in place
  - Apply pressure over a dressing
  - Prevent and reduce swelling
  - Provide support and stability for an extremity or joint
- Make sure that a bandage is not applied too tightly.

- There are several types of bandages, including:
  - Roller bandages
  - Triangular bandages
  - Adhesive tape
  - Adhesive strips

SKILL PRACTICE SESSION

- Have participants break up into small groups to practice applying dressings and bandages to hand, joint (elbow/knee), and foot.
- Review the Skill Scans on "Bandaging—Roller Bandage."
- Evaluate participant performance and remediate any problems.

ASSESSING PROGRESS

Have participants complete the "Learning Activities" at the end of the chapter in their manual. Answers to the Learning Activities are listed below.

Dressings and Bandages

1. Yes
2. Yes
3. No
4. Yes
5. Yes

Scenario:

Clean the wound and place a dressing over the wound. Secure the dressing in place with a bandage. You may also use adhesive strips for this type of wound.

Scenario:

Stop the bleeding with a sterile dressing. Apply a pressure bandage to help control the bleeding.

LESSON: BURNS

Lesson Objectives

After completing this lesson, participants should be able to:

- Identify three types of burns.
- Discuss how to determine burn severity.
- Explain how to care for thermal, chemical, and electrical burns.

Approximate Length: 10 minutes

Equipment for Skill Practice: None

SCENARIOS

Scenario: You are helping a fellow worker replace a battery when it explodes in his face, showering him with battery acid. You see that the acid is already causing burns to his face and arms that are blistering.

Scenario: You come into the office and see the custodian lying on the floor next to an frayed electrical wire. His face is pale, and his lips are blue.

TEACHING POINTS

Instructor's Note

Video segments cover many of the points in this lesson.

Burn Injury

- Burn injuries are classified as thermal, chemical, or electrical.
- Burns are described as first-degree (superficial), second-degree (partial thickness), and third-degree (full thickness).

Thermal Burn Care

- Immediately stop the burning process (water or smother).
- Check ABCs.
- Determine the extent of the burn ("Rule of Palm").
- Determine the parts of the body burned.
- Determine burn severity (first, second, or third degree).
- Determine if other injuries or medical problems exist.
- Seek medical attention as needed.

Additional Care for First-Degree Burns

- Administer ibuprofen to relieve pain (acetaminophen for children).
- After the burn area cools, apply a moisturizer such as aloe vera gel.

Additional Care for Second-Degree Burns

- Administer ibuprofen to relieve pain (acetaminophen for children).
- Do not break blisters.
- Apply a thin layer of Bacitracin™ after the burn cools (if <20% BSA).
- Cover the burn with a dry, nonsticking, sterile dressing.
- Seek medical attention.

Care for Third-Degree Burns

- Cover the burn with a dry, nonstick, sterile dressing.
- Care for shock.
- Seek medical attention.

Chemical Burns

- A chemical burn results from a caustic or corrosive substance.
- To care for a chemical burn:
  - Flush the area with water.
  - Remove contaminated clothing or jewelry.
  - Cover the burned area with a dry, sterile, dressing.
  - Seek medical attention immediately.

Electrical Burns

- An electrical burn or electrical shock may cause serious internal injuries.
- There are three types of electrical injuries: thermal, arc, and true electrical injury.
- To care for an electrical burn:
  - Make sure the scene is safe.
  - Check ABCs.
  - If the victim fell, check for a spinal injury.
  - Cover burn with dry, sterile dressing (look for entrance and exit burn wounds).
  - Care for shock.
  - Seek medical attention immediately.

ASSESSING PROGRESS

Have participants complete the "Learning Activities" at the end of the chapter in their manual. Answers to the Learning Activities are listed below.

Thermal (Heat) Burns

1. Yes
2. Yes
3. No
4. No

Scenario:

Stop the burn process by placing the arm in cold water.

Remove any clothing that is not stuck the wound.

Give ibuprofen.

Apply a thin coat of bacitracin if available.

Cover the burn areas with a sterile dressing.

Seek medical attention.

Chemical Burns

1. No
2. No
3. Yes
4. Yes

Scenario:

Flush the area with water for at least 20 minutes.

Remove clothing from arm.

Cover the burned area.

Seek medical attention.

Electrical Burns

1. No
2. Yes

Scenario:

Make sure the power to the trimmer is turned off.

Check ABCs.

Check the victim for burns and care for any you find.

Care for shock.

Seek medical attention.

LESSON: HEAD AND SPINAL INJURIES

Lesson Objectives

After completing this lesson, participants should be able to:

- Describe how to care for various types of head injuries.
- Identify various types of dental injuries and how to care for them.
- Demonstrate how to check a victim for a spinal injury.

Approximate Length: 15 minutes

Equipment for Skill Practice: None

SCENARIOS

Scenario: Several children are playing on a swing set. One child is hit on the forehead by a swing. The impact knocks the child down. He appears dizzy, confused, and weak. There is a bruise on his forehead.

Scenario: At the scene of a motorcycle accident, you do a scene survey and find the scene safe. You find the rider lying on his back. He complains of loss of sensation and can't move his toes.

TEACHING POINTS

Scalp Wounds

- A severe scalp wound may have an accompanying skull fracture, impaled object, or spinal injury.
- To care for a scalp wound:
  - Control bleeding by applying pressure with a dry sterile dressing.
  - If a fractured skull is suspected, apply pressure around the edges of the wound.
  - If you do not suspect a spinal injury, elevate the head and shoulders.

Skull Fracture

- Unless there is an obvious fracture, a skull fracture is difficult to determine without x-ray.
- To care for a possible skull fracture:
  - Monitor ABCs.
  - Cover wound with a sterile dressing.
  - Stabilize the victim's neck against movement.
  - Apply pressure around the edges of the wound to control bleeding.

Instructor's Note

See Action Guide, "Head Injuries."

Brain Injuries

- When the head is struck with sufficient force, the brain bounces against the inside of the skull.
- Signs of brain injury include altered level of responsiveness, headache, visual disturbance, unequal pupils, and seizure.
- When caring for a victim with a possible brain injury, you should:
  - Seek immediate medical attention.
  - Check ABCs.
  - Control any external bleeding carefully.
  - Keep the head slightly elevated if no spinal injury is suspected.

Eye Injuries

- To care for a penetrating injury to the eye:
  - Stabilize the object.
  - Cover the undamaged eye.
  - Seek medical attention.
- To care for a blow to the eye, apply ice for about 15 minutes.
- To care for a chemical burn to the eye:
  - Hold the eye open and flush the eye with water.
  - Loosely bandage both eyes with cold, wet dressings.
  - Seek immediate medical attention.
- To care for an eye knocked out of its socket:
  - Cover the eye loosely with a sterile dressing that is moist.
  - Protect the injured eye with a paper cup or similar object.
  - Cover the undamaged eye.
  - Seek medical attention immediately.
- To care for a foreign object in the eye:
  - Lift the upper lid over the lower lid.
  - Try flushing the object out.
  - Examine the lower lid by pulling it down.
- To care for eye injuries from light:
  - Cover both eyes.
  - Seek medical attention.

Instructor's Not
See Action Guide "Eye Injuries."

Nose Injuries

- Nosebleeds can be from the front of the nose (anterior) or to the back (posterior).
- To care for a nosebleed:
  - Place the victim in a seated position, with head slightly forward.
  - Pinch the soft parts of the nose together.
  - If bleeding persists, have the victim blow slightly.
  - Apply ice over the nose.
  - If bleeding cannot be controlled, or it appears the nose is broken, seek medical attention.

Dental Injuries

- To care for a knocked-out-tooth:
  - Have the victim rinse his or her mouth (if possible).
  - Place rolled gauze in the socket to control bleeding.
  - Save the tooth and seek dental or medical care immediately.
- To care for a broken tooth:
  - Gently clean the injured area.
  - Apply ice to the cheek.
  - Seek medical assistance.

> **Instructor's Note**
> *See Action Guide "Dental Injuries."*

Spinal Cord Injury

- Head injuries serve as a clue to possible spinal injuries.
- If you suspect a person has a head injury, also suspect a spinal injury.
- Signs of a spinal injury include:
  - Painful movement or inability to move the arms and legs.
  - Numbness, tingling, weakness, or burning sensations in the arms or legs.
  - Loss of bowel or bladder control.
  - Deformity of victim's neck.
- To care for possible spinal injuries, stabilize the head and neck.

> **Instructor's Note**
> *See "Skill Scan—Checking for Spinal Injuries," and Action Guide "Spinal Injuries."*

ASSESSING PROGRESS

Have participants complete the "Learning Activities" at the end of the chapter in their manual. Answers to the Learning Activities are listed below.

Head Injuries

1. Yes
2. Yes
3. Yes

Scenario:

Keep the victim from moving.

Control any bleeding.

Suspect a spinal injury and check for signs of a spinal injury.

Seek medical attention.

Eye Injuries

1. Yes
2. No
3. Yes

Scenario:

Flush the area with water for at least 20 minutes.

Try to keep the eye open.

Bandage both eyes.

Seek medical attention immediately.

Dental Injuries

1. No
2. No
3. Yes

Scenario:

Have the victim rinse his mouth.

Find the teeth and, if possible, try to place them back in their sockets carefully. If not possible, control bleeding and save the teeth.

Take the victim to the dentist immediately.

Spine Injuries

1. Yes
2. Yes
3. Yes

Scenario:

Make sure the scene is safe.

Keep the victim from moving.

Seek medical assistance.

LESSON: CHEST, ABDOMINAL, AND PELVIC INJURIES

Lesson Objectives

After completing this lesson, participants should be able to:

- Describe the care that should be given to a victim with chest injury.
- Describe the care that should be given to a victim with abdominal injury.
- Describe the care that should be given to a victim with a pelvic injury.

Approximate Length: 10 minutes

Equipment for Skill Practice: None

SCENARIO

Scenario: A 45-year-old repairman falls while carrying a replacement glass for a broken window. The new glass breaks in several jagged pieces. You find him lying on his back with a blood-soaked shirt. You see a lacerated abdomen with several loops of bowel protruding through the laceration.

Scenario: A person has been shot in the chest. A sucking sound is heard as the victim breathes.

TEACHING POINTS

Chest Injuries

- To care for possible broken ribs:
  - Help the victim find a comfortable position for breathing.
  - Support the injured area.
  - Seek medical attention.
- To care for an impaled objects in the chest:
  - Stabilize the object.
  - Seek medical attention.
- To care for a sucking chest wound:
  - When the victim exhales, seal the open wound with plastic wrap.
  - Tape it to the chest, with one corner untaped.
  - If the victim develops breathing difficulty, remove cover and reapply.
  - Seek medical attention.

Instructor's Note
See Action Guide "Chest Injuries."

Abdominal Injuries

- To care for a blow to the abdomen:
  - Place the victim in a comfortable position.
  - Seek medical attention.
- To care for a penetrating wound:
  - Do not remove any object impaled in the abdomen.
  - Cover any protruding organs with a moist sterile dressing or clean cloth.
  - Place a towel over the dressing to maintain warmth.
  - Seek medical attention.

Instructor's Note
See Action Guide "Abdominal Injuries."

Pelvic Injuries

- To care for a pelvic injury:
  - Place padding between the victim's thighs, and tie both legs together.
  - Keep the victim on a firm surface.
  - Seek medical attention.

ASSESSING PROGRESS

Have participants complete the "Learning Activities" at the end of the chapter in their manual. Answers to the Learning Activities are listed below.

Chest Injuries

1. No
2. Yes
3. Yes

Scenario:

Check the ABCs.

Have the victim take a breath and let it out.

Apply a cover to the wound with plastic wrap and tape 3 sides.

Seek medical assistance.

Abdominal Injuries

1. No
2. No
3. No
4. Yes

Scenario:

Check the victim's ABCs.

Cover any protruding organs with a moistened sterile dressing or clean cloth.

Place a towel lightly over the dressing to help maintain heat.

Seek medical attention.

Pelvic Injuries

1. Yes
2. No

Scenario:

Check the victim's ABCs.

Secure both legs together.

Seek medical assistance.

LESSON: BONE, JOINT, AND MUSCLE INJURIES

Lesson Objectives

After completing this lesson, participants should be able to:

- List signs of a possible bone fracture.
- Describe the care for a possible fracture.
- Describe the proper care for joint and muscle injuries.
- Describe the RICE (rest, ice, compression, and elevation) procedures for bone, joint, and muscle injuries.

Approximate Length: 10 minutes

Equipment for Skill Practice: None

SCENARIOS

Scenario: An electrician working on a ceiling fixture falls from his 10′ ladder. He complains about pain in his left lower leg. You look, feel, and find slight swelling when compared with the uninjured leg. You also note that the injured leg has a slight bend in it.

Scenario: A worker misses a step as he descends the warehouse stairs and strikes his knee on the landing. When you check the knee, you find a bony protrusion on the outside of the knee. It looks like the kneecap is displaced.

Instructor's Note
Video segments cover many of the points in this lesson.

TEACHING POINTS

Fractures

- Fractures can be either open (bleeding, bone protruding) or closed.
- Use the mnemonic D-O-T-S when examining an injury for a fracture.
- Signs of possible fracture include deformity, inability to use, grating, and mechanism of injury.
- To care for a possible fracture:
  - Examine the area using the mnemonic D-O-T-S.
  - Check circulation (pulse, skin color, and temperature), sensation, and movement.
  - Use the RICE procedure (Rest, Ice, Compression, Elevation).
  - Use a splint to stabilize.
  - Seek medical attention.

Instructor's Note
Splinting is presented in the next lesson.

Instructor's Note
See Action Guide "Bone Injuries."

Instructor's Note
See Skill Scan "Checking an Extremity's CSM."

Joint Injuries

- A dislocation occurs when a joint comes apart.
- The signs and symptoms of a dislocation are similar to those of a fracture.
- Care for a dislocation as you would for a fracture.
- A sprain results when ligaments and other tissues around a joint are injured.
- Because it is difficult to differentiate between sprains and fractures, care for a sprain in the same manner as you would a fracture.

Instructor's No
See Skill Scan: "RICE Procedure for an Ankle."

Instructor's No
See Action Guide "Ankle Injuries."

Muscle Injuries

- A muscle strain occurs when a muscle is stretched beyond its normal range of motion and tears.
- Signs of a strain include sharp pain and tenderness.
- A muscle contusion (bruise) results from a blow to the muscle.
- Use the RICE procedure to care for a contusion and a strain.
- Muscle cramps are a result of a muscle in uncontrolled spasm and contraction.
- To care for a cramp:
  - Stretch the affected muscle.
  - Relax the muscle by applying gentle pressure.
  - Apply ice.
  - Pinch the upper lip hard to reduce calf-muscle cramping.
  - Drink lightly salted cool water or a commercial sports drink.

Instructor's Not
See Action Guide "Sprains, Strains, Contusions, Dislocations."

ASSESSING PROGRESS

Have participants complete the "Learning Activities" at the end of the chapter in their manual. Answers to the Learning Activities are listed below.

Fractures

1. Yes
2. Yes
3. Yes

Scenario:

Check the ABCs.

Remove any clothing covering the injury site.

Examine the area using D-O-T-S.

Check CSM.

Use the RICE procedures.

Splint the extremity.

Dislocations and Sprains

1. Yes
2. No
3. Yes
4. Yes

Scenario:

Use the RICE procedure.

Muscle Injuries

1. No
2. No
3. Yes

Scenario:

Use the RICE procedure.

LESSON: SPLINTING THE EXTREMITIES

Lesson Objectives

After completing this lesson, participants should be able to:

- Describe the purpose of a splint.
- Identify various objects that can be used as splints.
- Describe and demonstrate how to apply a splint to an upper or lower extremity.

Approximate Length: 15 minutes

Equipment for Skill Practice: Splints, triangular bandages, roller gauze, tape

SCENARIO

Scenario: A worker has possibly broken his arm during a fall. He is in a remote area, and you need to get him to medical care.

Scenario: During a company softball game, a batter loses his grip while swinging at a pitch. The bat flies through the air and hits a nearby team member hard on the thigh. Although the skin is not broken, there is tenderness and some swelling.

TEACHING POINTS

Instructor's No

Video segments cover many of the points in this lessc

Splinting the Extremities

- A splint is used to help immobilize (stabilize) an injured body part.
- Splints can be commercial or improvised.
- Follow these guidelines when applying a splint:
  - Cover all open wounds.
  - Check circulation, sensation, and movement in the injured area.
  - Use a splint that will extend beyond the joints above and below the injury.
  - Apply splint firmly but not to affect circulation.

Instructor's Not

See Skill Scans for Splinting—Upper Extremities; Splinting—Elbow and Knee; and Splinting—Lower Extremities.

SKILL PRACTICE SESSION

- Have participants break up into small groups and move to the practice area.
- Have participants review the Skill Scans for Splinting—Upper Extremities, Splinting—Elbow and Knee, and Splinting—Lower Extremities.
- Have participants practice splinting arm and leg injuries.
- Evaluate participants and remediate any problems.

ASSESSING PROGRESS

Have participants complete the "Learning Activities" at the end of the chapter in their manual. Answers to the Learning Activities are listed below.

Splinting the Extremities

1. Yes
2. No
3. Yes
4. No
5. No
6. No
7. No
8. Yes

Scenario:

Assess the injury using D-O-T-S.
Keep the victim from moving his arm.
If he must be moved, apply a splint to stabilize the injury.

LESSON: SUDDEN ILLNESSES

Lesson Objectives

After completing this lesson, participants should be able to:

- Describe the signs and care for a heart attack.
- Describe the signs and care for breathing problems.
- Describe the signs and care for fainting.
- Describe the signs and care for seizures.
- Describe the signs and care for diabetic emergencies.

Approximate Length: 15 minutes

Equipment for Skill Practice: None

SCENARIOS

Scenario: A 50-year-old neighbor complains about chest pain after shoveling snow from his driveway. He says that it started about an hour ago and has not let up since. He is sure that it is just a little indigestion and feels dumb about talking about it. The pain feels like "something pressing on my chest" and is accompanied by feelings of nausea.

Scenario: An adult male suddenly collapses and falls to the floor in your store. He is having a seizure. His eyes are rolled back, his body is rigid, and he is shaking from head to foot. His head is pounding on the concrete floor.

TEACHING POINTS

Instructor's Not
Video segments cover many of the points in this lesso

Heart Attack

- A heart attack occurs when the blood supply to part of the heart muscle is severely reduced or stopped.
- Heart attacks are difficult to determine, and victims often deny the signs.
- Signs of a heart attack include:
    - Uncomfortable pressure, fullness, or pain in the center of the chest
    - Pain spreading to the shoulders, neck, jaw, arms, or back
    - Chest discomfort with lightheadedness, fainting, nausea, sweating, or shortness of breath
- To care for a victim with a possible heart attack:
    - Call EMS.
    - Monitor the victim's condition.

  - Help the victim to most comfortable position.
  - If the victim has heart medication (e.g., nitroglycerin or aspirin), assist him or her in taking it.
- Angina results when the heart does not get enough blood. Angina is brought on by physical exertion and is relieved when exertion stops.

Stroke (Brain Attack)

- A stroke results from a blocked or ruptured blood vessel in the brain.
- Signs of stroke include:
  - Weakness, numbness, or paralysis of one side of the body
  - Blurred or decreased vision
  - Problems speaking or understanding
  - Dizziness, loss of consciousness, or loss of balance
- To care for stroke:
  - Determine unresponsiveness and check the ABCs.
  - Position the victim in the recovery position.

Asthma

- Signs of asthma include coughing, cyanosis, difficulty breathing, and noisy breathing (wheezing).
- To care for asthma:
  - Keep the victim in the most comfortable position for breathing.
  - Assist with any asthma medication the victim may have (such as an inhaler).
  - Seek medical attention if the victim does not respond to the medication or is having an extreme asthmatic attack.

Hyperventilation

- This is rapid, deep breathing, often seen with emotional stress.
- Signs also include dizziness, numbness, and tingling.
- To care for hyperventilation:
  - Calm and reassure the victim.
  - Encourage victim to breathe slowly.

Fainting

- Fainting is associated with decreased blood flow to the brain.
- To care for fainting:
  - Prevent the victim from falling.
  - Help the victim lie down and raise the legs 8 to 12 inches.
  - Loosen tight clothing.
  - Seek medical assistance if the victim does not recover or has frequent fainting spells.

Seizures

- Seizures can result from various medical conditions, including epilepsy, poisoning, and hypoglycemia.
- To care for a seizure:
  - Protect the victim from injury.
  - Loosen any restrictive clothing.
  - Roll the victim onto his or her side to keep the airway clear.
  - As the victim begins to recover, offer your help.
  - Call EMS.

Diabetic Emergencies

- Diabetes is a condition in which insulin is either lacking or ineffective.
- There are two types of diabetes: Type I juvenile-onset or insulin-dependent and Type II adult-onset or non-insulin dependent.
- Very low blood sugar is called hypoglycemia or insulin reaction.
- Signs and symptoms of low blood sugar can have a sudden onset and include:
  - Staggering, poor coordination
  - Agitation
  - Pale color
  - Confusion and disorientation
  - Sudden hunger
  - Excessive sweating
  - Unconsciousness
- If the victim is a known diabetic and is still conscious enough and able to swallow, give him or her sugar.

- If the condition does not improve in 15 minutes (or if the victim is unresponsive), call EMS.
- When the body has too much sugar in the blood, hyperglycemia or diabetic coma can develop.
- Signs and symptoms of hyperglycemia often have a gradual onset and include
  - Drowsiness
  - Extreme thirst
  - Frequent urination
  - Flushed skin
  - Heavy breathing with fruity breath odor
- Care for hyperglycemia in the same manner as hypoglycemia.

Instructor's Note
See Action Guide "Diabetic Emergencies."

ASSESSING PROGRESS

Have participants complete the "Learning Activities" at the end of the chapter in their manual. Answers to the Learning Activities are listed below.

Sudden Illness

1. No
2. Yes
3. No
4. Yes
5. Yes
6. No
7. No
8. No
9. No
10. Yes
11. Yes

Scenario 1:

Talk to the victim and explain the consequences of not going to the hospital.

Scenario 2:

Have the victim rest and relax.

Place him on his side.

Seek medical attention.

Scenario 3:

Check ABCs.

Place in the recovery position.

Scenario 4:

Get everyone away from the victim.

Prevent the victim from injuring himself or herself.

Place the person in the recovery position.

Scenario 5:

Secure the vehicle and make sure it is safe.

Seek medical assistance immediately.

Check the ABCs.

Place the victim in the recovery position if unresponsive and breathing.

If responsive and able to swallow, give sugar.

LESSON: POISONING

Lesson Objectives

After completing this lesson, participants should be able to:

- Describe how to care for ingested poison.
- Describe how to care for a victim with possible alcohol intoxication.
- Describe how to care for carbon monoxide poisoning.
- Describe how to care for plant-induced dermatitis.

Approximate Length: 10 minutes

Equipment for Skill Practice: None

SCENARIOS

Scenario: You are at a party and see a person you know lying in the hallway unconscious. Right next to him is a prescription medicine bottle that belongs to another person at the party who gets migraine headaches. The bottle is empty.

Scenario: A person is found unresponsive in his car. The car is in the garage and the engine is running.

TEACHING POINTS

Instructor's Note

Video segments cover many of the points in this lesson.

Ingested (Swallowed) Poisons

- Most ingested poisons have low toxicity or are swallowed in small amounts.
- To care for a victim of an ingested poisoning:
  - Determine the age and size of the victim, what and how much poison was ingested, and when it was taken.
  - Corrosive/caustic poisons should be diluted with water or milk.
  - Call the poison control center if the person is responsive (EMS if the person is unresponsive).
  - Place the victim on his or her left side.
  - Give syrup of ipecac (induces vomiting) or activated charcoal (neutralizer) only if instructed to do so by poison control.
  - Save poison containers, plants, or victim's vomit to help identify the substance

Instructor's Note

See Action Guide "Swallowed Poison."

Alcohol and Other Drug Emergencies

- Helping a person under the influence of alcohol or other drugs can be difficult because the individual's behavior can be erratic (e.g., belligerent and combative).
- To care for a drug overdose (alcohol or other):
  - Look for any injuries.
  - Check ABCs and treat accordingly.
  - If unresponsive, place victim in the recovery position.
  - Seek medical assistance.
  - If the person starts to become violent, move to safety.

Carbon Monoxide Poisoning

- Carbon monoxide is colorless and tasteless, so victims are often unaware of its presence.
- To care for a victim of carbon monoxide poisoning:
  - Get the victim out of the toxic environment.
  - Seek medical attention.
  - Monitor the ABCs.
  - Place an unresponsive, breathing victim in the recovery position.

Plant-induced Dermatitis: Poison Ivy, Poison Oak, and Poison Sumac

- Most people cannot identify these irritating plants.
- Care for possible contact poison includes:
  - Cleaning the skin as soon as possible
  - Lukewarm water and colloidal oatmeal
  - Calamine lotion
  - Corticosteroid ointment
  - Physician-prescribed oral corticosteroid

ASSESSING PROGRESS

Have participants complete the "Learning Activities" at the end of the chapter in their manual. Answers to the Learning Activities are listed below.

Poisoning

1. Yes
2. Yes
3. Yes
4. Yes
5. Yes
6. Yes
7. Yes
8. Yes
9. Yes

Scenario 1:

Check the ABCs, contact poison control, and seek medical attention.

Scenario 2:

Check the victim's ABCs.

If the victim is breathing, place in the recovery position.

Monitor ABCs.

Scenario 3:

Reassure the victim.

Seek medical assistance.

Monitor the victim.

Scenario 4:

Remove the victim from the vehicle.

Check ABCs.

Seek medical assistance.

Scenario 5:

Clean the area.

Apply calamine lotion or corticosteroid ointment.

Seek medical assistance.

LESSON: BITES AND STINGS

Lesson Objectives

After completing this lesson, participants should be able to:

- Explain what rabies is.
- Describe the care for an animal bite.
- Discuss how to care for a snakebite.
- Describe how to care for insect bites and stings.

Approximate Length: 10 Minutes

Equipment for Skill Practice: None

SCENARIOS

Scenario: A mail carrier is shouting for help as he is attacked by a dog. The dog's owner calls off the dog and takes it inside the house. You help the victim and find several severe bite marks on the mail carrier's legs and arms.

Scenario: A fight breaks out at a bar and one person bites another person's ear, causing an avulsion.

TEACHING POINTS

Animal and Human Bites

- It is estimated that one of every two Americans will be bitten at some time by an animal or by another person.
- Rabies is a virus found in warm-blooded animals, spread through saliva.
- To care for a bite:
  - Report animal bites to the police or animal control.
  - Care for bleeding.
  - Clean the wound with soap and water.
  - Seek medical attention for cleaning, tetanus shot, or rabies vaccination if needed.

Instructor's Note
Video segments cover many of the points in this lesson

Instructor's Note
See Action Guide "Animal Bites."

Snakebites

- Only four snake species in the United States are poisonous.
  - Rattlesnake (pit viper)
  - Water moccasin (pit viper)
  - Copperhead (pit viper)
  - Coral snake
- Pit viper bites leave characteristic puncture wounds.
- To care for snakebite:
  - Get the victim away from the snake.
  - Keep the victim quiet.
  - Gently clean the bitten areas with soap and water.
  - Treat nonpoisonous snakebites as a minor wound.
  - In remote areas, use a Sawyer Extractor™ to apply suction for pit viper bites.
  - Wrap elastic bandage over the bite site and arm or leg for coral snake bites.
  - Seek medical attention.

Insect Stings

- Severe allergic reactions to insect stings can be life threatening.
- To care for an insect sting:
  - Check for a stinger and venom sac. If present, scrape them out (using a fingernail or plastic card).
  - Wash with soap and water.
  - Apply ice to slow absorption, relieve pain, and reduce swelling.
  - Consider topical steroid, pain medication, or antihistamine.
  - Assist the victim with his or her prescribed epinephrine kit if available.
  - Call EMS for signs of severe allergic reaction.

Spider Bites and Scorpion Stings

- To care for spider bites and scorpion stings:
  - Identify the spider if possible (size, color, markings, etc.).
  - Clean with soap and water or rubbing alcohol.
  - Apply ice.
  - Monitor ABCs.
  - Seek medical attention.

Embedded Ticks

- To care for an embedded tick:
  - Use tweezers to pull the tick straight off.
  - Wash with soap and water.
  - Apply ice.
  - Apply calamine lotion to help relieve any itching.
  - Periodically check the bite site for one month for a rash.

ASSESSING PROGRESS

Have participants complete the "Learning Activities" at the end of the chapter in their manual. Answers to the Learning Activities are listed below.

Bites and Stings

1. Yes
2. No
3. No
4. Yes
5. Yes
6. Yes
7. Yes
8. Yes
9. No
10. No
11. No

Scenario 1:

Clean the wounds.

Bandage the wounds.

Make sure the dog is evaluated for rabies.

Scenario 2:

Calm the victim.

Restrict movement.

Wash the bitten area.

Seek medical care.

Scenario 3:

Calm the victim.

Wash the site and remove any stinger.

Apply ice.

Help him or her to find and administer the epinephrine auto-injector.

Scenario 4:

Wash the area.

Seek medical advice.

Scenario 5:

Pull the tick straight out.

Wash the site area.

Seek medical care if rash develops.

LESSON: COLD-RELATED EMERGENCIES

Lesson Objectives

After completing this lesson, participants should be able to:

- Describe three types of cold-related injuries and how they are cared for.

Approximate Length: 5 Minutes

Equipment for Skill Practice: None

SCENARIOS

Scenario: In subfreezing temperatures during a snowstorm, a stalled truck is on the side of the road. Inside the truck is an elderly man. He tells you that his truck is out of gasoline. He has been stranded for hours. The man complains of numb fingers and cold feet.

Scenario: A 50-year-old man fell through the ice of a local pond during an attempt to rescue a dog. He was able to pull himself to safety. He is awake and has cold, pale skin. He has intense, uncontrollable shivering.

TEACHING POINTS

Instructor's Note

Video segments cover many of the points in this lesson.

Freezing Injuries (Frostbite)

- There are two types of freezing injuries: frostnip and frostbite.
- Frostnip is caused by water freezing on the skin surface.
- Frostbite occurs when temperatures drop below freezing and is more severe, involving deeper tissues.
- Signs of frostbite include:
  - White, waxy skin color
  - Cold and numb feeling in the affected part
  - As it progresses, the skin will feel hard and cold
  - During rewarming, the area will swell and discolor
- To care for frostbite:
  - Get the victim to a warm area.
  - Remove any items that could impair circulation.
  - Seek immediate medical attention.
  - Do not rub the affected part(s).
  - For hands and feet, place dry sterile dressings between toes or fingers and bandage loosely.
  - In remote locations, consider rapid rewarming using warm water.

Instructor's Note

See Action Guide "Frostbite."

Hypothermia

- Hypothermia occurs when body temperature falls and the body cannot produce heat as fast as it is being lost.
- The difference between mild and severe hypothermia is the core body temperature.
- Signs of hypothermia include:
  - Altered level of responsiveness
  - Shivering
  - Cool abdomen
- To care for hypothermia:
  - Stop further heat loss.
  - Handle the victim gently.
  - Replace wet clothing.
  - Rewarm gradually.
  - Call EMS.

> **Instructor's Note**
> *Normal oral and rectal thermometers cannot adequately measure hypothermia.*

> **Instructor's Note**
> *See Action Guide "Hypothermia."*

ASSESSING PROGRESS

Have participants complete the "Learning Activities" at the end of the chapter in their manual. Answers to the Learning Activities are listed below.

Frostbite

1. No
2. Yes
3. No
4. No
5. Yes

Scenario:

Remove the victim from the cold.

If there is no chance of refreezing, go ahead and warm the part.

Seek medical assistance.

Hypothermia

1. Yes
2. Yes

3. Yes
4. No
5. Yes
6. Yes

Scenario:

If possible, raise the heat; otherwise, move victim to a warmer location.

Monitor the victim.

Remove any wet clothing and replace with dry.

LESSON: HEAT-RELATED EMERGENCIES

Lesson Objectives

After completing this lesson, participants should be able to:

- Identify three types of heat-related emergencies.
- Describe the care for heat-related emergencies.

Approximate Length: 5 minutes

Equipment for Skill Practice: None

SCENARIOS

Scenario: A road crew is working on a very hot, humid day. A worker complains about being very thirsty, nauseous, and having a headache.

Scenario: Your neighbor has been working on the yard for hours during the warmest part of the day. He collapses in his yard. His skin is red and warm.

TEACHING POINTS

Instructor's Note

Video segments cover many of the points in this lesson.

Heat-Related Emergencies

- Heat emergencies include a range of disorders: heat cramps, heat exhaustion, and heat stroke.
- Heat cramps are painful muscular spasms that occur suddenly, usually immediately after exertion.
- Heat exhaustion is characterized by heavy perspiration with normal or slightly above normal body temperature.
- Heat stroke is a life-threatening condition in which the body temperature becomes extremely high, requiring rapid intervention.
- To care for heat-related emergencies:
  - Rest in a cool place.
  - If responsive, give cool water or a commercial sport drink.
  - Stretch any cramped muscle(s).
  - If altered level of responsiveness exists, raise legs 8 to 12 inches.
  - Remove excess clothing.
  - Sponge with cool water, fan the victim, or apply cold packs.
  - If unresponsive, or no improvement, seek medical attention.

Instructor's Note

See Action Guide "Heat-Related Emergencies."

ASSESSING PROGRESS

Have participants complete the "Learning Activities" at the end of the chapter in their manual. Answers to the Learning Activities are listed below.

Heat-Related Emergencies

1. Yes
2. No
3. Yes
4. No
5. Yes
6. No
7. No
8. No

Scenario 1:

Victim should stop what he is doing.

Move to a cooler location.

Drink cool fluids.

Scenario 2:

This victim may be suffering from heat stroke.

Victim needs to be moved to a cooler area.

Check ABCs.

Remove clothing.

Lower body temperature any way possible (fanning, water, or if available, cold packs).

Scenario 3:

Victim needs to rest and move to a cooler area.

Drink some fluids (water or commercial sport drink).

LESSON: RESCUING AND MOVING VICTIMS

Lesson Objectives

After completing this lesson, participants should be able to:

- Describe how to remain safe when attempting a water rescue.
- Describe how to remain safe at the scene of an electrical emergency.
- Describe what to do at the scene of a hazardous materials incident and other potentially unsafe environments.
- Describe the concept of triage.
- Explain situations in which a victim may have to be moved.

Approximate Length: 10 minutes

Equipment for Skill Practice: None

SCENARIOS

Scenario: You are the "lookout" for your co-worker who is operating in a confined space. He suddenly collapses to his knees.

Scenario: High wind has just collapsed a building room at your warehouse. At least a dozen workers have been hurt, some more than others.

TEACHING POINTS

Instructor's Note

Video segments cover many of the points in this lesson.

Water Rescue

- "Reach-throw-row-go" defines the safest approach for attempting a water rescue.
- Entering the water should be a last resort.

Electrical Emergency Rescue

- If high-voltage power lines have electrocuted a victim, the power must be turned off before approaching a victim.
- Wait for trained personnel with the proper equipment to cut or disconnect wires.

Hazardous Materials Incidents

- Stay well away and upwind from any area where there may be a hazardous materials emergency.

Motor Vehicle Crashes

- Most states require you to stop and help when you are involved in a crash.
- If you need to enter a vehicle, try the doors and windows first. Break a window as a last resort.
- Be safe: use your flashers.
- Do not remove the victim unless unresponsive and not breathing.

Instructor's Not
If calling 9-1-1 on cell phone, provide good directions because dispatchers will not automatically know your location (use mile markers or easily recognized building or street signs).

Confined Space

- A confined space is any area not intended for human occupancy, including trenches, tanks, silos, and vaults.
- A confined space may have or could result in a dangerous atmosphere.
- It requires special training and equipment to perform a rescue.

Triage: What to Do with Multiple Victims

- The process of prioritizing or classifying numerous victims is called triage.
- Various systems are in use today. All systems use the same categories to classify patients' conditions:
  - Immediate (highest priority, e.g., airway, breathing)
  - Urgent (second priority, e.g. burns without airway problems)
  - Delayed (low priority, e.g. minor wounds)
  - Dead (lowest priority, e.g., decapitated, no signs of circulation)
- Triage enables rescuers to classify victims according to who needs immediate attention and who can wait.

Instructor's Note
Show examples of triage tags or colored tape.

Moving Victims

- A victim should not be moved unless there is an immediate danger.
- The major danger in moving a victim with head or back injury is the possibility of aggravating a spinal injury.
- If you must move a victim with possible spinal injury, drag him or her in the direction of the long axis of the body.
- Other emergency moves include the human crutch, cradle carry, fireman's carry, pack-strap carry, and piggyback carry.

Instructor's Note
See Skill Scans "Drags," "One-Person Moves," and "Two/Three Person Moves."

SKILL PRACTICE SESSION

- Have participants break up into small groups to practice emergency moves.
- Review the Skill Scans on "Drags", "One-Person Moves", and "Two-/Three-Person Moves."

Instructor's Note

Only perform emergency moves that can be done easily and safely.

ASSESSING PROGRESS

Have participants complete the "Learning Activities" at the end of the chapter in their manual. Answers to the Learning Activities are listed below.

1. No
2. Yes
3. Yes
4. Yes
5. Yes
6. No
7. No

Scenario:

Scene safety is an issue; wait until professional help arrives and declares the area safe. If you must enter, perform an emergency move to remove the victim as quickly as possible.

LESSON: POST-COURSE CHECK AND COURSE REVIEW

Have participants return to the "First Aid IQ" that they completed at the beginning of the class and complete the "post-course" column. How many participants changed their answers and got them correct now that they have completed a first aid course? Discuss the answers to this activity with participants and then administer the final written exam.

Approximate Time: 5 minutes

SECTION 5: FIRST AID EXAMS

NATIONAL SAFETY COUNCIL FIRST AID EXAM A

Mark the correct answer on the answer sheet provided.

1. If you provide care to the best of your ability and within your standard of care, you can reduce the chance of a lawsuit claiming:
   a. negligence
   b. avoidance
   c. duty
   d. due regard

2. Which of the following actions is **not** one that a bystander should take?
   a. Recognize the emergency.
   b. Decide to help.
   c. Terminate care before help arrives.
   d. Assess the victim.

3. An unresponsive, breathing victim should be placed:
   a. in a seated position
   b. on his or her back
   c. face down
   d. on the side

4. The initial assessment is used to:
   a. gather medical history information about the victim
   b. determine if the victim has a broken wrist
   c. identify and correct immediate threats to life
   d. determine the degree of a burn

5. The first step used to control external bleeding is:
   a. pressure point
   b. elevation
   c. pressure dressing
   d. direct pressure

6. A child has been stung by a bee. Within minutes her face and tongue are swelling and she is having difficulty breathing. These signs and symptoms are associated with:
   a. seizure
   b. anaphylaxis
   c. asthma
   d. hypoglycemia

7. When caring for an amputated part, the part should be:
   a. placed in a freezer
   b. kept warm and dry
   c. kept at room temperature
   d. wrapped in plastic and stored on ice

8. A person has a serious cut on his arm. The purpose of a bandage is to:
   a. hold a dressing in place
   b. apply pressure
   c. control bleeding
   d. all of the above

9. The first step in caring for a thermal burn is to:
   a. cover the burn with a moist dressing
   b. elevate the burn area
   c. stop the burning process
   d. rub butter on the wound

10. When caring for a nosebleed, the victim should be positioned:
    a. flat on the back
    b. sitting back
    c. leaning forward
    d. head tilted back

11. When caring for an impaled object in the chest, you should:
    a. immediately remove the object
    b. carefully move the victim into the recovery position
    c. stabilize the object and control bleeding
    d. push the object in until resistance is met to stabilize it

12. When applying a splint for a possible broken forearm, the splint should be:
    a. applied tightly to reduce circulation
    b. extended beyond the wrist and elbow
    c. applied loosely to avoid further injury
    d. removed every 30 minutes to recheck the injured area

13. A 55-year-old female has a tight feeling in her chest. This feeling is getting worse, and now a pain is present in her arm. She is sweating and nauseated. She is likely suffering:
    a. seizure
    b. stroke
    c. heart attack
    d. fainting

14. When caring for a victim that is experiencing a seizure, you should:
    a. force an object in the victim's mouth.
    b. protect the victim from injury
    c. keep the victim flat on the back
    d. give water to drink

15. A person with low blood sugar will experience:
    a. flushed color
    b. altered level of responsiveness
    c. chest pain
    d. fruity breath odor
16. To care for ingested poison:
    a. Call the poison control center for a responsive victim.
    b. Induce vomiting for all poisons.
    c. Do a complete physical exam for a responsive victim.
    d. Dilute all poisons with water or milk.
17. Which of the following statements is true about bites and stings?
    a. Human bites are not as dangerous as animal bites.
    b. Apply ice to snakebite.
    c. Rabies is a disease spread from one animal to another through saliva.
    d. Care for a spider or scorpion bite by applying heat to the site.
18. A 40-year-old person is found lying in an alley in the winter time. He is cold, wet, shivering, and has an altered level of responsiveness. This victim should be cared for by:
    a. rapidly rewarming the body
    b. giving the victim something to eat
    c. replacing any wet clothing with dry clothing
    d. waiting 30 minutes to see if his condition improves before calling EMS
19. An electrician has been working on power lines in the heat of the day. While walking to his car after work, he collapses on the ground. He is unresponsive, with hot skin. How should you provide care?
    a. Give the victim an ice cold drink.
    b. Place the victim in ice water.
    c. Move the victim immediately out of the heat to a cool place.
    d. Wrap the victim in warm towels.
20. A situation in which a rescuer may have to perform an emergency move of a victim would be if a victim:
    a. has a broken fracture
    b. is in the middle of a highway
    c. is a child
    d. is dizzy

NATIONAL SAFETY COUNCIL
FIRST AID EXAM B

Mark the correct answer on the answer sheet provided.

1. You can care for an unconscious victim under what type of consent:
   a. expressed
   b. implied
   c. improvised
   d. assumed

2. All of the following are part of the scene survey, except:
   a. identify hazards
   b. determine the number of victims
   c. seek medical attention
   d. determine who is responsible for the incident

3. Of the following emergencies, which is considered an immediate threat to life?
   a. person with severe back pain
   b. person bleeding from his or her mouth
   c. person choking
   d. person screaming in pain

4. A pressure point should only be used to control bleeding:
   a. as the first measure to control bleeding
   b. when a tourniquet is not available
   c. if direct pressure does not work
   d. of the chest or abdomen

5. A condition that results when the body temperature falls because the body cannot produce heat as fast as it is being lost is called:
   a. hypertension
   b. hyperthermia
   c. hypothermia
   d. hypotension

6. When caring for a person in heat exhaustion, you should:
   a. give the victim ice cold drinks
   b. place the victim in ice water
   c. move the victim immediately out of the heat to a cool place
   d. have the victim walk around to avoid cramping

7. A powerful reaction to a substance that can occur within minutes or even seconds is known as:
   a. seizures
   b. anaphylaxis
   c. prophylaxis
   d. sensitivity

8. When caring for an amputated part, the amputation should be:
   a. stored directly on ice
   b. kept warm and dry
   c. kept at room temperature
   d. wrapped in plastic and then stored on ice
9. The first step in caring for a thermal burn is to:
   a. cover the burn with a dry dressing
   b. elevate the burn area
   c. stop the burning process
   d. rub butter on the wound
10. When caring for a penetrating wound to the abdomen you should:
    a. cover protruding organs with a moistened sterile dressing or clean cloth
    b. attempt to replace organs inside the abdomen
    c. cover protruding organs with a dry sterile dressing or cloth
    d. place the victim in a seated position
11. When caring for a nosebleed the victim should be positioned:
    a. sitting upright
    b. leaning forward
    c. leaning backward
    d. lying down
12. When using the RICE procedure, the "R" stands for:
    a. rotate
    b. run
    c. rest
    d. repeat
13. A life-threatening condition caused by heat is called:
    a. heat exhaustion
    b. heat stroke
    c. heat cramps
    d. heat discomfort
14. An example of a rigid splint would be:
    a. board splint
    b. blanket
    c. pillow
    d. all of the above
15. A condition that results when the blood supply to part of the brain is severely reduced or blocked is called:
    a. angina
    b. stroke
    c. heart attack
    d. diabetes

16. The first step in caring for a victim with possible carbon monoxide poisoning is:
    a. perform an initial assessment
    b. determine a SAMPLE history
    c. check ABCs
    d. remove the victim from the toxic environment

17. Which of the following statements is true about rabies?
    a. It does not affect humans.
    b. It is only found in areas with poor sanitary conditions.
    c. It spreads from one animal to another through saliva.
    d. It is only carried by bats and rats.

18. The D-O-T-S mnemonic is helpful in remembering:
    a. the signs of an injury
    b. past medical history
    c. steps in caring for an injury
    d. signs of illness

19. When caring for a victim that is experiencing seizures, you should:
    a. attempt to stick a bite block in the patient's mouth
    b. cushion the victim's head
    c. keep the victim flat on their back
    d. give the victim plenty of water to drink when he or she regains consciousness

20. A piggyback carry is an emergency move that can be used for:
    a. an unresponsive victim
    b. a victim with two broken arms
    c. a responsive victim
    d. all of the above

INSTRUCTOR ANSWER KEY
FIRST AID EXAMS

Answer Key—Exam A

1. A
2. C
3. D
4. C
5. D
6. B
7. D
8. D
9. C
10. C
11. C
12. B
13. C
14. B
15. B
16. A
17. C
18. C
19. C
20. B

Answer Key—Exam B

1. B
2. D
3. C
4. C
5. C
6. C
7. B
8. D
9. C
10. A
11. B
12. C
13. B
14. A
15. B
16. D
17. C
18. A
19. B
20. C

Exam Answer Sheet

Name______________________________ **Exam**__________________________ **Date**_______

Select the appropriate answer for each question and shade the circle.

1. A. ○ B. ○ C. ○ D. ○

2. A. ○ B. ○ C. ○ D. ○

3. A. ○ B. ○ C. ○ D. ○

4. A. ○ B. ○ C. ○ D. ○

5. A. ○ B. ○ C. ○ D. ○

6. A. ○ B. ○ C. ○ D. ○

7. A. ○ B. ○ C. ○ D. ○

8. A. ○ B. ○ C. ○ D. ○

9. A. ○ B. ○ C. ○ D. ○

10. A. ○ B. ○ C. ○ D. ○

11. A. ○ B. ○ C. ○ D. ○

12. A. ○ B. ○ C. ○ D. ○

13. A. ○ B. ○ C. ○ D. ○

14. A. ○ B. ○ C. ○ D. ○

15. A. ○ B. ○ C. ○ D. ○

16. A. ○ B. ○ C. ○ D. ○

17. A. ○ B. ○ C. ○ D. ○

18. A. ○ B. ○ C. ○ D. ○

19. A. ○ B. ○ C. ○ D. ○

20. A. ○ B. ○ C. ○ D. ○

APPENDIX A: INSTRUCTOR'S SLIDE SET

Table of Contents

APPENDIX B: TRAUMA SLIDE SET

Table of Contents

INSTRUCTOR NOTES

INSTRUCTOR NOTES

INSTRUCTOR NOTES

INSTRUCTOR NOTES

INSTRUCTOR NOTES

INSTRUCTOR NOTES

INSTRUCTOR NOTES

GREEN CROSS FOR SAFETY ®

National Safety Council ®

Instructor's Administrative Guide for

First Aid Institute Programs

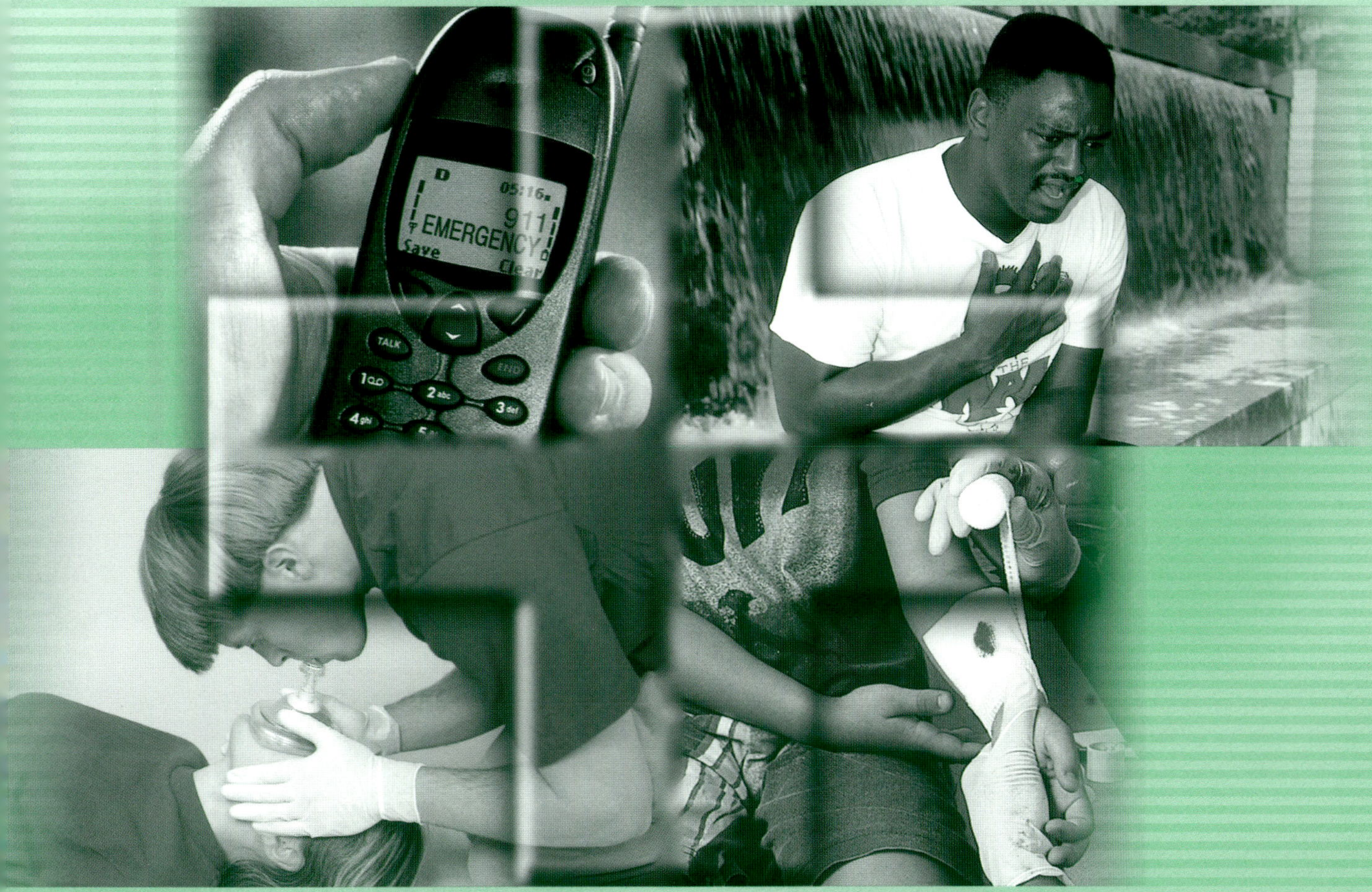

0-7637-1620-0

luct Number: 19658-0000

National Safety Council®

INSTRUCTOR'S ADMINISTRATIVE GUIDE FOR FIRST AID INSTITUTE PROGRAMS

JONES AND BARTLETT PUBLISHERS
Sudbury, Massachusetts
BOSTON TORONTO LONDON SINGAPORE

World Headquarters
Jones and Bartlett Publishers
40 Tall Pine Drive
Sudbury, MA 01776
978-443-5000
nsc@jbpub.com
Internet: http://www.jbpub.com/nsc/

Jones and Bartlett Publishers Canada
2406 Nikanna Road
Mississauga, ON L5C 2W6
CANADA

Jones and Bartlett Publishers International
Barb House, Barb Mews
London W6 7PA
UK

Printed in the United States of America

05 04 03 02 01 10 9 8 7 6 5 4 3 2 1

NATIONAL SAFETY COUNCIL®
INSTRUCTOR'S ADMINISTRATIVE GUIDE FOR FIRST AID INSTITUTE PROGRAMS

TABLE OF CONTENTS

Content	Page

SECTION 1: ABOUT THE FIRST AID INSTITUTE

INTRODUCTION

This manual provides National Safety Council Instructors with all the resources needed to conduct National Safety Council First Aid and CPR programs. These programs have been designed to provide course participants with the skills and knowledge to prevent and care for injuries and illnesses in an emergency.

NATIONAL SAFETY COUNCIL FIRST AID INSTITUTE

Through its First Aid Institute, the National Safety Council provides First Aid and CPR courses at various levels for training individuals internationally. National Safety Council programs consist of three elements:

- Flexible courses that utilize a variety of instructional audiovisual aids and student materials
- A network of training centers organized to deliver courses to industry and the general public
- Instructors authorized by the National Safety Council to deliver First Aid Institute courses

First Aid Institute Training Centers

The organization and operation of First Aid Institute training centers is described in the *First Aid Institute's Rules and Procedures Manual,* which every training center has.

A First Aid Institute training center:

- Follows all provisions of the National Safety Council's *Rules and Procedures Manual* and training center agreement
- Complies with all federal, state, and local laws, regulations, rules, and ordinances
- Is prohibited from conducting any first aid and/or CPR training other than that developed or offered by the National Safety Council
- Selects, supervises, and trains an adequate number of instructors and instructor trainers to meet the local demands
- Is responsible for assuring that high quality instruction is provided

- Maintains First Aid Institute student/provider training records and totals
- Procures all First Aid Institute materials from the National Safety Council, except as otherwise provided in its First Aid Institute training center agreement
- Confirms availability of equipment and supplies used to instruct courses
- Maintains training materials in good condition
- Assures each student/provider has student materials (student manual, evaluations, etc.)
- Assures course instructor's credentials are current
- Monitors courses to maintain quality
- Has representatives readily available during courses to answer questions
- Assures student course completion cards are issued at the end of the course
- Monitors instructors at least once each year
- Holds instructor update seminars annually
- Verifies current credentials of instructors who wish to be grandfathered into the First Aid Institute program
- Registers instructor development courses with the National Safety Council
- Communicates course/administrative changes to its instructor network in a timely manner
- Provides instructors with current student materials
- Cannot reproduce any National Safety Council materials
- Cannot provide training or sell First Aid Institute materials to the academic market when the course is part of a school curriculum and is taken for course credit

First Aid Institute Courses

The National Safety Council's First Aid Institute courses:

- Provide the public with accurate and easy-to-understand first aid and CPR procedures
- Promote an attitude of mutual understanding and cooperation so that first aid and CPR training is an important and successful activity for all concerned

All National Safety Council courses include the most up-to-date instructional materials. The National Safety Council actively solicits the widest possible authorized participation in this program on the part of all individuals; companies; military; federal, state, and local government centers; associations; and other groups.

First Aid Institute Instructors

As a National Safety Council Instructor, you are an integral part of successful course delivery. The National Safety Council's First Aid Institute trains instructors to deliver course material. As an instructor, you are responsible for ensuring that proper knowledge and skills are presented in all first aid and CPR classes. Instructors are responsible for:

- Assuring a safe, comfortable, non-threatening learning environment
- Making sure that all necessary course materials and equipment are available and in good working order
- Delivering current information according to National Safety Council guidelines
- Serving as a resource for course participants to answer questions and clarify course content
- Properly teaching the appropriate skills covered in the various National Safety Council courses
- Evaluating participants' knowledge and skills
- Submitting necessary course paperwork to the authorized training center
- Issuing course completion cards to those who successfully complete courses
- Teaching a minimum of two courses per year
- Assisting with instructor development courses

First Aid Institute Instructor Trainers

An instructor trainer is an instructor who has been authorized by the National Safety Council's First Aid Institute to train and monitor instructor candidates. An instructor trainer is not an employee or agent of the National Safety Council.

Instructor trainers have four primary responsibilities:

- Train candidate instructors according to First Aid Institute guidelines
- Monitor candidate and authorized instructors
- Ensure that knowledge of the courses that instructors are authorized to teach is consistent with the Instructor's Resource Manual and First Aid Institute requirements
- Teach at least two instructor development courses per year

"Grandfathering" Instructors

If a potential First Aid Institute instructor holds current first aid/CPR instructor/instructor trainer credentials from another national or state training organization, the instructor may be "grandfathered" as a First Aid Institute instructor, provided:

- The training center submits a completed instructor application (see Appendix K in the *Rules and Procedures Manual*) together with photocopies of current instructor credentials to the National Safety Council's First Aid Institute.

- The training center verifies current credentials of the instructor who wishes to be grandfathered.
- The training center orders the appropriate instructor development course packet for the candidate instructor and the candidate teaches two probationary courses within a twelve-month period to the training center's satisfaction.

Instructor Orientation for New and Renewing Instructors

Through instructor orientations, training centers ensure that all new and renewing instructors understand the First Aid Institute's policies and procedures. At a minimum, the orientation will include:

- Proper use of all First Aid Institute course materials
- Content contained in the First Aid Institute program that they will be teaching
- Correspondence from the First Aid Institute within the past twelve months regarding any program and administration revisions

Training centers must hold at least one annual meeting or refresher course for their instructors. These meetings update instructors on curriculum changes, state law modifications, and teaching techniques and provide them with an opportunity to review their skills.

Renewal/Recertification of Instructors

Instructor credentials are issued for a period of twelve months and bear an expiration date. They must be renewed annually or they become invalid. First Aid Institute instructors are required to teach (individually or as part of a team) at least two courses per year to maintain instructor status.

Renewal notices are sent to training centers prior to expiration. The National Safety Council issues an invoice when the renewal process is complete. The fee covers instructor authorization to teach all First Aid Institute programs in which the instructor has been qualified. Updated instructor credentials are mailed to training centers for distribution to instructors.

The instructor renewal fee also covers pertinent subscriptions that will be mailed directly to the instructor's home or designated address. Instructor credentials consist of a wallet card for the instructor and a file card for use by the training center. A training center representative must sign the wallet card and provide it to the instructor. The cards carry a code classification that is keyed to the courses an instructor is authorized to teach.

If a training center fails to renew an instructor's credentials within 30 days of expiration, the records for that instructor will be deleted from the National Safety Council's files. To reactivate the record, the training center must provide past documentation of the instructor's credentials. The training center will be invoiced for the appropriate recertification and reinstatement fees. Prepayment may be required.

Training Centers must notify the National Safety Council immediately when canceling or transferring instructor credentials. Sometimes an instructor who has stopped teaching for an extended period of time will request reinstatement. The training center administrator must determine the level of the instructor's skills and decide whether the individual should attend a full or partial instructor development course or some other type of orientation update.

Monitoring Courses

Supervision of courses helps ensure quality. All courses must be conducted according to current First Aid Institute Instructor's Resource Manuals and training center agreements. Periodically, the National Safety Council or its representatives will monitor courses. The National Safety Council requires training centers to monitor instructors.

Monitoring should include:

- Inspection of the actual classroom or facility
- Evaluation of the quality of instruction
- Verification of the instructor's credentials
- Evaluation of the instructor's adherence to the Instructor's Manual

Reports of such monitoring must be available to the training centers and instructors involved and filed with the National Safety Council. After reviewing the reports with the training center, the National Safety Council may take any corrective action it deems appropriate.

Instructor Status Revocation

The National Safety Council may revoke instructor status for disregarding any National Safety Council First Aid Institute policies, procedures, or standards, or for failing to perform stated First Aid Institute job responsibilities as required by the training center.

Course Fees

Training Centers face several considerations when establishing course fees. If fees need to be charged, they should be low enough to make the course widely available and to meet local competition, but high enough to make the program financially self-sustaining on a continuing basis. Training centers are authorized to establish their own fees or to waive fees altogether.

Copyright of National Safety Council Materials

First Aid Institute materials are copyrighted by Jones and Bartlett Publishers, with the exception of the Heartsaver FACTS program, which is copyrighted by Jones and Bartlett and the American Heart Association. You may not copy or otherwise reproduce any National Safety Council materials. If a training center becomes aware of any unauthorized duplication or use of copyrighted material, it must immediately contact the National Safety Council.

Trademarks and Logo Usage

The trademarks, trade names, and logos used by the National Safety Council are the sole property of the National Safety Council. The National Safety Council's marks, names and logos can only be used in the manner stated in "Use of National Safety Council Trademarks," in the First Aid Institute's *Rules and Procedures Manual.* Any reference to First Aid Institute courses must identify them as "the National Safety Council's First Aid Institute's courses." Additionally, anyone who wishes to use a logo with First Aid Institute courses must use the First Aid Institute design, also available in the First Aid Institute's *Rules and Procedures Manual.*

SECTION 2: TEACHING STRATEGIES

TEACHING TO OBJECTIVES

It is important for you, as an instructor, to know what to present in a particular course. You will also need to be able to address the specific needs of your audience. Although it may be difficult to meet everyone's needs, the information presented should be adequate for the majority of the class. You will not be able to be all things to all people at all times. The number of participants, time restrictions, available equipment, and facility limitations can pose challenges for you.

Some people get confused when *objectives* are mentioned. The term *objective* has been put through the mill—abused by some, misused by others, and unused by others. Objectives (or outcomes) must be carefully spelled out for the benefit of the learner and the instructor.

Objectives are the road maps that help learners know what their destination should be. They also provide the instructor with guidelines and direction for designing learning activities to move the learners in the right direction. Learning objectives describe the learning that is expected to occur during the course.

If you, the instructor, specify the course objectives, and the learners attain those objectives, effective learning will occur. When people contribute their experiences to a situation, they may carry learning above and beyond that specified in the objectives.

A behavioral objective means that some observable change is to take place as a result of the training provided. Such an objective identifies not what the instructor will be doing, but rather what the learner will have learned or will be able to do upon finishing the course.

For most courses, there are two basic objectives for learners:

1. Be able to recognize a specific problem (e.g., heart attack, fracture) through various signs and symptoms
2. Be able to describe and/or apply proper procedures to care for the problem

How much material should be covered in a specified time period and the manner in which it should be presented differs from person to person. This is especially true with adults, who bring different personal and professional goals, requirements, attitudes, and needs to each learning situation. Consequently, a particular course outline or objectives that work well for one group of participants may not work as well with another group.

As the instructor, you must constantly be aware of your pace and then be prepared to speed up or slow down as needed. You must be flexible, your outline must be flexible, and you should be ready to modify your program to meet the needs of the group. Your outline should be the servant, not the master.

TEACHING METHODS

If objectives provide the road map for the learning destination, teaching methods provide the vehicle to reach the destination. The number of participants and their backgrounds, time restrictions, available equipment, and the facility will also affect the teaching method that is used.

Various teaching methods can be used in first aid and CPR programs:

- Lecture
  Lectures are necessary in certain situations, such as when initially discussing a new skill. Lecturing is a traditional teaching method, but it limits instructor-participant interaction and does not always create the most effective learning environment.
- Discussion
  Material can be presented by involving participants in discussions. This allows for good group interaction and allows participants to learn from each other.
- Group Activities
  Participants can work in small groups to solve a problem or determine a course of action to a given scenario. This method also creates good interaction.
- Demonstration
  Step-by-step techniques demonstrated by the instructor help participants understand proper care procedures. Videos should be used to show proper care techniques, and ensure standardized demonstrations from class to class.
- Skill Practice Sessions
  Participants usually learn more from actual hands-on practice. Providing participants with time to practice skills greatly enhances their understanding and ability to perform when needed.
- Case Studies
  In case studies, participants are presented with a situation that they need to solve. Participants are then asked to analyze the situation. In their analysis, they identify what went well and what could have been done differently. They also identify and discuss the principles being presented.
- Role Playing
  In role–playing, participants assume various roles in different situations and attempt to deal with the problem facing them. This method provides for greater interaction; however, it will not be effective if participants are shy and not willing to actively participate.

As an instructor, you need to identify the best method to use for your training group. You will also benefit by using various teaching methods. Try some of the following suggestions:

- Explain what you will cover and how much time you anticipate spending on the topic.

- Keep the course interesting, and keep it moving. Participants remember information that is presented in an interesting, challenging, and even entertaining way. Making the best use of audio visual aids will help keep the course interesting.
- Make the participants responsible for their own learning. Give them enough information, but don't tell them where to dot the "i's" and cross the "t's".

SECTION 3: FIRST AID INSTITUTE COURSE COMPONENTS

COURSE COMPONENTS

National Safety Council Programs include a variety of educational components to allow for flexibility in course delivery and teaching styles. Course components include written materials such as participant and instructor manuals, as well as audiovisual aids such as videos, slides, and CD-ROMs. The use of additional audiovisual aids should enhance, not replace, those provided for each First Aid Institute course.

Participant's Manual

Each National Safety Council First Aid and CPR course has a participant's manual. The participant's manual provides the participant with the latest information and skills for that particular course. The participant's manual provides:

- Information on recognizing, caring for, and preventing injuries/illnesses
- Skill scans that depict pictorially how to perform certain skills
- Caution boxes that describe what "not to do"
- Photographs/illustrations that provide current images of important concepts and procedures, including proper care steps
- Action Guides that provide algorithms for care steps
- End-of-chapter activities that help participants assess the level of their understanding of the topic.

Instructor's Resource Manual

In addition to this Instructor's Administrative Guide, each National Safety Council course also includes an Instructor's Resource Manual that has the lesson plans and participant exams for specific courses.

Videos

National Safety Council courses have videos that present key information and demonstrate the fundamental skills taught in the courses. Videos are designed to help create consistency in course delivery and skills demonstration. First Aid Institute videos are closed-captioned for the hearing-impaired.

Slides

35mm color slides are available for first aid and CPR to help enhance course delivery. These slide sets contain photographs of real emergencies, illustrations, and PowerPoint presentations.

CD-ROMs

CD-ROMs are available that contain lesson plans, PowerPoint presentations, and images from chapters from the texts.

Teaching Packages

Teaching packages are available that contain the Instructor's Administrative Guide, Instructor's Resource Manual(s) with lesson plans and exams, and video(s) for various courses.

SECTION 4: CONDUCTING NATIONAL SAFETY COUNCIL COURSES

FIRST AID INSTITUTE COURSES

The information presented in this section is generic for all First Aid Institute Courses. First Aid Institute courses are designed for three broad categories of audiences:

- Community, including business and industry, as well as family
- Professionals who have a duty to respond
- Academic

The following National Safety Council courses are available:

- Good Samaritan
- First Aid (Adult)
- Pediatric First Aid
- CPR (Adult, Child, Infant)
- Pediatric CPR
- CPR for the Professional Rescuer
- First Aid and CPR, Standard
- First Aid and CPR, Advanced
- Pediatric First Aid and CPR
- Wilderness First Aid
- Heartsaver FACTS
- First Responder
- Automated External Defibrillation
- Bloodborne Pathogens

Course Participants

Participants in National Safety Council First Aid and CPR courses include new parents, schoolteachers, day care workers, business and industry employees, emergency response groups, ski patrols, lifeguards, and many others. It is important for participants to enroll in courses that best meet their needs. As an instructor, you can help individuals select appropriate courses.

Course Length

Each National Safety Council course has a recommended minimum course length required to cover the objectives of each course. Many governing bodies use these times and content to determine the training time needed for employees.

You should be familiar with the time required for the course(s) you are teaching. When determining a class schedule, you should remember that class times do not include breaks or lunch periods. As the instructor, you should also be familiar with your audience and be aware of additional time that may be needed to meet participants' needs.

Recommended Class Size

In order to ensure proper training and supervision, an appropriate class size is important. Class size will depend on several factors, including:

- Type of course
- Number of instructors
- Number of participants
- Teaching method
- Equipment availability

In order to provide a positive learning experience and ensure adequate practice time, the recommended maximum class size for first aid and CPR classes is 10 participants for each instructor. For larger classes there should be an additional instructor for every 10 participants. In order to most effectively teach the CPR/AED portion of the Heartsaver FACTS course, the American Heart Association requires 1 instructor for every 6 students.

Classroom Environment

As an instructor, you need to make sure that the classroom environment where you are teaching is adequate for proper course delivery. An inadequate classroom environment may affect the ability of participants to get the most out of a National Safety Council course. When selecting a course site, consider the following issues:

- Acoustics — The facility should have proper acoustics so that both the participants and the instructor can actively interact without difficulty.

- Floor space — Most courses involve skills that participants must practice. To run skill-practice sessions you will need sufficient floor space for participants to practice skills without any safety hazards.
- Electricity — Most courses will require a video or some other type of audio-visual equipment. There should be proper access to electrical outlets with minimal safety concerns. Avoid the use of extension cords. If extension cords are used, they should be secured to minimize any tripping hazard.
- Restrooms — Restrooms should be available for participants to use. Avoid situations where participants have to travel far to reach restrooms.
- Lighting — Proper lighting is important to ensure a proper learning environment. A dimmer switch to control lighting is advantageous when showing videos or slides.
- Accessibility — The room should provide easy access to carry equipment in and out as needed. The ability to establish a separate area for skill practice is desirable. Depending on the location and audience, the facility should also have handicap access.

Course Material and Equipment

To properly run National Safety Council courses, you will need the proper course materials and equipment. A general list of items needed to conduct a course is provided below:

Classroom Needs

- Proper tables and seating arrangements
- VCR and TV
- Slide projector and screen
- Computer projection system
- Spare bulb for slide projector
- White board or easel with newsprint
- Markers, pencils
- Name tents/badges
- Barrier devices (face masks or face shields)
- Cleaning supplies
- Manikins as needed for course
  - Adult manikins
  - Child manikins
  - Infant manikins

- First aid supplies as needed for course
  - Splints
  - Roller bandages
  - Gauze pads
  - Triangular bandages
  - Medical exam gloves (latex, nitrile)

Participant Needs

- Specific course manual
- Pen or pencil

Instructor Needs

- Specific course manual
- Specific Instructor Resource Manual
- Participant roster
- Exam answer sheet
- Audiovisual items (video, slides, CD-ROM)
- Course completion cards

Customizing Courses

If any of the First Aid Institute's courses do not fit a specific audience's need, contact the National Safety Council to see if a program can be designed or modified. This also applies to language translations. Please direct your inquires to:

Manager, Emergency Response and Aquatics
National Safety Council
First Aid Institute
1121 Spring Lake Drive
Itasca, IL 60143

Helping Participants Overcome Disabilities

The Americans with Disabilities Act bars discrimination against the handicapped in places of public accommodation. Individuals with physical or mental disabilities can not be denied full and equal enjoyment of the goods, services, facilities, advantages, or accommodations offered to the public.

As an instructor, you may be presenting a course to participants who are disabled, including those who are hearing-impaired, legally blind, partially paralyzed or lacking full use of limbs, or with other physical limitations. If the disabled individual can successfully meet the course objectives, he or she will receive a course completion card.

Instructors are expected to make reasonable accommodations for those with disabilities to ensure the best opportunity for learning. Instructors can adapt their teaching methods and techniques for these individuals to perform skills. For example, a person with only one arm can not be expected to perform standard adult CPR using two hands. Instead, this person can use one hand to compress the chest.

SECTION 5: COURSE COMPLETION

SUCCESSFUL COURSE COMPLETION

In many instances, participants desire to receive course certification as part of a job requirement. In order to earn a National Safety Council Course Completion Card, participants must successfully complete a written examination and demonstrate competency in the skills taught in the course.

Written Requirements for Successful Course Completion

All written examinations for National Safety Courses are multiple-choice exams and require a minimum passing score of **80%**. Any participants who have difficulty reading can complete an oral exam by having the instructor read the examination verbally.

If a participant fails the written exam, he or she should be given the opportunity to review the exam. The instructor should clarify any areas of confusion the participant may have. The participant should be given a second chance to pass the written exam. If a participant is not able to complete the written exam successfully on the second attempt, the participant should repeat the course.

Practical Requirements for Successful Course Completion

In addition to the written requirements for successful course completion, participants must also be able to demonstrate the required skills for each course. Instructors need to make sure that participants can meet the objectives for each skill.

Practical skills should be evaluated in a non-threatening, positive manner. Practical skills can be evaluated while participants practice, during a group check, or individually.

Participant Remediation

Remediation must be given to those students having a difficult time answering questions or completing the necessary skills. Remediation continues until the instructor is satisfied that the student understands why the question or skill was missed, what the correct answer or action should be, and how to perform the skill. Only then can a successful completion card be issued. Remediation includes:

- Monitoring and mentoring to identify the student's weaknesses
- Reviewing missed questions with the student
- Additional skill practice

Issuing Course Completion Cards

Participants who successfully complete a course taught by an authorized instructor are eligible to receive a National Safety Council Course Completion Card from the local training center. The certificate is a two-part document. The main record indicates the course title, date of completion, expiration date, hours of instruction, and participant information. An employer or other party that needs to maintain course completion records can keep this section on file. The other section is a detachable wallet card for the participant to keep. See *Section 7: Forms* for a sample of a Course Completion Card.

The following course names should appear on course completion cards issued to participants:

- Adult CPR
- Pediatric CPR
- Adult and Pediatric CPR
- Professional Rescuer CPR
- Standard First Aid
- Advanced First Aid
- Pediatric First Aid
- Wilderness First Aid
- Bloodborne Pathogens
- Automated External Defibrillation
- First Responder
- Heartsaver FACTS

Certification for participants who complete a CPR course is valid for up to two years. The First Aid course card is valid for up to three years. Participants who complete a First Aid and CPR program receive two cards: a CPR card valid for up to two years and a First Aid card valid for up to three years. Participants completing AED or Bloodborne Pathogens courses receive a card valid for one year. Participants completing the Heartsaver FACTS course receive a card valid for two years.

In some instances, participants may be taking a first aid or CPR course just to become familiar with the skills needed in an emergency or to expand their knowledge. These individuals may not desire a Course Completion Card and will not need to complete any written or practical skills evaluation.

Replacement of Lost Cards

Replacing lost, damaged (torn), or incorrect (misspelled name, inaccurate dates, wrong instructor number, etc.) cards is the responsibility of the training center. Course rosters should be consulted to verify participant attendance before issuing a duplicate card. Any course card that is destroyed in the printing process must be returned to the National Safety Council's First Aid Institute for replacement.

SECTION 6: AFTER THE COURSE

COURSE WRAP-UP

After completing a course, instructors must complete the necessary paperwork required by the training center. Participants should complete a course evaluation at the end of the course. These evaluations should be turned in to the training center.

Instructors must complete the course roster and submit it along with any fees to the training center. Training centers may require additional paperwork, so instructors should be familiar with the requirements of their training center.

Training centers should keep a copy of the course record. It is important to keep proper records of courses taught in case any questions arise.

Evaluation

Instructors should be able to answer these questions at the completion of the course:

- Did participants meet the course objectives?
- Did participants' behavior change?
- How successful were the learning activities?

If the participants did not meet the objectives, and the participants are not better prepared now than they were before, what was the point of the course? Without course evaluation, instructors will not know how well they and the participants performed.

Course evaluations should include (1) evaluation by the instructor, (2) evaluation by the participants, and (3) evaluation of the participants through performance or testing.

Evaluation by objectives will measure whether participants achieved the goals of the course. Participants either met the course objectives or they did not. If the participants met the objectives, this success can be proven to anyone who is interested, and the participants can feel secure in their new competency. Evaluation by objectives also allows the instructor to judge the value of the instruction.

In evaluating participants, instructors should focus on the objectives of the skill and make sure that the participant is proficient, even if not necessarily achieving mastery. Use the progress log found in *Section 7* of this administrative manual to keep track of participants as they complete each skill.

SECTION 7: FORMS

COURSE FORMS

The following forms are available in this section for use with your courses:

- Exam Answer Sheet
- Course Evaluation
- Sample Course Roster
- Sample Course Progress Log
- Sample Course Completion Card

Exam Answer Sheet

Name______________________________ **Exam**__________________________ **Date**______

Select the appropriate answer for each question and shade the circle.

1. A. ○ B. ○ C. ○ D. ○

2. A. ○ B. ○ C. ○ D. ○

3. A. ○ B. ○ C. ○ D. ○

4. A. ○ B. ○ C. ○ D. ○

5. A. ○ B. ○ C. ○ D. ○

6. A. ○ B. ○ C. ○ D. ○

7. A. ○ B. ○ C. ○ D. ○

8. A. ○ B. ○ C. ○ D. ○

9. A. ○ B. ○ C. ○ D. ○

10. A. ○ B. ○ C. ○ D. ○

11. A. ○ B. ○ C. ○ D. ○

12. A. ○ B. ○ C. ○ D. ○

13. A. ○ B. ○ C. ○ D. ○

14. A. ○ B. ○ C. ○ D. ○

15. A. ○ B. ○ C. ○ D. ○

16. A. ○ B. ○ C. ○ D. ○

17. A. ○ B. ○ C. ○ D. ○

18. A. ○ B. ○ C. ○ D. ○

19. A. ○ B. ○ C. ○ D. ○

20. A. ○ B. ○ C. ○ D. ○

NATIONAL SAFETY COUNCIL COURSE EVALUATION

Instructor: ______________________________ Date: __________

Course Name: ___________________________ Location: __________________

Please rate the following questions using the following system:
1 = Strongly agree 2 = Agree 3 = Disagree 4 = Strongly Disagree

The information presented today will be very useful.	1	2	3	4
The text was easy to understand.	1	2	3	4
The skill practice sessions were very useful.	1	2	3	4
The instructor was well prepared.	1	2	3	4
The instructor was able to hold the class' attention.	1	2	3	4
The audiovisual materials were appropriate.	1	2	3	4
The equipment was in good working order.	1	2	3	4
The course length was appropriate.	1	2	3	4
The classroom environment helped learning occur.	1	2	3	4
I am more confident in my ability to respond to an emergency.	1	2	3	4
I would recommend this class to someone else.	1	2	3	4
My reasons for taking this class were met.	1	2	3	4

Please answer these additional questions:
Did the course meet your expectations? If "no," please explain.

What did you like the most about this course?

What did you like least about this course?

Any additional comments you would like to share?

Name: (Optional) ____

NATIONAL SAFETY COUNCIL SAMPLE COURSE ROSTER

Page ____ of ____

Name of Sponsoring Training Center: ______________________

Course Name: ______________________ Course Length: ______________________

Instructor(s): ______________________ Instructor Number(s): ______________________

Start Date: ______________________ End Date: ______________________

Course Location: ______________________ Number enrolled: ______________________

Course Name: ______________________ Number passed: ______________________

Student's Name(Print)	Social Security # (optional)	Address (include Zip Code)	Pass/Fail	Completion Card #

SAMPLE COURSE PROGRESS LOG

Course: ______________________ Instructor: ____________________ Date: __________

Participants	Victim Assessment	Adult Rescue Breathing/CPR	Child Rescue Breathing/CPR	Infant Rescue Breathing/CPR	FBAO—Adult/Child	FBAO—Infant	Bleeding Control/Caring for Shock	Bandaging	Splinting—Upper Extremity	Splinting Lower Extremity	Emergency Moves	Written Exam(s)

SAMPLE COURSE COMPLETION CARD

National Safety Council®

Course Completion Date:
Course Expiration Date:

Name
Address
Address
City, State, Zip

Training Agency:
Instructor Name:
Instructor Number:

FIRST AID INSTITUTE®

Security Control No.
234921

FIRST AID INSTITUTE

Automated External Defibrillation Course

CERTIFICATE OF COMPLETION

Mary Smith

This certifies that the person named
above has successfully completed the
National Safety Council's Automated External Defibrillation course

THIS DOCUMENT IS VOID IF REPRODUCED

National Safety Council®

Founded in 1913, the National Safety Council is a non-governmental, not-for-profit international public service organization devoted to protecting life and promoting health.

***Our mission:** to educate and influence society to adopt safety, health and environmental policies, practices and procedures that prevent and mitigate human suffering and economic losses arising from preventable causes.*

You have the power to save a life

5M600 Printed in the U.S.A. 19649-0000

National Safety Council®

Mary Smith
has completed the National Safety Council's
Automated External Defibrillation Course

Course Completion Date: January 1, 2000
Course Expiration Date: January 1, 2001

Gerard F. Scannell, President
Instructional Hours: 4 Hours

ILLINOIS TRAINING AGENCY
TRAINING AGENCY

Barbara Caracci — Instructor Name
983485 — Instructor Number

Security Control No. 234921

Keep this card for your records. Void if reproduced.

INSTRUCTOR NOTES

INSTRUCTOR NOTES

INSTRUCTOR NOTES